The Educational Resource Library Asks that you
please return your library materials when you are
done with them. If they have been helpful to you,
they will help another. If you would like to
purchase this title, please contact the librarian and
she can assist you with your purchase.
This Library copy is not for sale.

 Vail Valley Medical Center

Your Genes, Your Health

Books by Aubrey Milunsky, M.D., D.Sc.

Know Your Genes
Choices, Not Chances
How to Have the Healthiest Baby You Can
Heredity and Your Family's Health
Your Genetic Destiny, Perseus Publishing

And Medical Texts (as Author, Co-Author, or Editor)

The Prenatal Diagnosis of Hereditary Disorders
The Prevention of Genetic Disease and Mental Retardation
Coping with Crisis and Handicap
Clinics in Perinatology
Advances in Perinatal Medicine
Genetics and the Law (3 Editions)
Genetic Disorders and the Fetus: Diagnosis, Prevention and Treatment (6 editions)

Your Genes, Your Health

A Critical Family Guide That Could Save Your Life

Aubrey Milunsky, MD, DSc

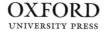

OXFORD
UNIVERSITY PRESS

OXFORD
UNIVERSITY PRESS

Oxford University Press, Inc., publishes works that further Oxford University's
objective of excellence in research, scholarship, and education.

Oxford New York
Auckland   Cape Town   Dar es Salaam   Hong Kong   Karachi
Kuala Lumpur   Madrid   Melbourne   Mexico City   Nairobi
New Delhi   Shanghai   Taipei   Toronto

With offices in
Argentina   Austria   Brazil   Chile   Czech Republic   France   Greece
Guatemala   Hungary   Italy   Japan   Poland   Portugal   Singapore
South Korea   Switzerland   Thailand   Turkey   Ukraine   Vietnam

Copyright © 2012 by Aubrey Milunsky, M.D., D.Sc.

Published by Oxford University Press, Inc.
198 Madison Avenue, New York, New York 10016

Oxford is a registered trademark of Oxford University Press
Oxford University Press is a registered trademark of Oxford University Press, Inc.

Library of Congress Cataloging-in-Publication Data

Milunsky, Aubrey.
  Your genes, your health : a critical family guide that could save your life / Aubrey Milunsky.
    p. cm.
  Includes bibliographical references and index.
  ISBN 978-0-19-979207-8 (hardback : alk. paper)
  1. Medical genetics—Popular works. I. Title.
  RB155.M55 2011
  616'.042—dc22   2010049059

Printing number: 9 8 7 6 5 4 3 2 1

Printed in the United States of America
on acid-free paper

TO JEFF.

For the joy of being your Dad.

For the pride in your achievements.

For the admiration of you as a father.

If, of all the words of tongue and pen,
The saddest are, "It might have been,"
More sad are these we daily see:
"It is, but hadn't ought to be."

FRANCIS BRET HARTE
in "Mrs. Judge Jenkins"

CONTENTS

PREFACE

Have you ever read a book that could save your life or that of a loved one? This might be it! If you harbor a particular gene mutation that was destined to cause you serious illness, disability, or even death, and there were actions to take that would enable you to avoid, prevent, ameliorate, or treat unwanted consequences, wouldn't you want to know? If you had children (or plan to have) or living parents and the knowledge of this gene mutation would help them too, wouldn't you want to know? This book is dedicated to the proposition that you would want to know and that to know is to care.

For most, recognition of risk is a prelude to action. Imagine you were crossing a street and suddenly realized that an out-of-control truck was hurtling toward you and that there was no escape. If you had been forewarned and had spotted the truck before crossing the street, you could have taken evasive action and avoided a catastrophe. Similarly, if you were standing on the street corner watching a loved one cross the street and saw the truck bearing down, would you not automatically yell out a warning? Silence and inaction are the alternatives but can result in tragedy and loss, much as I have witnessed these many decades seeing patients and families echoing what now is an all-to-familiar refrain—"If we had only known."

Now, with the continuing resolution of the human genome, we have an enormous amount of new information about our genes that enable us to avoid, prevent, and treat an ever-increasing number of genetic disorders. We know that our body structure and function result from the action of our genes with some environmental influence. Indeed, every genetic and non-genetic disease is influenced, caused, regulated, or modulated by our genes, as is our body's response to environmental factors such as viruses, bacteria, X-rays, temperature, diet, medications, carcinogens, and even trauma.

Gene discovery has revealed that you—indeed, all of us—unwittingly carry a significant number of harmful genes that may remain hidden for a lifetime. Many, however, eventually make their presence known in us or a loved one. There are a large number of examples discussed in this book that include many specific genetic disorders caused by single or multiple harmful genes that involve particular organs or systems. Manifestations wrought by these gene mutations or variations include cancer, heart disease, birth defects, mental retardation, infertility, recurrent miscarriage, diabetes, hypertension, obesity, Alzheimer's disease, depression, schizophrenia, epilepsy, drug actions and reactions, as well as allergies. Gene mutations found especially (but not only) in our ethnic or racial group are given special emphasis, as are the susceptibility genes that cause or contribute to the development of autism, and the common disorders to which we all fall victim.

The first seven chapters help the reader establish a factual understanding of chromosomes and genes, the various ways genetic disorders are transmitted and the options for avoidance or prevention. Chapters that follow recount the histories of many families whose experiences serve as important lessons. For virtually all genetic disorders discussed, there is potential involvement in reproduction, effects in children and adults, and options for avoidance, prevention, and treatment. Hence, the family stories of disease and destiny, pain and certainty, and the power of prediction all meld into life's mosaic and are not presented in a systematic categorical way. Placement of Chapter 25, (which discusses treatment options) towards the end of the book is necessary if the reader is to comprehend the vast range of genetic disorders for which therapeutic approaches now exist. The final three chapters represent very common disorders overwhelmingly caused by the interaction of multiple genes and environmental factors.

This book is not, however, an encyclopedia of genetic disorders. Realization that our genomes are made up of more than 3 billion bits of DNA, that there are almost 20,000 entries in the key genetic disorders database,[1] and more than 21,500 recognized protein-coding genes (thus far) gives pause to any author. Rather, my intention is to focus on patients and families my son[2] and I have seen in consultation. My purpose throughout is to share my long and extensive experience and the lessons learned from those for whom I have had the privilege of providing care. I have, of course, been careful not to divulge any clues that enable recognition of any individual or family. Many will recognize a genetic disorder in their families for the first time after reading this book. The likely reason is that the vast majority of people with a genetic disorder have not

---

1. Called Online Mendelian Inheritance in Man
2. Jeff Milunsky, MD, Professor of Pediatrics and Genetics and Genomics, and Co-Director of the Center for Human Genetics at Boston University School of Medicine

consulted a clinical geneticist. If this book helps remedy that situation, lives will be saved for some and health secured for many.

You need no prior knowledge of genetics or biology to understand the facts and lessons outlined here. I have selected individual patients and families whose histories, often poignant, help communicate quintessential facts and messages over a wide range of genetic disorders. The emerging lessons can be applied to many disorders in the same category, without discussing each in turn. I have used italics to describe patients and families, shaded boxes for commentary on the specific cases, and normal print to provide additional factual and up-to-date information on the disorders discussed. The Index will prove helpful in seeking information on a subject that is not confined to a single chapter, and the Appendix provides a number of tables with more detail about certain genetic disorders.

Reading about the families I describe with specific selected genetic disorders will undoubtedly alert many to potential risks that they had never recognized or known and to the important steps they now need to take. I have purposefully not provided a detailed list of genetic disorders in the Table of Contents, as that would inevitably lead the reader to familiar or special interest topics and miss one of my main goals. Specifically, I hope that readers will recognize for the first time that certain health issues in one or more family members, not previously thought of as genetic, are directly pertinent to their lives and health. You may also suddenly realize that the family of a close friend is unknowingly at risk, and your action in drawing their attention to the information could be life-saving.

I want to be sure that any idea you might have that your genetic destiny is pre-ordained and that you can do nothing about it is forever dispelled. You should know your three-generation family history where possible, be cognizant of your ethnic origins, opt for indicated gene tests, take preventive actions, determine your genetic susceptibilities, establish appropriate surveillance for you and your loved ones, and seek pre-emptive treatment where possible. This book will empower and encourage you to *KNOW YOUR GENES, SECURE YOUR HEALTH, AND HELP SAVE YOUR LIFE.*

ACKNOWLEDGMENTS

The information in this book represents a distillation of facts and concepts published over many decades in thousands of scientific papers. It is with great respect and awe that I acknowledge all the scientists and physicians whose work I have admired and relied on. Facts and concepts are, however, insufficient in the practice of medicine. It is from the thousands of patients I have seen that I learned the importance of humanity, empathy, and understanding of the human condition. I acknowledge with gratitude and humility the lessons my patients have taught me these many decades.

In retrospect, I believe that I and my colleagues graduated from the University of the Witwatersrand Medical School in Johannesburg, South Africa, during a golden era of medical education. A remarkable number of graduates in those years emigrated and achieved success in many countries. Dr. Gerald Gilchrist in 2004 published his (informal) survey of South African academic pediatricians in the United States and found 65 full professors of pediatrics in the United States, all from our Medical School. This, of course, does not account for the many others in similar positions in internal medicine, surgery, and other specialties.

These successes were not the result of chance. We were fortunate in having remarkable and outstanding basic science and clinical teachers. Although all influenced my growth and development, there were a few whose imprint molded my life in medicine and to whom I am eternally grateful.

Phillip V. Tobias, Dean and Professor of Anatomy, Emeritus, world-famous anthropologist, and one of the world's leading authorities on the evolution of mankind. He was subsequently nominated for the Nobel Prize. He unwittingly planted the idea of genetics in my head. It was from him that I first felt the excitement of discovery from research well-done. His lectures were akin to a symphony in words. He is one of the finest orators I have ever heard.

Sydney Brenner, then Lecturer in Physiology and later Nobel Prize winning scientist, who became the head of the Medical Research Council Laboratory of

Molecular Biology (and later Molecular Genetics) in Cambridge, England. In 2000 he was appointed Distinguished Professor in the Salk Institute in La Jolla, California. From him I later realized that I had learned to question and look beyond the "obvious."

D.J. DuPlessis, the late Dean and Professor of Surgery, for whom I worked as a resident and who taught me the art of incisive and logical thinking so valuable at the bedside. By example, he conveyed the importance of discipline of thought and action that have guided me through my life in medicine.

Solomon E. Levin, Professor of Pediatrics and a superb cardiologist who taught me the basic and finer points of pediatrics and pediatric cardiology. Even more important, he encouraged my nascent interest in research. My very first two published papers were with him. He couldn't have known that the pleasure and pride of those papers powered my creative engine, resulting (thus far) in more than 400 published scientific communications and 24 written and edited books. By example, I learned from him humility, sensitivity, and the benefits to a child of a gentle reassuring voice and hand.

Harry C. Seftel, Professor of Medicine, for whom I worked as a resident (and Registrar in that system), who taught me that there were no limits to the acquisition of knowledge. To this day, his encyclopedic knowledge of medicine has left me feeling insufficiently knowledgeable, despite being board-certified as a specialist in three separate disciplines (internal medicine, pediatrics, and medical genetics). His diagnostic acumen remained as a beacon and a standard for me to achieve in a lifetime of medicine.

While I could never have hoped to emulate the collective brilliance of my teachers and mentors, I acknowledge with gratitude the limited abilities I gleaned from their efforts. I do know that I have been a worthy carrier who has also shared their passion for medicine and science.

My grateful appreciation is extended to Seema Jamal, M.Sc., LGC, CCGC, one of our outstanding genetic counselors, who read the entire manuscript and made important recommendations. Multiple iterations of the manuscript were made possible only through the superlative efforts of Sheila Kelly, Jessica Storozuk, and Marilyn McPhail. Thanks, too, are extended to my wife Laura, for her love, support, understanding, and fruitful discussion.

Your Genes, Your Health

WHY AND WHAT YOU SHOULD KNOW

If you aimed to reach a critical destination, in all likelihood you would seek and establish the needed information and directions. If that destination was your health, would you do less for anything so precious? Because genes determine our physical being and influence our every function, logic dictates that we would be well-advised to at least understand the quintessential facts that govern our lives and health.

Every aspect of health and all disease is controlled, regulated, modulated, or influenced by your genes, so there is much you should know and can do. Contrary to what you might have expected, your genetic destiny is not preordained. True, you are born with a set of genetic blueprints that dictate the structure and function of your body.

Notwithstanding this irrevocable fact of nature, you are not a hapless victim inevitably bound to suffer the inexorable consequences of any flawed genes you may have inherited.

Despite the fact that we all harbor some disadvantageous or harmful genes, fortunately, the results of their dysfunction can frequently be remedied. Needless to say, we also inherit advantageous genes that endow protection against infections and convey many beneficial traits.

My purpose here is to focus on genetic disorders (frequently unrecognized) and predispositions in individuals or families with the express aim of prevention, avoidance, amelioration, or treatment. The Office of Rare Diseases at the National Institutes of Health estimates that about 1 in 12 people have 1 of the 7000 diseases listed as rare. In China at least 10 million are living with rare diseases. Some know that their specific disorder is genetic but, as is more often the case, have no idea of its genetic basis or the mode of inheritance. The question that should always be asked is: "To what extent is my disorder or illness genetic?" It will quickly become apparent in reading about the families and disorders described here that there is a genetic cause or component for all disorders, even those that are acquired. Examples abound. The way our bodies respond to infection is genetically controlled. How we react to medications and how our bodies respond to trauma depend on gene action.

There is much in this book you need to know, and many reasons why that could save your life and secure your health and the lives of all your loved ones. To know is to care and caring takes time and effort.

WHY YOU SHOULD KNOW

Quite simply, the reason you should know about your genes is that you care about yourself and your loved ones, wish to secure your and their health, and, where possible, save lives.

We are all fortunate living in the golden era of human genetics. While in the past we might have been able to clinically establish a genetic diagnosis, the true genetic basis remained elusive. Now, as a consequence of the Human Genome Project—an international, successful effort that mapped and discovered the structure of almost all human genes—we are able with increasing frequency and precision to determine the genetic basis of a disorder. This has been no small feat and has been compared in its significance to the splitting of the atom and walking on the moon! The personal and direct implications are likely to benefit us more than the other two historical feats.

All illnesses have a genetic component, and many result from a mutation in a single gene (such as cystic fibrosis, Huntington's disease, sickle cell disease, hemophilia, and muscular dystrophy) or alterations (called variations or polymorphisms) in a number of genes. Thus far, almost 20,000 genetic disorders or inherited physical or biochemical traits caused by single defective genes have been catalogued. Many of the common illnesses to which we may fall victim result from variations in multiple genes and interaction with one or more environmental triggers (such as pollen, viruses, or vitamin deficiency). When we decide to start a family, we each share an average 3% to 4% risk of having a child with a birth defect, mental retardation, or a genetic disorder. A March of Dimes Global Report on birth defects in 2006 estimated that more than 7 million babies are born each year with either a congenital abnormality or a genetic disease. That risk escalates to 7% to 8% by the age of 7 or 8 years, while a surprising number of defects with which we are born manifest for the first time in middle age or later (*see* Chapters 9 and 19). Birth defects (better called congenital malformations) are the leading cause of death in the newborn and account for 30% to 40% of hospital admissions to children's hospitals. In 2007 in the United States, about 1 in 5 newborn deaths resulted from congenital malformations. In China, 2008 figures indicated that congenital malformations accounted for 11% of deaths in childhood. The prevalence of mental retardation in Western populations approximates 3%, the causes of which to an important extent are genetic. It is important to know that a genetic disorder may be inherited or arise anew or simply involve the cell's genetic machinery.

The advent of DNA technology has spawned accurate diagnostic tests previously not possible. Now these remarkable tests enable us to identify carriers of certain genetic disorders and provide opportunities for very early prenatal diagnosis or pre-implantation genetic diagnosis.[1] These tests have the power to diagnose and predict the presence of a genetic disorder that might only manifest many decades later.

Although in the past it was possible to estimate personal risks of being a carrier or even being affected by a certain genetic disorder, DNA tests today frequently provide precise answers. Failure to recognize the availability of carrier or diagnostic tests may result in depriving you or a loved one of the opportunity to avoid a serious genetic disorder or miss out on a critical treatment that could secure health or even prevent a sudden death. Genetic tests may enable definitive recognition of risk and provide options, including prenatal diagnosis, pre-implantation genetic diagnosis, artificial insemination by donor, predictive testing, and adoption.

People are frequently unaware that quite different diseases or birth defects in the family are actually linked and all result from a single gene mutation. Multiple examples are discussed in the chapters that follow. Cancers affecting different organs in various family members might all have a common genetic basis. Sudden unexplained death might be due to an easily diagnosed genetic condition with available treatment. The rupture of a blood vessel resulting in a stroke or a fatal hemorrhage might have been anticipated and caught in time by anticipatory DNA testing. A family history of certain cancers might require surgery on a child barely a few weeks of age, given the anticipatory power of DNA testing. Recurrent miscarriages may well indicate genetic issues that inform future risks and options. Vitamin supplements taken just prior to and

---

1. Preimplantation genetic diagnosis enables detection of single gene defects from a single cell extracted from the embryo when it is merely between 8 and 16 cells in size! This test is performed after conception in a laboratory dish (called in vitro fertilization or IVF) and requires placement of the selected normal embryo into the hormonally prepared womb.

immediately after conception enable the avoidance of some 70% of conceptions developing the birth defect spina bifida.

The incidence of epilepsy is estimated to be about 1% of the population in industrialized countries, while about 3% will experience a seizure at some time in their lives. Close to one-third of those affected can have the cause determined by DNA or other genetic or neurological tests. Simple observations of birthmarks may provide clues to serious genetic disorders and should never be ignored. Carriers of certain genetic disorders may also show symptoms and signs of a disorder that can require treatment.

Certain genetic traits will make a person seriously susceptible to certain foods, ingestion of which could prove fatal, or in some rarer disorders, each child born to an affected mother would have the same disorder. Serious hemorrhage, presenting either as a stroke or a bleed elsewhere in the body, may signal the presence of a treatable bleeding disorder. On the other hand, sudden death caused by a clotting disorder presents opportunities for avoidance, surveillance, and life-long successful management. There are many other treatable genetic disorders where the remedies may prevent mental retardation developing, banish episodes of recurrent abdominal and joint pain, help avoid infection and early death, save life by preemptive surgery, and enable pursuit of a healthy life despite a genetic burden.

These examples are explored throughout this book in the stories of families I have seen whose often poignant experiences illustrate the critical need for everyone to be well-informed about their family history. Opportunities for avoidance, prevention, and treatment of genetic disorders largely stem from the new advances in genetic technology and other biomedical advances. There are endless reasons why you should know your genes. A guide to what you should first find out is the basis for our next discussion.

WHAT YOU SHOULD KNOW: YOUR FAMILY HISTORY

Every cell in our bodies houses at least 21,500 protein-coding genes, not much more than the total 20,000 or so genes in the lowly roundworm. It should come as no surprise that most of these genes are beneficial, but some are positively harmful. Fortunately, the defective genes we carry are mostly cryptic—hidden and frequently never revealed in our lifetime. These are usually recessive genes that rarely impair health, but when mated with a partner's similarly defective gene, offspring with serious disease or defects may emerge. Dominant genes in particular may only wreak havoc in midlife or even later, despite being detectable as early as the eight-cell embryo. So gathering information about defective genes needs to be culled from your family history.

Yet important details about the health of close relatives is often difficult to gather. Witness the roughly 50% of marriages that end in divorce, the number of single mothers, the physical (and emotional) distance between close relatives, and adoptions. Further confounding every effort to discover vital information is the noncommunicating family and estranged families. Grandparents or parents who have hidden or not shared important health information or knowledge of nonpaternity complicate matters even more.

Quite often during a genetic evaluation I have pressed couples to seek and to find vital information in their families. Not infrequently, one or the other have returned and unabashedly echoed a common refrain: "I didn't know, I didn't know." I've also been startled by the many couples I have seen who have no idea about their ancestral origins.

Others, upon questioning, have stated that they didn't know what happened to their grandparents, because they had died when the patients were still "young." When asked about whether their parents have told them about the fate of their own grandparents, the simple answer is often no. When I inquire whether they had actually asked their parents about their own grandparents, their answer was again a simple negative.

Making acquisition of factual information difficult is the natural reluctance to question a family member who has experienced the loss of a child or an untimely death of a family member. This natural sensitivity and empathy is easy to understand. In such circumstances, I have advised patients to enlist the help, for example, of a grandparent or a mother, explaining the critical reason for the inquiry. This has often proven successful, but not always.

For those whom I hope are in the majority, what needs to be known is rather clear. First, you should reach for a pencil and paper and draw a diagram of your family tree (pedigree). You could use the symbols shown in Figure 1.1 to construct your family pedigree and use the example shown in Figure 1.2. You should enter the names of individuals below their symbols. Alternatively you could proceed online using My Family Health Portrait (www.familyhistory. hhs.gov), which was developed by Dr. Richard H. Carmona, 17th Surgeon General of the United States. He also declared that every year there will be National Family History Day on Thanksgiving.

The ancestral origins should be noted for each side of the family. From time to time, in trying to discover the cause of a serious and even rare genetic condition, suspicion has fallen on common ancestral origins of a member of

Pedigree Symbols

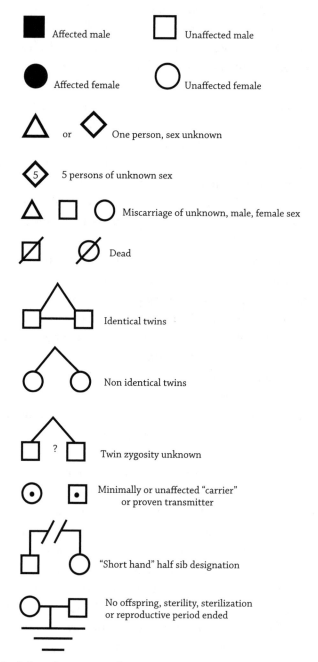

FIGURE 1.1 Symbols used to construct a family pedigree.

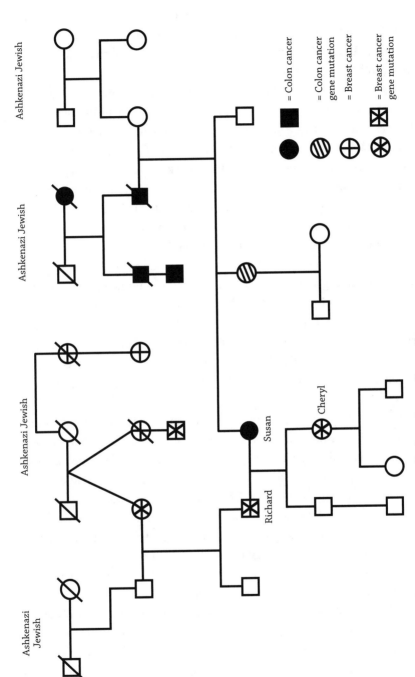

Ashkenazi Jewish

Ashkenazi Jewish

Ashkenazi Jewish

Ashkenazi Jewish

= Colon cancer

= Colon cancer gene mutation

= Breast cancer

= Breast cancer gene mutation

Susan

Cheryl

Richard

FIGURE 1.2   Richard and Susan's family pedigree (for discussion, *see* Chapter 8).

the mother's and father's grandparents or great-grandparents having "lived" in the same town in a distant country. Rare genetic conditions are not infrequently the result of mutated recessive genes that quietly make their way down the ancestral tree, only to meet an ancestral genetic mate that results in an offspring with a serious genetic disorder.

In the same way, ethnicity should be documented, given the realization that there is no ethnic or racial group without some type of genetic burden. Simply on the basis of ethnicity, a host of different genetic carrier tests are recommended (Chapter 15). Consanguinity is also an important cause of rarer genetic disorders and is often suspected when there are known first-cousin marriages or uncle–niece unions. In fact, in Saudi Arabia, the Arab Emirates, and some other Arab countries, consanguinity rates are 25% to 70%. High rates of consanguinity also occur in India and Pakistan, with the same consequences of an increased rate of serious birth defects and mental retardation.

Clear determination from which side a particular disorder has emerged is of major importance, given the different patterns of inheritance. For the most part, given solid family information about a specific genetic disorder, pedigree analysis can reveal the mode of inheritance and the likely risks for individual family members being at risk. The various modes of inheritance are explored in Chapter 6. Determination that there has been paternal inheritance may, in some genetic disorders, indicate the likelihood of earlier onset of more severe disease.

Information about anyone having recurrent miscarriages or having experienced a stillbirth is important for the clues that information provides about causation, risk, and explanations for subsequent defects. Certainly as much information as possible should be ascertained about birth defects and mental retardation in any family member. Of particular importance is the nature of the evaluation that might have been done with special reference to what tests were done and whether a diagnosis had been established. Similarly, information about the genetic defect or fetal abnormality that resulted in pregnancy termination should be obtained and documented. Prolonged infertility is a further risk factor that needs to be considered.

It is critical to obtain accurate information about family health disorders. Simply knowing that grandma had "stomach cancer" is unhelpful. Was the diagnosis cancer of the ovary, colon, uterus, pancreas, stomach, liver, or intestine? The genetic risks and available tests will differ according to the precise answer. "My cousin had muscular dystrophy" may not help either. There are many forms of muscular dystrophy, and once again, a precise answer will inform both risks and future options as well as what special DNA tests might be useful.

Those who have been adopted often have no idea of their ethnic origin or their family history. Moreover, they mostly never get to know if serious genetic disease occurs later in the parent(s) who gave them up for adoption. There should be uniform requirements that a child's ethnicity and extant family history be disclosed at the time of adoption. Moreover, newborns and children in the adoption process should be subject only to genetic tests or screening performed routinely for all children.

Knowledge about how a diagnosis was made may be critically important. Was there a biopsy or a DNA test, rather than simply a "blood test"? Was there an autopsy? Who has the report? Obtaining a copy of an autopsy report may, on occasion, prove extremely valuable. Autopsy reports are usually accurate, although sometimes genetic disorders are not actually noted, especially when the cause of death was not a particular genetic disorder. Note, however, that death certificates are notoriously misleading or incorrect and have to be interpreted with caution.

Photographs of an affected family member may end up being crucial. I recall an out-of-state couple who came for a consultation concerned about their risks of having a child affected with muscular dystrophy. The wife said that her grandmother had muscular dystrophy, but she could not provide a specific name for the type of muscular dystrophy she had. She was, however, able to obtain a photograph of her grandparents that had appeared in the local newspaper. On their return visit, my inspection of the photograph revealed a definitive diagnosis from the appearance of their grandmother whom they had said had some difficulty swallowing. She had the dominantly inherited oculopharyngeal muscular dystrophy. Subsequent targeted DNA tests confirmed that the mutated gene had indeed passed along to the grandchild, who had come for the consultation. She had a 50% risk of transmitting this disorder to each of her own children. Fortunately, prenatal diagnosis was available and the fetus proved to be unaffected.

Parents who have a child with serious birth defects or mental retardation may spend years consulting different physicians in seeking to understand the cause of their child's disability. Eventually, after much anguish and often enormous cost, parents may be too exhausted to continue, more especially given the realities of success. For major birth defects and significant mental retardation, a cause may not be established in at least 40% of cases, and with milder forms of mental retardation, that figure might approach 60%. The need to know the cause may never cease. During the last year, I was consulted by three sets of parents who requested that their search be resumed. The common theme for all three families was the hope that new genetic technology might now provide a long sought-after answer. The first family's son was moderately to severely retarded and 40 years of age. After all those years, they still were hoping to find an answer because their daughter, now in her 30s, wished to have children and was concerned about her risk of having a child with the disorder that affected her brother. We were able to only perform a few DNA tests because of insurance limitations and failed to establish a diagnosis. The second couple's son was 45 years old and severely retarded. Once again, the search had been spawned by the desire of their daughter to begin a family. This time, a chromosomal micro-array (*see* Chapter 5) revealed a deletion in the brother's single X chromosome. We determined that his sister was not a carrier and not at risk of having an affected child. The third couple were grandparents who had raised their granddaughter and were concerned about her future health, because their daughter had died at age 32 years from colon cancer. Our studies of the DNA that they had obtained and banked with us 15 years previously, when their daughter was dying, provided the opportunity to exclude mutations in the most important and common colon cancer genes.

The occurrence of a sudden death in the family is unfortunately not rare. In Chapter 9, important details about sudden death occurring at any age in different families is discussed. Of importance to other family members is the precise result of the autopsy, if one is performed. For years, I have advocated that during every medical autopsy (noncriminal) a 1-centimeter square sample of liver should be taken and frozen without preservative for potential future DNA studies on behalf of the family. This sample could literally remain frozen, or where facilities are limited, DNA can be extracted and banked frozen in tiny vials for decades. I have seen families eternally grateful for that step having been taken and subsequently benefiting family members. One recurring and disturbing observation is that autopsy reports may never find their way back to the family, who also may not realize the importance of the findings. Families should be sure to obtain the autopsy report, which may only materialize many months after the loss of a loved one.

Hemorrhage at any age may occur in any organ and cause serious complications or even death. In the brain, the diagnosis might be a stroke or a ruptured aneurysm,[2] which can be life-threatening or the cause of permanent disability.

---

2. A small balloon-like dilatation along the course of an artery

Serious bleeding may also occur in the lung, the intestinal tract, and the kidneys. Bleeding into joints, muscles, and skin may cause considerable pain and discomfort and, together with nose bleeds, signal the presence of a hereditary bleeding disorder (*see* Chapter 17). Easy bruising and frequent nosebleeds should not be ignored. Knowledge about family members with any unexplained or recurrent bleeding episodes should initiate inquiries with the aim of determining if there is an inherited bleeding disorder within the family. On the other hand, clotting (thrombosis) may also occur in any organ. Once again, thrombosis in blood vessels of the brain could result in a stroke, while clots coming from the legs (due to deep vein thrombosis) may lodge in the large blood vessels to the lung with the potential of causing sudden death (caused by pulmonary emboli). Any clotting disorder in a family member requires evaluation to determine whether or not there is a diagnosable genetic clotting disorder (*see* Chapter 17).

I have discussed some of the most important reasons why you should get to know your family history and what information you should seek. It is desperately sad to encounter patients who have ignored their family history, only to discover too late that there were specific gene tests available whose early use would have been lifesaving. I have repeatedly seen siblings and cousins, uncles and aunts, and even parents, whose lives were lost or placed at serious risk because of failure to pay attention to genetic disorders in the family. Worse still is the failure to communicate the diagnosis of a serious genetic disorder in a child and later witness the devastating realization by the parents (and other family members) that one of their own was affected, but they had failed to warn close relatives about the risks and available tests.

Consultation with a medical geneticist should be sought if and when there are concerns about the genetic basis of any disorder.[3] The importance of all the fact-gathering described above will become clear as you read about the families and their various genetic disorders described in this book. As mentioned earlier, chapter headings do not reveal specific genetic disorders, as each family history could be yours without you ever having realized it.

---

3. A medical geneticist in the United States can be identified through the American College of Medical Genetics (www.acmg.nct), in Canada through the Canadian College of Medical Geneticists (www.ccmg-ccmg.org), in the United Kingdom through the British Society for Human Genetics (http://www.bshg.org.ukl), and in Europe through the European Society of Medical Genetics (http://www,eshg.org/)

TOO MANY OR TOO FEW CHROMOSOMES

Under the high-powered microscope and after staining, tiny zebra-like striped threads can be visualized in almost all cells. These tiny threads are housed in every cell's center of operations, called the nucleus.[1] The nucleus is the control center of the cell as well as the receptor of messages and the repository of our blueprints (genes), which we inherit from our parents and grandparents. The blueprints determine cell function and the characteristics we pass to each of our children. These tiny threads, called chromosomes, are made up of chemical compounds, the most important component of which is deoxyribonucleic acid (DNA)—the substance of which genes are made.

More than a century ago, it was noticed that when a special dye was added to a cell at a critical point in its formation, thread-like structures of protein would take up the stain, becoming easier to see. They were, therefore, called chromosomes, from the Greek words *chroma* (meaning "color") and *soma* (or "body"). As early as the late nineteenth century, chromosomes were already considered the likely carriers of hereditary factors.

All of the information necessary to direct the formation and function of a human being or any other living thing—from bacteria, to plants, to elephants—is contained in these complex, thin threads. The chromosomes are, in turn, composed of genes, which are the units of heredity. Single genes are so small that they remain invisible, even when viewed through the most modem instruments, including the electron microscope.

You receive half of your chromosome complement from your mother and half from your father. In other words, the genes constituting your chromosomes are equally contributed by both parents. In turn, you will pass along half

---

1. The exception is mature red blood cells, which are devoid of a nucleus.

of your chromosomes and genes to each of your own children. You have 46 chromosomes in every cell—23 contributed from each parent.

The number of chromosomes and their structure vary greatly among living organisms. Chimpanzees and gorillas have 48 chromosomes per cell. We have only known since 1956 that humans have 46 chromosomes in every cell.

Experienced cytotechnologists can view the chromosomes of a cell, visually identify and check each chromosome under the microscope for structural integrity, and, of course, determine the number of chromosomes present. The visual examination is followed by photographing a number of cells and then, with available special computer software, pairing the parental chromosomes for a final definitive analytic conclusion.

Each chromosome can be distinguished from another, not only by size but by using various staining techniques that create horizontal bands or cross-striations that enable precise identification. This banding or zebra-like pattern along each chromosome is represented by 550 bands that are usually examined in routine analysis. It is now possible, however, to examine chromosomes at an earlier stage in cell division when they appear longer under the microscope. When these chromosomes are stained, between 800 and 1,400 bands (some say even as many as 5,000) can be visualized, thereby making it possible to detect very small defects. These high-resolution chromosome-banding techniques allow recognition of minor differences between individuals.

The mother's and father's contributed chromosomes to a cell are analyzed by matching and pairing and then are numbered from 1 through 22, with the last pair being the female (X) or male (Y) chromosomes that determine gender. Females have two X chromosomes, and males have one X and one Y chromosome.

It is therefore possible to distinguish between chromosomes—particularly between the structural differences that are commonly seen between individuals for chromosomes 1, 9, 16, and the male Y chromosome. These common chromosome differences, called polymorphisms, can be used to trace an individual chromosome through a family. I recall a prenatal diagnosis I made some years ago, in which a rather odd-looking Y chromosome was found in the fetus. To exclude the possibility of a potential structural abnormality, I requested a blood sample from the husband to check his Y chromosome. That study showed a completely different Y chromosome. This gentleman, who was a merchant seaman, had spent much of his time away from home and it did not take much for him to calculate the implications!

The chromosomal polymorphisms[2] have also been used to determine the parental origin of individual chromosomes such as the extra chromosome number 21 that appears in conditions such as Down syndrome.[3] From chromosome or DNA studies, we know that the extra number 21 chromosome in Down syndrome, for example, originates from the mother in about 95% of cases and from the father in about 5%.

SPERM AND EGGS

The cell from which the egg (ovum) originates has the usual 46 chromosomes.

Creation of the ovum requires splitting of all the chromosome pairs so that one of each pair occupies the future ovum, constituted by 23 single chromosomes that will pair up with the 23 contained within the sperm, which originated via the same process (called meiosis). In this process, which in fact involves another step with division and duplication, errors may occur either in the first or second steps. A particular chromosome could be "sticky" and adhere to the chromosome from which it was duplicated. The consequence would be the presence or absence of a whole extra chromosome constituting the complement of the future egg or sperm. If that extra chromosome is a number 21, then the two number 21 chromosomes in the egg (more common) will meet the sperm, carrying one number 21 chromosome, at fertilization, resulting in a fertilized egg with three number 21 chromosomes. This is the classical outcome for Down syndrome (called Trisomy 21). This same "sticky chromosome" process (called nondisjunction) can theoretically occur with any chromosome but is most common by far with chromosomes 21, 18, 13, 16, and X. Trisomy 16 invariably ends in miscarriage or fetal death. Trisomies 18 and 13 are associated with profound mental retardation, serious birth defects, and early death, and numerical abnormalities involving the X chromosome are associated with syndromes discussed in the next chapter. Absence of any non-sex chromosome is almost always lethal in the embryo and rarely compatible with long-term survival. A missing X chromosome will result in Turner syndrome in surviving females (*see* Chapter 3).

---

2. Today, DNA markers enable determination not only of individual chromosome origin but even segments of actual genes within the chromosome structure.

3. Named after an English physician, John Langdon Down, who described the features of this condition in 1866.

The fact that most of us are born healthy seems a miracle, when one considers the human embryo soon after fertilization. A study of human embryos at about the eight-cell stage and analyzed in the course of in vitro fertilization (IVF) revealed that only 9% had a normal set of chromosomes in each cell.[4] Abnormalities of chromosome number were rife and included chromosome pairs derived entirely from one parent. Moreover, major structural chromosomal abnormalities (*see* Chapter 4) were observed in 70% of all embryos examined! Embryos were from young healthy fertile couples undergoing IVF for genetic disorders unrelated to chromosomal disorders. Thankfully we can conclude that we are spared from being born defective by abnormal embryos not implanting in the womb, not developing, or being rejected by the mother's body in very early pregnancy.

During the pairing process within the developing egg or sperm, tiny segments of chromosomes or genes may skip over or interchange with their sister chromosome.

Moreover, besides this process, called recombination, two chromosomes may break, and the broken pieces, like musical chairs, simply exchange places (called a translocation).

Consequently, there are two categories of chromosome abnormalities—numerical (too many or too few chromosomes) or structural rearrangements.

NUMERICAL CHROMOSOME ABNORMALITIES

The most common non-sex chromosome abnormality results from the extra number 21 chromosome, resulting in Down syndrome (also called Trisomy 21). The tendency to have "sticky" chromosomes increases with a woman's age, as do the risks of bearing a child with a trisomy, such as Down syndrome, Trisomy 13, or Trisomy 18. The precise cause of the "stickiness" remains uncertain. It is startling to realize that almost 1 in 200 human **conceptions** (not live births) have Trisomy 21. The number of genes recognized thus far on chromosome 21 exceeds 400, which, therefore, occur in triplicate in this disorder. Overexpression of some of these genes undoubtedly leads to the intellectual disabilities and physical defects encountered in Down syndrome.

---

4. Another study showed that eggs from women younger than age 24 years had 8.5% with chromosomal abnormalities, but for women between 40 and 44 years, 39.5% showed abnormalities. This probably explains the main reason for "infertility" in women with advancing age.

Gunter and Helga had carefully planned their professional lives and the 2-year spacing between their three children. Their children were 18, 16, and 14 when Helga discovered her unplanned fourth pregnancy. Then, at 42 years of age, she and Gunter were initially shocked by recognition of this fourth pregnancy. They had intense discussions about abortion and decided against pregnancy termination. They did, however, follow the recommendations of Helga's obstetrician in agreeing to have a prenatal genetic study, given her age and the associated increased risk of having a child with an extra chromosome, especially chromosome 21, which results in Down syndrome.

Prenatal chromosome studies revealed that the fetus had Trisomy 21 (Down syndrome). Once again, they had intense discussions about pregnancy termination and came for a genetics consultation. They knew little about this condition and needed a full description, including a detailed perspective on the short- and long-range implications of having a child with Down syndrome.

I described the common features, signs, and associations in Down syndrome, as noted in Table 2.1. The facial features, although the least problematic, frequently receive earliest attention. These include the flat face; small jaw; upslanting eyes; epicanthal folds (in corners of the eyes); small, low-set ears; flat bridge between the eyes; and a short, broad neck with excess skinfolds. Poor muscle tone makes for a floppy infant. Frequent but not invariable findings include some incurving of the fifth fingers and toes, a single crease across the palms, and a wider than usual gap between the first and second toes. More importantly, short stature is a constant, as is mild-to-moderate learning disability or mental retardation.

Besides the physical features and characteristics, about 50% of those with Down syndrome have heart defects, frequently requiring surgical repair. Not all of the heart defects can, in fact, be fully repaired, and a few may prove fatal in infancy. Eye abnormalities are common, including crossed-eyes, strabismus, poor eyesight, and other more minor eye problems. About 20% of those with Down syndrome require orthopedic attention, the most important issue being due to the lax ligaments. This is especially the case at the top of the spine, where vertebral instability[5] (vertebral slipping) has the potential for damaging the spinal cord. The risk of leukemia is at least 20-fold higher compared to children with normal chromosomes. That risk translates into a 2% to 2.7% actual risk by age 30 years.

Cancer of the testes is more frequent in Down syndrome, whereas the likelihood of solid tumors is generally reduced. Premature aging makes a 30- to 40-year-old with Down syndrome look much older. However, and more important, the frequency of early onset Alzheimer's disease is greatly increased. By age 60 years, between 50% and 70% of those with Down syndrome develop dementia.

We had an intense and extensive discussion about coping with a child with Down syndrome in the family. Decades of experience learning from the many families involved provided the necessary insights into the issues that could be anticipated. Given that both Gunter and Helga had professional careers, it was important to consider the new medical and special education needs that would require time, effort, and finances. The additional stress could involve their personal lives, as well as having effects on their other children. Careful thought was necessary about the ultimate lifetime care that would be required, as life expectancy is an average of 55 to 60 years. Inevitably, continuing care would be necessary either by siblings, government, or other organizations. Lifetime oversight would be required.

Helga and Gunter, after careful consideration, decided to keep the pregnancy. I subsequently saw the baby, who did in fact have a major heart defect that fortunately was later surgically repaired. The family subsequently moved out of Massachusetts, and I never saw them again.

DOWN SYNDROME

The incidence of Down syndrome averages about 1 in 733 births in the United States[6] but is likely to approximate 1 in 1,000 among populations where pregnancy termination for this condition is more common. Helga's risk for having

---

5. Called atlanto-occipital subluxation.
6. More than 5,000 infants are born with Down syndrome each year in the United States.

Table 2.1 Down Syndrome: Common Features and Associations

Major Features

Typical facial appearance (upslanting eyes, flat facial profile, epicanthal folds, short nose with depressed nasal bridge)
Brachycephaly (foreshortened head)
Mental retardation/learning disability
Hypotonia
Growth retardation
Abnormal dermatoglyphics (creases on palms and soles)
Congenital heart defects
Hyperflexible joints
Dysplasia of the pelvis
Dysplasia of mid-phalanx of fifth finger
Short stature (<5 feet)

Minor Features

Eye disorders (strabismus, cataracts, nystagmus)
Hearing impairment
Ear and respiratory tract infections
Dental problems
Diastasis recti (splayed abdominal muscles)
Duodenal atresia
Imperforate anus
Wide gap between first and second toes
Incurved fifth fingers and toes
Abnormal gait

Other Medical Problems

Premature aging
Alzheimer's disease
Alopecia areata (hair loss)
Immune disorders
Obstructive sleep apnea
Atlantoaxial joint instability or subluxation (skull–spine joint)
Diabetes
Obesity
Epilepsy
Hirschsprung's disease (bowel obstruction)
Celiac disease
Leukemia
Testicular cancer
Hypothyroidism
Decreased life expectancy

a child with a numerical chromosome disorder (especially 21, 18, 13, and X) approximated 3%.

Prenatal genetic studies are recommended routinely for women pregnant at age 35 years or older, given the escalating risk that eventually rises to 7% to 10% by the age 45 years. However, the vast majority of offspring conceived and born with Down syndrome are delivered by mothers **under** age 35 years. As a consequence, maternal serum screening (*see* Chapter 7) was developed to recognize pregnancies at increased risk and to offer prenatal chromosome studies. In this way, detection of between 80% and 94% of all pregnancies where the fetus has Down syndrome is achievable.

Notwithstanding ethnic origin, all children with Down syndrome have easily identifiable features, regardless of the chromosome type.[7] About 94% of cases have the extra number 21 chromosome, 3% to 4% have a translocation (*see* Chapter 4) involving chromosome 21, and 2% to 3% have a mixture of normal cells and some with Trisomy 21 (called mosaicism).

With early intervention, speech therapy, and special education, those with Down syndrome can lead meaningful lives but will require care and oversight for life. A number of associations are particularly important in the care of those with Down syndrome. Diabetes, thyroid disease, celiac disease, arthritis, and periodontal gum disease are all more common, as is a tendency to obesity. Hearing loss (mainly caused by the high frequency of ear infections); eye abnormalities such as cataracts, glaucoma, crossed-eyes; and major refractive errors (found in about 61%) are all important. The greater susceptibility to infection remains a major cause of morbidity and mortality among those with Down syndrome. Epilepsy occurs in about 5% to 10% of cases.

My experience with Down syndrome has been extensive and of long duration.

The genetics laboratories that I directed in the late 1960s and 1970s were in the grounds of the Walter E. Fernald State School, where about 400 of the 2,000 residents had Down syndrome. In the subsequent decades, there were endless genetic evaluations and counseling with special reference to prenatal diagnosis. Families shared their experiences and the many challenges they confronted.

---

7. Features of Down syndrome are clearly evident in an Egyptian sculpture dating to the first century BC, recognized by my colleague Professor Christos Bartsocas and shown in a book entitled *Genetics and Malformations in Art* by J. Kunze and I. Nippert, published in Berlin by Grosse Verlag, 1986.

Three different families over time related a similar story. Upon arriving home, they were horrified to discover blood "all over the house" and immediately thought there had been an accident or worse. Each of these families discovered their young teenage daughter with Down syndrome having her first menstrual period, which had occurred without warning and of course was not understood by any of them.

A number of families have described their teenage boys with Down syndrome who lacked any sexual inhibitions. Besides masturbating in public, they would often inappropriately touch and grope their female siblings or mother.

One family, who eventually decided to have their daughter with Down syndrome placed in a state residential school for the handicapped, discovered to their horror that another non-Down syndrome patient had impregnated their daughter. Their daughter was discovered to be pregnant at a stage beyond 6 months, her attendants thinking that she had just put on weight. She delivered a child, who also had Down syndrome. The medical literature records a few dozen such examples, with about 50% of cases resulting in the birth of a child with Trisomy 21. Some parents have resorted to tubal ligation before any such eventuality. Males with Down syndrome have not been reported as fathering a child.

Apart from the children with Down syndrome, I've heard stories concerning their siblings. Several families reported female teenagers who complained that they were being stigmatized and were not being dated because of a younger sibling with Down syndrome. This was distressing, for the siblings, but nevertheless real, requiring consideration of all possible consequences, psychological and otherwise.

I have seen a few families in which one or more siblings of the child with Down syndrome became juvenile delinquents, ultimately complaining that they were completely ignored given the time, effort, and money being devoted to their younger sibling with Down syndrome. There is just so much time in the day where parents are torn between their duties to care for the entire family and the demands of a handicapped child. There appear to be no easy solutions, but parents in these unenviable situations will have to be keenly aware of the needs of all their children.

I have encountered many families in which the siblings of a child with Down syndrome have subsequently pursued health-related careers and who have been clearly influenced by their experience with Down syndrome in their own homes. Those that I have had the good fortune to meet have demonstrated outstanding compassion and understanding of the less able among us.

I have been consulted by a very large number of couples planning pregnancies where one of them has had a sibling or cousin with Down syndrome. The thematic inquiry in this selected but large group of couples was to determine their risks and the options for avoidance of Down syndrome. The partner with this history invariably sought a way to avoid reliving their past experience.

Finally, while working in London in the mid-1960s, I recall the publication of a book by Nigel Hunt. Hunt had Down syndrome but nevertheless was able to put together the book entitled *The World of Nigel Hunt*. He was the son of a school principal and demonstrated what good care, learning, and education could do for those with Down syndrome. Whether or not he was a mosaic for Down syndrome remains unproven.

OTHER TRISOMIES

Virtually all chromosomes have been found in triplicate, mostly in the very early, spontaneously miscarried, abnormal embryo/fetus or (much less frequently) in the stillborn or liveborn infant. Two important trisomies involve chromosomes 18 and 13. Key features for both include severe defects of brain, heart, eyes, face, spine, intestine, kidneys, and limbs. Both these disorders are associated with advancing maternal age but may occur in women of any age. Extremely few fetuses with trisomies 13 or 18 survive during pregnancy. For the few that do, the average survival for Trisomy 13 is about 3 days and for Trisomy 18 about a week. Although fewer than 5% of these infants survive to age 1 year, some are very long-term survivors with profound retardation and other birth defects. Generally, the risk of recurrence to a mother younger than age 35 years following conception of offspring with trisomies 21, 18, or 13 approximates 1%. Older mothers' risk depends on age and can reach 7% to 10% by age 45 years. Prenatal chromosome diagnosis (*see* Chapter 7) is recommended for all women who are age 35 years or older or who have previously had a child with a chromosome abnormality.

MISCARRIAGE AND STILLBIRTH

You may be surprised to learn that as many as one-third of all recognized pregnancies end in miscarriage. Even more startling, an estimated 78% of all conceptions do not result in a live birth. About 22% of miscarriages occur at the time of the first expected menstrual period after conception, even before pregnancy has been detected.

Among the most common causes of miscarriage are chromosome disorders in the developing embryo or fetus. About 1 in 10 sperm and 1 in 4 mature eggs have a chromosome abnormality, and up to half of the ova of women with infertility have chromosome defects. Remarkably, chromosome defects occur in some 8% of all pregnancies (about 1 in every 13 conceptions). Miraculously, the body is able to detect and reject more than 99% of them. About 50% of the embryos or fetuses miscarried in the first 3 months of pregnancy have some type of chromosome disorder.

In couples who experience miscarriage repeatedly, there is an increased likelihood that one of the partners carries (but in most cases is not affected by) a chromosome defect. After two miscarriages, there is a 1% to 3% likelihood that one member of the couple carries a chromosome defect that is being passed on to the embryo. After three miscarriages, that likelihood increases to 3% to 8%. At this point, it is standard medical practice to recommend blood chromosome analysis of both partners. If a chromosome abnormality is in fact detected in one partner, the couple's risk of bearing a chromosomally abnormal child can be determined. This risk is rarely more than 20% and is usually only about 1%. Fortunately, prenatal diagnostic tests are available and are recommended for all pregnancies when one partner carries or has a chromosome defect.

Given the body's remarkable ability to detect and reject chromosomally defective embryos and fetuses, the frequency of such defects drops from a high of about 78% at about 2 weeks of pregnancy to about 3% at 16 weeks and to 0.5% in live-born infants. Stillborns and babies who die in the first weeks of life have a 6% to 11 % frequency of chromosome defects. It is therefore critically important to check the chromosomes of every stillborn baby (even if no physical defects are found), not only to determine the cause of stillbirth but also to detect any potential risks to future pregnancies and to identify appropriate options, including future prenatal testing.

Fortunately, the remarkable efficiency of the body in recognizing and rejecting defective embryos or fetuses results in very few babies actually being born with these disorders. For example, about 75% of pregnancies with Down syndrome do not result in a live birth. Notwithstanding the efficiency of the body, chromosome abnormalities still occur with a frequency of about 1 in every 156 live births (0.65%). About 0.4% of live-born babies have a **serious** chromosome defect, and an additional 0.25% carry a chromosome defect that may later have repercussions when they begin childbearing. All chromosome defects can be detected in early pregnancy so that parents can consider the option of elective abortion. Moreover, being aware of your family history may prompt chromosome tests before pregnancy, which could provide early warning of significant risk. Early warning permits the issue of elective abortion to be circumvented in favor of other options.

Clearly, having too many non-sex chromosomes almost invariably causes serious or fatal disorders. In contrast, having too many or too few sex chromosomes do not portend as ominous a future, as discussed in the next chapter.

3

X'S AND Y'S

THE SEX CHROMOSOMES

Zoey's first marriage was a disaster. She had met Eric at a baseball game and was immediately taken by his lively personality and apparent fun-loving nature. He was also sports-loving and an excellent ice hockey player, who she heard later enjoyed a scrap on the ice. They married after a short courtship. Zoey soon discovered that Eric probably suffered from manic depressive disorder and that he was more often anxious, depressed, and angry than happy. Within months of marriage, it became clear that he was verbally and physically abusive, and the marriage ended after she miscarried her first pregnancy. Zoey promised herself that she would never marry again after that traumatic relationship.

About 15 years later, and well into her successful accounting career, she met Victor—a quiet, introspective, tall, and rather gangly man. He was the manager of a furniture store and a bachelor. After more than a year of courtship, Zoey invited Victor to come and live in her apartment. Zoey was already 38 years old, and as she said, since "the clock was ticking," she decided to try for a pregnancy once again.

I got to see this couple in consultation after they had tried in vain to achieve a pregnancy for more than a year. The consultation with me was precipitated by the discovery that Victor had no sperm in his semen.[1] Victor's family history provided no clues, and there were no recognizable

---

1. Called azoospermia. An important and relatively common finding in men (with either no sperm or a severely reduced sperm count) is a tiny deletion in the long arm of the Y chromosome, simply diagnosed by a DNA study on a blood sample. A second important reason for the lack of sperm is a genital form of cystic fibrosis. Hence, if a chromosome study is shown to be normal, DNA studies for cystic fibrosis mutations and the Y deletion study are recommended.

factors that could impact conception in Zoey's family. She had experienced one miscarriage but had a normal menstrual history and was shown to ovulate regularly.

Victor's personal history assumed significance during my physical examination. He had always been the tallest boy in the class, had very few friends, and had always been reticent and very much a loner. In elementary school, he had considerable difficulty with arithmetic and performed below average in all other subjects. After puberty, he recalled being teased unmercifully about his large breasts, resulting in his systematic avoidance of all sports. He finished high school and completed a 2-year Associate's degree in a community college and then went to work at the furniture store.

When I examined Victor, he was a pleasant, quiet, and awkward fellow who towered above me with his height of 6'4". His enormously long arms, when measured, gave a wingspan equal to his height! His breasts were indeed prominent, but the most striking finding was particularly small testes. His penis was entirely normal. The findings on examination and his history made for a clinical diagnosis of Klinefelter syndrome, a disorder in which a male has an extra female (X) chromosome.[2] The absence of sperm is characteristic in this condition and is due to a failure of sperm production by the testes. The clinical diagnosis was confirmed by a blood chromosome study, which revealed the extra X chromosome, resulting in his having not the usual 46 but a total of 47 chromosomes because of his XXY chromosome complement.

Zoey was tearful on hearing the news. I advised that there was a possibility that a single sperm could be harvested via needle aspiration from Victor's testes. The chance of success, however, was very small. Moreover, it would be possible to pick up a sperm that might have two rather than one sex chromosome. If the sperm had XX chromosomes, the offspring would be born with one of Zoey's sex (X) chromosomes to make up a triple X female (discussed later in this chapter). If the sperm housed an

2. Named after Harry Klinefelter, who described the typical signs of this chromosome disorder in 1942.

XY chromosome complement, then a male offspring with Klinefelter syndrome would be conceived and born.

Alternative options that we discussed included artificial insemination by donor (more than 20,000 babies born in the United States have been conceived by this method each year). Neither was interested in adoption and reluctantly decided to live their lives without children.

Zoey and Victor returned to see me some 5 years later, after he had undergone a unilateral mastectomy. While showering, Victor had discovered a lump in his right breast, which he apparently ignored for at least 6 months. Only when he mentioned this finding to Zoey did she insist on him seeing a surgeon. That appointment was quickly followed by a biopsy, which revealed breast cancer. A mastectomy was performed within days thereafter. Fortunately, no evidence of the cancer having spread was found. Victor's physician had referred him to me for the consultation, since Victor's late mother had a history of breast cancer.

This all happened long before DNA studies were available, and the only recourse was to advise about the importance of surveillance in his other breast for the rest of his life. Men with Klinefelter syndrome have a very much greater risk of developing breast cancer than men with a normal set of chromosomes.[3] However, his late mother had had cancer in both of her breasts, and this fact translated into a possible 50% risk for Victor, reflecting a probable dominantly inherited additional condition, which is covered in Chapter 6. They subsequently moved to the West Coast, and I never heard from them again.

KLINEFELTER SYNDROME

Klinefelter syndrome is common and occurs in about 1 in 576 males, with 6,000 to 7,000 born each year. It is likely that there are many more than 200,000 males with Klinefelter syndrome in the United States alone. The vast majority have remained undiagnosed, consistent with the conclusion of a large Danish National Registry study that showed less than 10% of the expected diagnoses had been made before the age of puberty. Not surprisingly, then, men mostly come to medical attention because of issues related to infertility.

3. A National Cancer Institute study of 4,501,578 men 18-100 years of age found 642 with breast cancer. Men with Klinefelter syndrome had an almost 17-fold increased risk.

About 80% of affected men have the extra X chromosome in all their cells. The other 20% have variations that include most commonly a mixture of normal (XY) and XXY cells (called mosaicism), or they may have three or four X chromosomes and even an extra Y chromosome. Possession of three, four, or more X chromosomes invariably spells serious mental retardation. Occasionally, there may also be a structurally abnormal X chromosome. Rarely, a male may be born with two female (X) chromosomes, one of them having the male determining gene (SRY), normally housed in the Y chromosome, embedded within it! The symptoms and signs are those of Klinefelter syndrome. Those with mosaicism have the best chance of normal sperm recovery and successful fertilization. Sperm recovery might require needle aspiration from the testes, after which fertilization can be accomplished in a tissue culture dish by directly inserting the sperm into the egg (a procedure called intracytoplasmic sperm injection).

Couples who choose intracytoplasmic sperm injection have the opportunity of checking the embryo via preimplantation genetic diagnosis (*see* Chapter 7). This procedure allows the selection and transfer of normal embryos into the womb. Those who are unable to obtain or benefit from preimplantation genetic diagnosis have the opportunity of checking the fetal chromosome status at either 11 weeks (by chorion villus sampling) or 15 to 16 weeks (by amniocentesis study; *see* Chapter 7). At both these stages, the option is to continue or terminate the pregnancy. Clearly, genetic counseling is recommended for all men with this syndrome and especially if a pregnancy is being planned.

Victor's childhood was characteristic for Klinefelter syndrome in that he was tall, had significant learning problems, was socially and behaviorally disadvantaged, and developed prominent breasts after puberty. Although some reduction of intellectual ability has been reported primarily resulting from deficits in language and executive function, mental retardation is not usually a feature. While speech, language, and learning difficulties as well as behavioral problems may hamper educational achievement in boys with Klinefelter syndrome, the majority have perfectly normal IQs, and at least one has been reported with a genius-level IQ of 145. On the other hand, men with Klinefelter mosaicism commonly show few or no clinical symptoms or signs. After puberty, the small testes and absent sperm almost invariably lead to the chromosome diagnosis of this syndrome.

Men with Klinefelter syndrome have an increased frequency of developing diabetes and heart disease, as well as chest and intestinal disorders. Of particular importance is their higher risk of developing breast cancer or non-Hodgkin lymphoma. Men with Klinefelter syndrome should, therefore, learn to palpate their breasts so they can recognize any deviation from normal over a lifetime of expected surveillance.

The frequent absence of a diagnosis in Klinefelter syndrome is distressing, as there is an effective treatment—namely, regular male hormone (testosterone) administration—that restores self-confidence, energy, and self-esteem and improves libido (sexual drive) as well as bone density in these men who may have spent endless years of unhappiness and self-doubt. Generally, men affected by this syndrome tend to be reticent, passive, and low key. Mental illnesses, both neuroses and psychoses, are more common among them, as are periods of depression and of mania. Sexual behavior is normal, and homosexuality is not a consequence.[4]

Females, too, may be born with an extra X chromosome—the triple X female. Invariably, either as babies or as adults, they have a normal appearance. On close examination, their heads might be slightly smaller in relation to their height, and on occasion there may be slightly incurved fifth fingers and toes, low-set ears, and poor coordination. As in Klinefelter syndrome, learning disorders are common for a condition that occurs in about 1 in 1,000 females. Again, just as in Klinefelter syndrome, the overwhelming majority of triple X women have never been diagnosed.

In childhood, this disorder might be detected only incidentally as part of an evaluation for disorders of speech, language, and learning. Some reports indicate a decrease in the average IQ in this group, but just as in all genetic disorders, the range of symptoms and signs can be wide. While the learning disorders in childhood require early intervention, in adulthood, mental illness appears to occur more frequently in this group of women. Triple X females tend to be passive and immature (again with a wide range) and may have difficulty in forming interpersonal relationships, frequently experiencing psychological problems. Psychosis or schizoid personality is more frequent than in XX women.

Menstrual difficulties are relatively common and include late onset of periods, scanty or skipped periods, infertility or sterility, and early onset of menopause. Triple X women have a normal sex life and may bear male or female offspring who may be born with an extra X chromosome (XXX or XXY).

---

4. Homosexuality and transvestism are not associated with abnormalities in the sex chromosomes.

TURNER SYNDROME

Not infrequently, females may be born with a missing X chromosome and manifest a range of symptoms and signs that collectively are called Turner syndrome[5] (Table 3.1). The frequency of this sex chromosome abnormality among females at birth is between 1 in 1,500 and 1 in 2,500. For the overwhelming majority of **conceptions** with a missing X chromosome, the outcome is lethal. A remarkable 99% of conceptions with this type of chromosome complement are miscarried or die during pregnancy. In at least two-thirds of such pregnancies, obstetric ultrasound findings suggest the diagnosis. Thick folds in the

Table 3.1 The Most Common Features and Disorders Associated With Klinefelter Syndrome

Common Features[1]	Associated Disorders[2]
Small testes, normal penis	Obesity in adulthood
Sterility/infertility	Diabetes mellitus
Feminine build	Varicose veins and leg ulcers
Excessive breast development in 50%	Rheumatoid arthritis
Tall stature (especially long legs)	Lupus erythematosus
Personality/character trait disturbances	Germ-cell tumors
Emotional/behavioral problems	Early tooth decay
Psychiatric/sexual problems	Erectile dysfunction
Various nervous system abnormalities	Breast cancer
Osteoporosis (thin bones)	Predisposition to clot
Delayed speech	Leukemia/lymphoma
Attention deficit disorder	
Learning disorders	
Fine tremor	

[1] An affected individual might not have every listed feature.
[2] Because the majority of males with Klinefelter syndrome have never been diagnosed, the frequency of these associated disorders is unknown.

5. This syndrome was named after Henry Turner, an Oklahoma endocrinologist, who described its features in 1938. Since earlier cases had been described in Europe, this condition is usually called the Ullrich-Turner syndrome.

Table 3.2 Turner Syndrome[1]: Common Features and Associated Disorders

Major Features

Short stature
Webbed neck
Primary gonadal failure/sterility/infertility
Cubitus valgus (increase carrying angle at the elbows)
Congenital heart defects

Minor Features

Excess skin folds on back of the neck
Widely spaced nipples
Low posterior hairline
Ptosis (droopy eyelids)
High arched palate
Pigmented nevi
A distinctive type of nail curvature
Lymphedema (puffiness) in the dorsum of hands and/or feet
Short fourth metacarpal bones (in wrists)

Other Medical Problems

Deficit in spatio-visual organization
Cognitive disabilities
Behavioral problems
Psychiatric problems (depression/schizophrenia)
Osteoporosis (increased risk of fractures)
Hypothyroidism (Hashimoto's thyroiditis)
High blood pressure
Bicuspid aortic valve
Coarctation (narrowing or stricture) of the aorta
Dilatation of the aorta
Celiac disease
Kidney structural abnormalities
Carbohydrate intolerance
Hearing loss

[1] Only some features are present in any one individual.

neck, swelling of the body, and heart or kidney abnormalities are the primary observations that raise the possibility of this disorder. Prenatal genetic studies of fetal chromosomes enable a precise diagnosis.

In about one-third of affected babies, puffiness of the back of the hands and feet are obvious. Webbing of the neck is frequently present, but only noticed in some, months or years later. Heart defects occur in at least 50% of cases. Dramatic narrowing or constriction of the aorta (called coarctation) is critically important and may require urgent surgical correction. This vascular abnormality occurs in about one in five people with Turner syndrome. About 50% have an abnormality of the aortic valve (bicuspid aortic valve). Structural abnormalities of the kidneys, such as a horseshoe kidney, are common. The vascular and kidney abnormalities, including those of the urinary tract, contribute to an increased likelihood of high blood pressure, which would, in turn, need to be monitored. Certainly, once a diagnosis has been achieved, an echocardiogram (ultrasound of the heart) and an ultrasound of the kidneys should be performed routinely. These studies later enable demonstration that the uterus does not develop fully and the ovaries remain simply as streaks of tissue. Consequently, the vast majority of women with this disorder are infertile or sterile; do not have functional ovaries; have no menstrual periods; and, without hormone treatment, do not develop breasts. Short stature is also the rule. Growth hormone therapy is usually offered between ages 2 and 5 years. Unfortunately, this treatment is by injection and may continue for some years, but it may be possible to add about 3 to 4 inches (about 8–10 centimeters) to an individual's height.

Among those with Turner syndrome, only about 50% have a pure chromosome complement with a missing X. About 15% have a normal set of female chromosomes mixed with cells having a single X (called mosaics). In about 4%, there is a mixture of single X cells and cells containing normal male (XY) chromosomes. Females who harbor a male (Y) chromosome mixed with their cells possessing a single X chromosome have a markedly increased risk (about 12%) of developing tumors[6] in the streaks of ovarian tissue. Surgical removal of these tissues is therefore indicated as soon as a Y chromosome has been detected.

The various structural defects of the second X chromosome are also seen in other manifestations of Turner syndrome, with various associated disorders and complications being more or less common. Diminished function of the thyroid gland (hypothyroidism) occurs in 15% to 30% of women with Turner syndrome. Given that frequency, all should be checked every 1 to 2 years. Ear infection is common and should be anticipated and briskly treated, as should hearing loss (especially of high frequency sound). Various autoimmune disorders are common and include ulcerative colitis, Crohn's disease, celiac disease,

---

6. Called gonadoblastomas

and diabetes. British, Australian, and Belgian studies document the frequent lack of continuing medical care of women with Turner syndrome. This is positively unwise given the host of medical issues that do occur and for which treatment is available.

About 50% of girls with Turner syndrome need special education, especially for mathematics and handwriting. Typically, some impairment of perceptual and spatial thinking has been noted with special reference to geometry, left-to-right directions, and solving arithmetic problems. In one study of 6,483 females with schizophrenia, Turner syndrome was found with a threefold greater frequency (about 3%) than in the general female population.

Preadolescent girls have been reported with an increased frequency of attention deficit hyperactivity disorder (ADHD). Observations in some studies show affected adolescents to be more anxious and depressed, more socially withdrawn, and shy and insecure. However, with a supportive environment, none of these issues should interfere with the development and fulfillment of an enjoyable life with a normal lifespan.

This was the second marriage for both Manuel and Consuela, and neither had children. Their obstetrician had recommended prenatal genetic studies in view of Consuela's age (38 years) when she first became pregnant. The primary concern was the maternal age-related increased risk for Down syndrome. This test is routinely offered to all women pregnant at age 35 years or older. They both readily accepted the offer of amniocentesis at 16 weeks of pregnancy and waited anxiously for the results 10 days later.

Our studies showed that the fetus did not have Down syndrome but unexpectedly had a chromosome complement with an extra Y chromosome (XYY). My request that they both return for a consultation to discuss these results was responded to immediately.

I explained at length the mechanism by which the extra Y occurred and the characteristic features and other aspects that could be anticipated in the XYY male. At birth, there are no definitive characteristic features that distinguish XYY boys from those with a normal chromosome set. The most common findings relate to the development of learning disability and behavioral difficulties. Language delays are common, and about 50% of these boys require special education classes, focused primarily on their reading and spelling difficulties. Their IQ scores are on average some 10 to 15 points below the average for XY boys. Although there is considerable variability, most IQs are within the average range. There may, however, be an increased likelihood of pervasive developmental disorder, compounded by attention deficit disorder and impulsive behavior. Problems with impulse control, including temper tantrums in early childhood, are not unusual. An increased frequency of antisocial behavior has been reported among XYY adolescents and adults. A propensity to commit "silly" crimes is noteworthy (such as breaking into house when the residents are home). Property offenses constitute the majority of criminal convictions for XYY males.

XYY boys are typically tall and sometimes have rather severe facial acne at puberty and beyond. These boys are fertile and otherwise have a normal puberty. Early educational and psychologic intervention is important and may ameliorate some of the learning and behavioral difficulties usually encountered later. By this time in the consultation, Consuela was weeping uncontrollably. She seemed no longer interested in even listening to the other information that I was ready to offer.

I then discussed the availability of pregnancy termination, should they so wish. The husband responded first by saying that he did not want to bring a criminal into the world. He said that he had read that XYY males were aggressive, violent, and antisocial and that many were in prison. When I asked how he came to know this type of information, he stated for the first time that both he and Consuela were FBI agents!

Consuela's immediate response was that she would not terminate this pregnancy, upon which they literally began shouting at each other. I had to stand up and insist they settle down, return home, and discuss the pros and cons of continuing or terminating this pregnancy. This they agreed to do and would return in a week or less for further discussions or any further assistance I could provide.

Klinefelter syndrome, triple X females, and XYY males are almost invariably diagnosed prenatally purely inadvertently. Down syndrome, Trisomy 18 and Trisomy 13, Klinefelter syndrome, and Triple X all increase in frequency with advancing maternal age. But not so for XYY males and females with Turner syndrome. Mostly maternal age-related studies reveal a sex chromosome abnormality that was not being sought and, consequently, these unexpected diagnoses cause considerable angst, despite the fact that mental retardation is not a feature of any of these numerical chromosome abnormalities. XYY men do have an increased risk of having offspring with Klinefelter syndrome or even XYY male offspring, and hence, prenatal diagnosis would be recommended for their partners in all pregnancies.

XYY MALES

About 1 in 1,000 males are born with the XYY chromosome complement, and the vast majority have never been diagnosed. Diagnostic studies may be initiated because of learning and behavioral difficulties in childhood or for developmental problems with speech, coordination, and learning difficulties. Inadvertent prenatal diagnosis may, however, be the most common way XYY males are recognized.

Manuel, however, had read correctly about the earlier history of what was known about the XYY male at the time. In the early 1960s, research scientists in Edinburgh, Scotland, questioned whether abnormal sex chromosomes might predispose individuals toward deviant behavior. They studied the chromosomes of male prisoners who were mentally subnormal and being held in special high-security institutions after committing various crimes of violence. Some 6.1% of the 196 males studied showed abnormal chromosomal patterns. Of these males, 3.6% were XYY males—many times the expected incidence of 1 in 1,000 males. Manuel apparently was not aware that subsequent studies have shown that XYY males are not more likely than other males to commit crimes of violence. There does remain data, however, that XYY males find themselves in trouble with the police considerably more often than XY males. This ultimately may be due to immature personalities, weak self-concept, social maladjustment, and occasionally borderline-normal intelligence.

There have been at least six criminal trials in which the defendant has raised his abnormal XYY chromosome set as a basis for a plea of insanity. This defense refers to the legal concept that defines the extent to which accused or convicted individuals may be relieved of criminal responsibility because of mental disease at the time the crime was committed. Usually the defense has to demonstrate that the accused was indeed suffering from a "mental disease." Moreover, a relationship must be established between this mental disease and the alleged criminal act.

The insanity defense based on the XYY chromosomal pattern was first raised in April 1968 in France. The defendant, Daniel Hugon, was accused of murdering a 65-year-old prostitute in a Paris hotel. Chromosome studies done after he attempted suicide revealed his XYY chromosome complement. Nevertheless, he was found legally sane and was convicted of murder.

In the same year, 21-year-old Lawrence Hannel came to trial in Australia, charged with the stabbing death of his 77-year-old landlady. Again, the plea of insanity based on his XYY chromosomes was offered. The jury, after only 11 minutes of deliberation, delivered a not-guilty-by-reason-of-insanity verdict, and Hannel was committed to a maximum security hospital until "cured."

Ernest D. Beck, a 20-year-old farm worker with XYY chromosomes, was tried in Bielefeld, West Germany in 1968. The court in this case accepted the prosecution's argument that Beck was fully aware that he was committing murders, even though he might not have been able to control his impulses to kill. Beck received the maximum sentence of life imprisonment for the murder of three women.

In April 1969, Sean Farley of New York, a 6-foot, 8-inch 26-year-old male, pleaded not guilty on the grounds of insanity to the alleged brutal murder and rape of a 40-year-old woman in an alley near her home. On cross-examination, the prosecutor established that it was possible to live a normal life despite possession of XYY chromosomes. The jury found Farley guilty of murder in the first degree. Other convictions have been obtained, despite the individual's contention of being an XYY male. It would appear clear at this time that chromosomes cannot be held culpable for criminal behavior.

Manuel and Consuela returned 5 days later for a follow-up consultation. Consuela had decided that she would, after all, terminate the pregnancy.

There is considerable variability between countries regarding pregnancy termination for sex chromosome abnormalities. Many factors impact this decision and include religious belief, education and economic factors, number of previous pregnancies, preceding infertility, maternal age, and the knowledge, expertise, and specialty of the health-care provider of genetic counseling.

MOSAICISM

In the process of cell division, which follows soon **after** fertilization of the egg, a mixture of normal and abnormal cells with two different complements of chromosomes may emerge. One with a normal set may be mixed with one having an extra (missing, abnormal, or rearranged) chromosome. The individual born with this mixture of cells (which may predominate in one organ or another) has what is described as chromosomal mosaicism. For example, the brain, the genital organs, the blood, and the skin may have cells with too many chromosomes, with all the other organs having normal cells.

The more normal cells present, the greater the likelihood of approaching normality or ameliorating the effect of the extra chromosome. Hence, with a Trisomy 21 type of Down syndrome, mosaicism with an overwhelming presence of normal cells may make for a milder form of that condition.

Mosaicism of the sex chromosomes are common, which is not the case for non-sex chromosomes. Those men or women with sex chromosomes mosaicism may experience problems with infertility or recurrent miscarriages. Structural rearrangements of both non-sex and sex chromosomes vary in their implications from irrelevant to grave. Knowledge about any such rearrangements in the family history must not be ignored and should certainly be communicated to all family members, as outlined in the Chapter 4.

4

CHROMOSOME REARRANGEMENTS

Simon was the product of Minnie's fourth pregnancy. She and her husband Harold had tried repeatedly to achieve a pregnancy and had consulted with their local family doctor. He had recommended the usual folic acid supplementation (to avoid spina bifida) and provided progesterone hormone tablets to help retain a future pregnancy. The delivery of Simon was precipitous and chaotic. Millie was 36 weeks along in her pregnancy when she suddenly went into labor and was rushed to the hospital. She barely made it into the labor ward, where she promptly delivered. Initially, Simon did not breathe, was blue and floppy, but fortunately had a heart rate of 110 per minute. Minnie thought that it took forever to have the resuscitation team of pediatricians (neonatologists) arrive to help Simon. She did acknowledge that the nursing staff and midwives had given him oxygen and "squeezed" his chest.

The hospital notes of the neonatologists clearly indicated that Simon had a rather unusual appearance. When he was finally weighed, they noted a weight of 5 pounds 2 ounces, but the size of his head was noticeably small. Moreover, his forehead was high, the space between his eyes flat, above which there was a prominence, giving him the appearance of a Greek helmet. His eyes were widely spaced and cross-eyed, with droopy eyelids. His ears were rather low-set, and his lower jaw was particularly small. A heart murmur was audible and a defect between the lower chambers of the heart (ventricular septal defect) was determined later. This hole in the heart closed spontaneously some months later. Simon's development was abysmally slow, and by his second year, it was clear that he was going to be severely retarded.

My involvement began with a request from Harold and Minnie's attorney, whom they had hired to sue the hospital and the doctor for their alleged *failure to provide appropriate and timely resuscitation for Simon and thereby prevent the resulting brain damage. Review of the medical record with special reference to Simon's features made it clear that a chromosome study should have been done. Harold and Minnie lived in a small town distant from major hospitals and they had not consulted a geneticist. No chromosome or other genetic studies had been done, so I recommended such a study to the plaintiff attorney. He duly made arrangements for that analysis and, sure enough, a tiny deletion in the short arm of chromosome 4 was detected. Further studies of both parents revealed that Minnie carried a chromosome translocation (an exchange between chromosomes 4 and 10), but in a balanced form (see discussion below). It was noteworthy that Minnie's sister had suffered two miscarriages thus far and had no living children. Recommended studies later showed that Minnie's sister also was a balanced carrier of the same translocation.*

The features the neonatologist described in her notes about Simon were typical for a well-recognized birth defect syndrome.[1] In this microdeletion syndrome (discussed in Chapter 5) involving the short arm of chromosome 4, severe mental retardation can be expected. The plaintiff's attorney, upon hearing the results of the chromosome analysis, declined to take Harold and Minnie's case. Legal issues aside, it would have been indicated to test Harold and Minnie's chromosomes after Minnie had suffered three miscarriages. After three early pregnancy losses, there is between a 3% and 8% likelihood that one parent carries a chromosome abnormality, which, in those cases, may explain the recurrent losses. Prior determination of Minnie's chromosome abnormality (a balanced translocation between chromosomes 4 and 10; see discussion below) would have led to a recommendation for prenatal genetic studies via chorion villus sampling or amniocentesis studies (*see* Chapter 7) at 11 or 16 weeks of pregnancy, respectively. This would have enabled these parents to have had the choice of deciding whether to have a child with severe birth defects and mental retardation with a truncated life span. Moreover, discovery of Minnie's translocation would have immediately led to the recommendation to test both her brother and sister. Her sister,

1. Wolf-Hirschhorn syndrome

being a carrier of the same translocation, was saved from being faced with the unexpected birth of a child with a syndrome characterized by severe mental retardation and birth defects. She had the option of prenatal diagnosis in every future pregnancy.

It is unnerving to realize that the protein scaffold and linked genes forming our chromosomes may break. Such an event occurring in one or two (rarely more) chromosomes have greater significance if they occur during formation of the egg or sperm. Breakage at that critical moment could result in transmission of the broken chromosome(s) through fertilization, into the new embryo. Serious health implications may also follow chromosome breakage in bone marrow cells or in cancerous tumors.

WHEN CHROMOSOMES BREAK

About 1 in 120 newborns have some type of chromosome breakage, usually called a structural rearrangement. There are often no health consequences. However, birth defects, mental retardation, or certain cancers may occur if the break or breaks interfere with the function of one or more genes, or if genes are literally lost or duplicated. The various structural rearrangements that may occur differ in their effects on our body's structure and function and include translocations, deletions, duplications, and inversions.

Translocations

The most common rearrangement is when two different chromosomes snap and the broken pieces, as in the game of musical chairs, simply exchange places and reattach. This process is called translocation. Half of all cases occur spontaneously when the sperm or egg is being produced. The other 50% are directly inherited from one parent and passed through the generations. Implications differ depending on which two chromosomes are involved. For example, an inherited form of Down syndrome is caused by a translocation between chromosome 21 and another, most often a chromosome 14. When the chromosome pieces change places without any piece being lost in the exchange, the process is called a **balanced translocation** and occurs in about 1 in 500 individuals. Almost all the balanced translocations that occur are not associated with any health consequences. However, for those balanced translocations that are not inherited, there is about a 6% risk that a tiny sliver of chromosome material, not visible by routine microscopy, may be lost. The consequence could be mental retardation, birth defects, or both. When brand new (not inherited) translocations occur—for example, in a fetus or someone with mental retardation or birth defects—a chromosomal microarray is now offered (*see* Chapter 5). Moreover, there is also an increased risk of chromosome "stickiness" (nondisjunction) and hence a slightly greater risk than random of having a child with an extra chromosome (e.g., Trisomy 21 type of Down syndrome).

The chromosome with the translocated piece is vulnerable, so during formation of the egg or sperm or during fertilization, a break may occur again at the original site, this time of only one chromosome. The piece broken off may then literally disappear. This deletion virtually always results in serious birth defects/mental retardation, as happened with Harold and Minnie's son, Simon. Not all deletions are visible under the microscope, especially those that occur near the gene-rich tips of every chromosome.

In yet other examples, the chromosome piece that exchanged places during a translocation may duplicate, thereby yielding three identical pieces when the similar segment from the unbroken chromosome is taken into account. These three segments (called partial trisomy) almost always result in birth defects or retardation. Structural rearrangements with translocations resulting in deletions or duplications are termed **unbalanced translocations**. A parent who carries a balanced translocation is therefore at risk of having a child either with a balanced or an unbalanced translocation, the latter resulting in partial trisomy, a deletion, or a duplication.

For reasons that remain unclear, parental origin of a translocation can influence the future risk of having a child with an unbalanced translocation. Women who carry a balanced translocation involving chromosomes 14 and 21 have an 11% to 15% risk of having a translocation-type Down syndrome child. Men carrying the same 14/21 translocation have a 2% to 4% risk of the same outcome. An intriguing recent report concludes that most <u>new</u> translocations are of paternal origin.

Sex Chromosome Translocations

Because males develop normally with only a single X chromosome, you may wonder why females have two. Much of the Y chromosome is inert and, at least thus far, appears to have no genes that threaten survival. The second X in the female, you may be surprised to learn, is largely (but not completely) silenced in a process that occurs around the second week following conception. This process, called genetic inactivation, is random (either X chromosome is inactivated). In all descendant cells, this same inactivated X chromosome continues, each X "remembering" its permanent state of activation or inactivation. The inactivated segments are nonfunctional.

Translocations occurring between an X chromosome and any other are well-recognized. Usually the normal X will be preferentially inactivated. Hence, if the translocation somehow disrupts or interferes with the expression of a gene on the X chromosome, or the particular X chromosome involved in the translocation has a disease-causing gene, that female will have the genetic disorder.

Deletions and Duplications

Small segments of chromosomes containing one or many genes may literally be deleted or duplicated, potentially resulting in mental retardation, birth defects, or specific genetic disorders. However, to everyone's amazement, use of the chromosomal microarray has revealed that all of us have many deletions and duplications throughout our genomes (*see* Chapter 5). This obviously means that various genes are deleted or duplicated, apparently without causing a genetic disorder and probably accounting mostly for the physical (and maybe mental) differences among us. An excess number of deletions or duplications (now called copy number variations) involving genes that function primarily in the brain seem highly relevant in conditions such as autism and schizophrenia (*see* Chapter 19).

Deletions may occur anywhere along the length of any chromosome, be visible under the microscope, or be so tiny and beyond resolution of the microscope. Microscopically visible deletions mean that multiple contiguous genes have been deleted, possibly resulting in multiple genetic disorders in the same person. In one such case, a boy with a large deletion in the short arm of his X chromosome had Duchenne muscular dystrophy and three other genetic disorders simultaneously. Ironically, while living with this burden, he was killed in an automobile accident!

A significant number of newly recognized microdeletion and microduplication syndromes have been recognized since the introduction of the chromosomal microarray test. Most have been associated with variable symptoms and signs including mental retardation, learning disabilities, speech and language delay, autistic behavior, seizures, and birth defects (*see* Chapter 5).

Many years ago, I was consulted by a mother who brought her infant in for a "check-up." She said that she had become concerned when the plumber, on a service call, asked her when she got her new cat. Only then did she register that her baby truly did mewl like a cat. Examination of the baby revealed a rather round face with some minor unusual features. I suspected a then newly recognized disorder, and the chromosome analysis showed a tiny deletion of the short arm of one chromosome 5. The condition called the Cri-du-chat syndrome (cry-of-the-cat syndrome) was hardly known then, so I added it to the medical literature.[2] Unfortunately, this disorder is characterized by severe mental retardation, and the second consultation was overwhelmingly sad.

Tiny hidden deletions may occur along the length of any chromosome—especially gene-rich regions at the tips, which are capped by specialized DNA that seals the chromosome and prevents its fusion with any other chromosome. Special techniques (such as FISH; see below) now enable detection of tiny deletions either tucked immediately below these chromosome caps (called telomeres) or elsewhere. Microdeletions and microduplications now rank as important causes of unexplained mental retardation. In those situations where evaluation has not revealed a precise diagnosis in an individual with mental retardation, autism, or birth defects, a chromosomal microarray test reveals the cause in 10% to 20% of cases showing a hidden deletion or duplication (Chapter 5), as we have also found in our center studies.

Inversions

Any one chromosome may break in two places and have the freed piece turn upside down and reattach. These inversions frequently have no health consequences but on occasion may be associated with infertility, recurrent miscarriage, or an increased risk of birth defects or mental retardation because of vulnerability at the break site. Again, about half of these are inherited, the remainder arising spontaneously.

New inversions (not inherited) may occur at critical locations and the break may, in fact, be within a gene, thereby causing it to dysfunction. Such was the case of a handsome Japanese boy who was born deaf with different colored and

---

2. Milunsky A & Chitham R. (1966) The Cri-du-Chat syndrome. *J Ment Def Res* 10:153.

wide-set eyes. The report of his case in a medical journal immediately focused the search we were on for the gene causing this condition, called Waardenburg syndrome. We were indeed successful in discovering the culprit gene (called *PAX3*) and publishing our findings.[3] History was also made by other scientists and physicians tipped off by newly occurring inversions, pointing, as examples, to genes for breast cancer and polycystic kidney disease. Other forms and consequences of chromosome breakages occur and fortunately are much rarer.

CLUES SUGGESTING A REARRANGEMENT

We usually have no idea whether we have been born with a balanced chromosomal rearrangement, such as a translocation or an inversion. Each year in the United States alone, more than 8,000 children are born with balanced rearrangements and more than 2,500 with unbalanced chromosomes. Important clues arise mostly in connection with reproduction. Women who experience repeated miscarriages may find that either they or their partners are balanced translocation carriers or that one has a chromosome anomaly or harbors an inversion. After two miscarriages occurring in the first 3 months of pregnancy, the likelihood is between 1% and 3% that either partner has a structural chromosomal rearrangement. After three losses, the risk escalates to between 3% and 8%. After three unexplained losses, blood chromosome analysis is invariably advised for both partners.

Couples experiencing problems in achieving a pregnancy also have an increased risk that either partner carries a chromosomal rearrangement. Evaluation for infertility should always include a blood chromosome analysis for both partners. Other clues follow the prenatal detection of a fetus with anatomical defects, a child born with birth defects, or one who subsequently manifests developmental delay or mental retardation. In all of these situations, chromosomal analysis of the fetus, the child, and/or the parents may reveal the precise rearrangement.

FUTURE RISKS

The carrier of a structural chromosomal rearrangement has an increased risk of bearing a child with birth defects or mental retardation. That risk depends

---

3. Baldwin CR, Hoth CF, Amos JA, da-Silva EO, & Milunsky A. (1992) An exonic mutation in the HuP2 paired domain gene causes Waardenburg syndrome. *Nature* 355:637.

on which parent is a carrier and the location of the break(s), as discussed earlier. For most translocations, risks of having a child with mental retardation or malformations are less than 10% and usually around 1%, except for mothers carrying a translocation involving chromosome 21, as discussed earlier.

For some uncommon inversions, an individual's risk for having a child with birth defects or mental retardation range between 1% and 10%. All of these structural rearrangements when visible under the microscope are detectable prenatally.

"FISHING" FOR CHROMOSOMES

Detection of specific deletions or duplications have been facilitated by the technique employing FISH.[4] The fine structure of DNA constituting the thousands of genes that make up our chromosomes can be probed with tiny fragments of DNA tagged with a chemical signal that fluoresces in the dark. This technique is based on first unfurling the DNA helix and then having the prepared piece of DNA (called a probe) find its complimentary mate, very much like a jigsaw puzzle piece being placed in the right position. Once joined with its mate, the location of this tiny DNA probe can be seen under the fluorescent microscope.

FISH is used often for a quick analysis (called Rapid-FISH) of the common fetal numerical chromosome abnormalities involving chromosomes 13, 18, and 21, as well as the X and Y sex chromosomes that are found in amniotic fluid cells. These cells are aspirated for prenatal diagnosis tests. This valuable approach is possible because of the availability of chromosome-specific FISH probes, enabling one to distinguish one chromosome from another. Unlike routine chromosome analysis, which requires a cell to be caught in the middle of cell division, FISH analysis can be achieved even in nondividing cells. Absence of a FISH probe signal reveals a missing gene or gene segment, thereby facilitating a diagnosis of a so-called "microdeletion syndrome." Visualization of the probe signals in duplicate enables a diagnosis of a microduplication syndrome. Using a cocktail of such probes, it is possible to literally "paint" individual chromosomes by using DNA fragments that are highly specific for a particular chromosome or a region within it. Different colors can be generated and allow remarkable photographic evidence of exquisitely tiny chromosomal regions. This ability also allows precise recognition of the origin of tiny additional

---

4. Fluorescent *in situ* hybridization

chromosome fragments. About half the time, these unusual findings are familial and of no significance. The other half may have potential implications for mental retardation or birth defects. Curiously, such extra fragments are more commonly derived from chromosome 15.

CHROMOSOMAL BREAKS AND CANCER RISKS

Thankfully, the vast majority of inherited translocations raise no additional risks of cancer. However, chromosomal breakage leading to translocations may develop spontaneously or through stimulation by a cancer-causing chemical in the environment.

Acquired translocations are especially prone to arise in the bone marrow. As a consequence of two broken chromosome segments exchanging places and reattaching, an ominous development may occur. For example, the juxtaposed new fragment on a different chromosome brings into contact pieces of two genes that then could fuse. This gene fusion then may produce a cancer-stimulating protein, which in turn activates specific cells, mostly in the bone marrow, to grow out of control and therefore become cancerous (e.g., leukemia). Another mechanism arising from a translocation may operate by landing control genes close to other promoting genes, thereby orchestrating uncontrolled cell growth, which is really the induction of malignancy.

The vast majority of such translocations in the bone marrow induce leukemias and lymphomas of various types. The most common translocation is between chromosomes 9 and 22, which ultimately leads to chronic myeloid leukemia and acute lymphoblastic leukemia. Various other translocations are well-known to cause specific types of leukemia or lymphomas.

There are certain well-recognized translocations that may initially be recognized prior to the development of any malignancy. Discovery in these circumstances is frequently based on a family history of a specific tumor. The chromosome break usually involves a gene that, when defective (mutated), leads to the development of a hereditary tumor. Three important examples include the 11/22 chromosome translocation, which may increase the risk for breast cancer, and the 3/6 translocation predisposing to certain bone marrow cancers. Hence, take note of your family history, be aware of specific cancers, and seek genetic evaluation and counseling and, if recommended, chromosome analysis. In this way, appropriate surveillance can be initiated, baseline studies done, and very early diagnosis made, thereby facilitating pre-emptive life-saving treatment.

Other rearrangements that interrupt the normal structure and alignment of genes along chromosomes may also result in the development of a cancer. Once again, involvement of a key gene in a specific location could result in a predictable tumor. An important example that is not infrequently inherited involves a gene on the long arm of chromosome 13. The following poignant case illustrates some important lessons in this regard.

L.M., who was blind, came to her obstetrician for prenatal care. He never inquired about the cause of her blindness. He provided routine care and treatment, pregnancy progressed without incident, and labor and delivery were uneventful. The child, when born, appeared healthy and was discharged from the hospital with the mother.

When the child was about 9 months old, her father observed a peculiar whitish appearance behind the pupil of one eye. Upon consulting an eye specialist, the parents discovered that the child had a malignant eye tumor called retinoblastoma—a cancer that was shortly thereafter also found in the baby's other eye. Despite treatment efforts with anti-cancer drugs and radiation, the child's eyes had to be removed to save her life.

In this case, the obstetrician failed to inquire about the cause of the mother's blindness. He would have learned that her eyes had also been surgically removed when she was an infant. She had been adopted in early childhood, and she was unaware that her own eyes had been removed because of tumors.

Referral to a clinical geneticist would have revealed involvement of chromosome 13 and the realization of dominant inheritance with a 50% risk of bearing a child with this disorder (*see* Chapter 8). Prenatal diagnostic studies would have been an option for this mother.

Equally egregious was the action of the pediatrician who also failed to have an eye specialist perform an eye examination under anesthesia shortly after birth and repetitively every 3 months thereafter for at least 5 years. This surveillance, instituted because of the mother's history, would have enabled a very early diagnosis of the retinoblastoma tumor, facilitating immediate treatment, which had a 90% likelihood of not only saving the child's eyes but also ensuring reasonably good vision.

Know your family history, and if there are any serious illnesses in the family that could possibly be genetic, telephone a clinical geneticist to determine if a consultation is necessary. The name of a board-certified clinical geneticist can be obtained by contacting the American College of Medical Genetics, or the name of a board-certified genetic counselor can be obtained from the National Society of Genetic Counselors.

BLUEPRINTS

YOU AND YOUR GENES

It is mind-boggling when you think about it. You were created by the joining of your father's sperm and mother's egg, each carrying the genetic messages or blueprints of your forebears. The single fertilized cell, which underwent endless divisions and multiplications to make you, housed your complete set of genes— somewhere between 26,000 and 30,000 (the current best estimate after the completion of the Human Genome Project). We have 99.9% of our genes in common. No advanced knowledge of biology is necessary to form a basic understanding about your genes and what may happen when things go awry.

WHAT IS A GENE?

Your genes are held together within a two-stranded spiral scaffold (called the double helix) of proteins and other elements. They are tightly coiled and packed into the holding scaffold to constitute each of your chromosomes. To give you some idea how tightly these genes are coiled, if they were unraveled from a single cell, they would measure a few yards. The total length of **all** chromosomes in a cell **together** measures less than a half a millimeter—less than 0.02 of an inch!

Your genes regulate, modify, control, promote, enhance, or otherwise influence all of your body's structure and function. Whether you are tall or short, fat or thin, fair or dark-skinned, have certain facial characteristics, suffer from allergies, or actually are affected by a genetic disorder—all are functions of your genes with environmental interactions. Your genes will largely determine your body's characteristics, your various susceptibilities or resistance to certain diseases, how you react to medications, and whether you will transmit certain genetic disorders or, sadly, fall victim to one (or more) of them.

Although each gene is too small to be seen with the naked eye, by chemically extracting genes from cells, you can actually see a white, stringy, and sticky substance. This stringy mass of genes, or DNA, is really constituted by very long fibers, tightly compacted within the chromosome structure. These long DNA fibers, which actually consist of two strands, coil around each other in a clockwise spiral (the double helix). Each strand of DNA is composed of long chains of molecules, called nucleotides, which are made up of sugar, phosphate, and nitrogen, also called bases. Together, these substances constitute nucleic acids, of which there are two. The one with the sugar ribose is called ribonucleic acid, or RNA. The other, with a different sugar, deoxyribose, is referred to as deoxyribonucleic acid, or DNA. All the chromosomes, and hence the DNA, constitute the nucleus and are held within a "bubble," the nuclear membrane, which in fact has tiny holes throughout, making it porous. The liquid (called cytoplasm) that bathes the nucleus contains the RNA.

A gene is constructed like a ladder or spiral staircase, the two strands or "sides of the ladder" having connections like "rungs" of a ladder made up of these bases that are always connected to each other in the same way. There are only four possible bases (or nucleotides). Each is referred to by its capitalized first letter: Base A (called adenine) always pairs up with base T (called thymine), and base G (guanine) is always paired with base C (cytosine). In RNA there is a slight difference in that base A pairs up with another base called base U (Uracil).

Incredibly there are about three billion of these base-pairs. The largest chromosome (1) has about 249 million base-pairs of DNA, whereas the smallest (21, not 22 as would be expected) has about 48 million. The X chromosome, of great importance because of its role in many severe X-linked diseases, has about 154 million base-pairs of DNA. Individual genes seem to range in size from a few hundred to more than 2 million base- pairs. The defective gene causing Duchenne muscular dystrophy is enormous, at 2,400,000 base-pairs!

We have been considering the structure of genes and how a change (mutation) even in a single base may cause disease. Imagine, then, everyone's surprise when it was only recently shown that throughout all of our genomes, many variably sized slivers and segments of DNA were either missing (deletions) or duplicated—and we are still normal! These structural changes (now known as copy number variants [CNVs]) may delete or duplicate whole segments of DNA, possibly encompassing multiple genes or parts of genes, probably accounting for some of our diversity. More important, CNVs that involve key genes are already recognized as having a causal role in complex genetic disorders, including mental retardation, autism, schizophrenia, psoriasis, Crohn's disease, obesity, systemic lupus erythematosus, and amyotrophic lateral sclerosis (Lou Gehrig disease).

In both autism and schizophrenia, recurring deletions in many of those affected involve genes that have important functions in the brain (especially regarding connectivity; *see* Chapter 19). For both of these complex disorders, a larger-than-normal number of CNVs have been discovered. Besides their potential causal role, CNVs may well create or convey genetic susceptibilities. Duplication or deletion of a gene might enhance or reduce the activity of its protein product. A good example is one particular gene (*CYP2D6*), responsible for activating certain drugs, such as codeine or tamoxifen (used to prevent breast cancer). Breast feeding mothers taking codeine (which the body breaks down into morphine) could, by virtue of this genetic susceptibility, rapidly secrete the morphine into their milk, placing their babies at risk.

We all have thousands of CNVs—both deletions and duplications—in our genomes.

Finding any of these in someone with mental retardation, autism, or a genetic disorder immediately raises the question of significance. Most CNVs are simply inherited and when the transmitting parent(s) are unaffected, no significance can be attached. However, when neither parent harbors the newly observed CNV(s) in the affected person, the genes contained within the CNV(s) become prime suspects and subject to further intensive studies.

GENOME-WIDE ASSOCIATIONS

Confronted by an overwhelming 3 billion bits (bases) of information, how do geneticists find their way through this mass of data? Maps became the tool of choice.

First, by tagging individual bases spread out through the genome (like milemarkers on a highway), small blocks of genes were identified (called haplotypes) and a map constructed (called HAP-MAP). These blocks of genes are, of course, transmitted through generations. When a gene of interest was suspected, examination of the HAP-MAP determined the linkage to the disorder in question. In other words, was the gene with its mutation lodged within a specific block of genes and only linked to the affected individuals within the family?

The second approach was to focus on individual bases (also called single nucleotide polymorphisms [SNPs]) and to construct linkage maps, which again facilitated more refined linkage to specific genetic diseases. This approach focused the search for a culprit gene but did not resolve the precise causal mutation, until actual gene sequencing was performed.

The third approach followed discovery of the many CNVs we all have, and the construction of "normal" CNV maps that now aid in the interpretation of deletions/duplications observed in the course of a diagnostic study. The precise mechanism by which CNVs arise remains uncertain. An environmental or genetic influence may have a role in view of a striking report about identical twins. Notwithstanding the expectation that such pairs would have identical DNA, researchers have found differences in CNVs between them!

From all these linkage and mapping studies, endless genetic disorders and common traits have usually been linked to a handful of SNPs. These SNP "signatures" point to faulty genes that contribute to or directly cause a complex genetic disorder. Discovery of a SNP "signature" in an individual implies a susceptibility to and therefore risk of developing a specific genetic disorder or reacting adversely to an exogenous agent (e.g., medication, smoking, toxin, etc.).

There is an extensive list of disorders and traits recognized thus far by genome-wide association studies. It is likely that all disorders involving multiple genes will eventually end up on that list. Remember, these studies reflect statistical risks but do **not** make a diagnosis. Their recognition may ultimately lead to the development of new therapeutic approaches and the provision of advisory policies regarding diets, medications, and other environmental exposures.

HOW DO GENES FUNCTION?

Imagine a train with many coaches. Our genes are made up of many functioning coaches (called exons). The intervening connections between "coaches" are called introns. The exons and introns are simply continuous stretches of DNA located within a gene. Each exon is made up of a chain of nucleotides linked together in a pattern that we received from our parents and earlier ancestors. Such a pattern could be TTTAAAAAGGCT. Just three of these nucleotides are needed to construct a single amino acid. Multiple amino acids together make a protein. There are only 20 amino acids from which all proteins are made. Each exon, like a factory, makes amino acids, using three bases at a time to specify the amino acid made.

Introns, long considered "junk DNA" because they do not code for proteins, are now recognized to have important roles in gene-silencing. In addition, variants within introns have associations with the risks of developing adult-onset diabetes (type 2) and hypertension. Introns also exert their influence on gene splicing, which results in the formation of different proteins (isoforms) from the same gene.

The process by which genetic information is transmitted involves separation of the two DNA strands and copying (called **transcription**) of the strand forming a molecule (called RNA), which in turn carries the genetic information as a messenger out of the nucleus into the surrounding fluid (cytoplasm). Following transcription, the messenger RNA molecule undergoes further processing in which the exons are spliced together following removal of the intervening introns. In the cytoplasm, the joined exons are transported to tiny factories (called ribosomes), where the information contained is translated into a protein. In fact, even after this translation into protein, further modification or processing can occur, adding to or cutting down the structure of the protein. The completed protein that is made folds itself into a precisely determined shape, depending on its constituent amino acids. Its physical and chemical structure is key to its proper function. In hemophilia, for example, the presence of the Factor VIII protein can be demonstrated, but it is functionally inactive. Remarkably, only just over 1% of DNA actually works to make proteins!

The genetic code, then, is the set of bases we have inherited that make up to 20 amino acids. These, in turn, join to form a protein that executes all the functions of a gene. It is the proteins that build our bodies and make them function. Much of this book addresses the consequences of defects that occur in the pathway just described or in the chromosomes.

Your genes produce between 250,000 and 1 million proteins, which drive the body's chemical reactions and build you physically and functionally. In turn, thousands of byproducts (such as cholesterol) result from these reactions. Given the incredibly complex interactions from genes, between genes, transcription, protein manufacture, and function, it is no surprise that a fault anywhere along this chain has the potential for causing a genetic disorder. It should be clear that we all inherit the same key set of genes that make us human and that genetic disease can result if there is a defect (mutation) in a gene that has a major role in an organ (e.g., muscle), resulting in muscular dystrophy or a function (e.g., blood sugar) causing diabetes.

ERRORS IN THE CHAIN

You will recall that the four bases are referred to by their initials (A, G, T, and C) and a chain (or gene) is actually like a series of letters that might look as follows: TATAATGAAATTCATCCATTAG. The TATA set indicates the start of a gene, the adjacent ATG points to the position of the first building block (amino acid) of a protein, and the TAG signals the end of the working part of the gene and therefore the end of the protein.

Even the smallest "spelling" error in the DNA chain may cause grievous or fatal genetic disease. These errors, or defects (called mutations), may involve one or more letters (bases) in the chain, and there can be a number of different types. For example, a single base change (a G instead of a T) could occur, but even with this change an amino acid can be formed that does not alter the function of a protein. This single base change (called a *point mutation*) may occur without any effect on health. This so-called type of *silent mutation* is not rare, accounting for 20% to 25% of all possible single base changes.

More likely, however, in 70% to 75% of cases, a single base mutation leads to the formation of a different amino acid and an altered protein. This so-called "*missense mutation*" may lead to a severe reduction in the protein or even a complete loss of its function. In about 2% to 4% of single base changes, the fault may lead to shortening of the DNA chain that codes for the protein, which in turn results in abrupt termination by this so-called "*nonsense* mutation" and again leads to a flawed protein devoid of structure or function. More than a single base in the DNA chain or sequence can be involved. A small piece of DNA may be inserted, deleted, or duplicated within the gene or DNA sequence. Such mutations are called *insertions*, *deletions*, or *duplications*— all resulting in potentially serious deficits in the manufactured protein. If a mutation occurs that involves the insertion or deletion of bases that are not multiples of three, a serious disruption of the DNA sequence or reading frame occurs (called a *frame-shift mutation*) with abnormalities or absence of the protein product. In cystic fibrosis, the deletion of only 1 of 1,480 amino acids is the most common mutation resulting in the most severe form of this disease. In Duchenne muscular dystrophy, a common deletion occurs in almost two-thirds of those affected.

Another class of mutations identified are termed unstable. These *dynamic mutations* consist of repetitive three-letter sequences (triplets), which, in a stuttering fashion, appear in excess of the normal expected number within a gene. This form of mutation, which is especially relevant to diseases of the brain and nervous system (*see* Appendix 3), is subject to expansion into larger numbers of triplet repeats; the larger the number, the more severe the disease and the earlier its onset.

Gene mutations can be inherited directly from one or both parents or arise spontaneously in the egg or sperm. Thereafter, that mutation would be transmitted through future generations. The origin of many dominant genetic disorders are new mutations that frequently account for about half of all such disorders. For some disorders, the vast majority arise through new mutations, such as for Achondroplasia (characterized by dwarfism, a relatively large head, and bony abnormalities), where about 7 of 8 have their origin in new mutations. Precisely how gene mutations occur in humans remains uncertain. We do know that tobacco products, ultraviolet light, X-rays, toxic chemicals (such as aflatoxins), radon gas, naturally occurring radioactive compounds, and viruses may cause mutations.

Our cells are constantly barraged by internal and external agents that damage DNA. These assaults on our DNA may result in mutations that lead to genetic disease, cancer, or death unless the damage is properly repaired. Incorrect repair will not spare us the consequences. Fortunately, our cells have evolved mechanisms for DNA repair that are initiated by DNA signaling that damage has occurred. Where repair has not occurred or been imperfect (e.g., mismatched), a range of untoward consequences are seen. These include mutations that lead to cancers, immune disorders, degenerative diseases of the brain and nervous system, infertility, cardiovascular disease, and premature aging. Understanding of the body's DNA damage response has revealed promising avenues for novel treatments of cancer and other disorders.

THE GENE TEAM

Although the gene is the leader, there is always an entourage that facilitates function. Certain letters (bases) in the DNA chain that abut the sequence of letters, which constitute the gene, make up the *promoter*. The role of the promoter is to fix the site at which the copying (transcription) of the gene is initiated as well as to control the quantity of the messenger (RNA). The promoter may extend for several thousand bases, the most important of which are the 100 or 200 close to the gene. Situated within about two dozen base-pairs of the start of a gene is another sequence of letters (quaintly called the "TATA Box") that is involved in the precise localization of the start of transcription of the gene. A little further away there is another sequence of letters (referred to as the CCAAT Box) that, if present, is also involved in securing efficient transcription.

Next in the entourage are the **enhancers**. These DNA sequences are not close but nevertheless increase transcription from a neighboring gene. Some enhancers in fact only exercise their control in specific tissues. **Silencers** are DNA sequences that reduce transcription of the gene. Promoters, enhancers, and silencers interact through signals, although separated by thousands of base-pairs, in transcribing DNA.

From lessons learned in the study of the common bacterium *Escherichia coli*, we now know about genes that control activity of structural genes in determining the amount of a gene product. These are the so-called "control genes." The operation of these **controllers** are, in turn, regulated by more distantly located genes (called regulator genes) that produce a protein that turns a gene on and off (called a **repressor**). Therefore, structural genes may only function when the regulator is switched off by the repressor gene.

Many of these control and regulatory genes as well as the designer genes are switched on to function briefly in directing embryo development. They work in a coordinated sequential cascade regulating the step-wise development of the embryo. Key steps in development that these transcription factors control include separation of tissues into head and tail, arm from leg, and so forth; development of specific organs; and control of the movement of cells to form such organs and their specialization into a particular tissue, such as brain, kidney, and so on. Thereafter, they are switched off permanently, almost never to function again. Rarely, in the face of certain cancers, one or more of these genes may be switched on again to produce embryonic proteins that are detectable in the blood of an adult cancer victim.

GENE FAMILIES

Genes sometimes occur in clusters, particularly when they have similar structures and functions. For example, a cluster of genes on chromosome 6 involves our body's reaction to foreign proteins, such as after an incompatible blood transfusion or upon receiving a transplanted heart, kidney, or other organ. These so-called "human leukocyte antigen" or major histocompatibility genes also make us susceptible to infections and certain diseases (such as ankylosing spondylitis, a form of rheumatoid arthritis of the spine). Besides an unknown number of single genes, several gene families with architectural or designer codes play key roles in the development of the embryo. Most of these genes produce specific proteins that initiate transcription. These so-called "transcription factors" switch genes on and off, thereby activating or repressing the expression of a gene.

Designer Genes

Genes that arrange the body's architecture fall into this category. There are at least three such gene families that dictate the development of body structures such as a leg or an eye. For example, genes that dictate the formation of the eye can be placed in another location, turned on, and function to produce the structure of an eye. Precisely this has been shown in the fruit fly, with an eye developing on a leg! In a similar vein, a gene has been discovered in the mouse that can be induced to grow active hair follicles, raising (for the first time) the possibility of a cure for baldness. These designer genes dictate the fate of a cell and along which axis it moves. They are fundamental to all species and have been found to be highly conserved through many species from the fruit fly, to the mouse, to humans. Given their critical role in development of the early embryo, it is not surprising that a mutation in any of them may have profound consequences. For example, the defective gene we discovered,[1] which causes deafness, widely spaced eyes, eyes of different color, and a white frontal patch of hair (Waardenburg syndrome), is also found in the mouse. Incidentally, there are about 16 different genes responsible for eye color.

A sex-determining gene, which encodes a protein with a specific motif, has been discovered in the tiny worm *Caenorhabditis elegans*, the fruit fly, and in the human. Remarkably, the conserved human counterpart was not located on a sex chromosome but on chromosome 9. This is the very site at which a gene mutation is found in the human, resulting in sex reversal! Other defects in these designer genes may be so serious as to be lethal within weeks of conception or to cause defects of the face, skull, kidneys, limbs, digits, and even absence of the iris (colored portion) of the eye.

GENE PROGRAMS

Programmed Cell Suicide

The truism that death is part of life finds no better witness than exists in gene function.

Sculpting the inner cavities (heart, bowel) and channels (e.g., arteries, veins) requires programmed cell death. In the embryo, for example, the

---

1. Baldwin CT, Hath CF, Amos JA, da-Silva EO, & Milunsky A. (1992) An exonic mutation in the HuP2-paired domain gene causes Waardenburg's syndrome. *Nature* 13(355):590.

hand develops as a pad, the fingers firmly knitted together. Around 10 weeks of pregnancy, the cells binding the fingers and toes together begin to die, allowing separation of the digits. This programmed cell death (called apoptosis[2]) is controlled by specific genes. A mutation in such a gene would interrupt the programmed cell suicide, and a child would be born with one or more fingers stuck together (syndactyly). Curiously, the second and third toes are the digits most frequently partially stuck together (webbed), and this is often inherited from one parent.

Defects in genes that control programmed cell death also have a role in the evolution of cancer (*see* Chapter 8). Apoptosis has a key role in modulating the number of cells, especially where turnover rates are high (e.g., bone marrow). Failure of apoptosis, for example, would allow an increase in the number of cells (e.g., B-lymphocytes), as seen in chronic lymphocytic leukemia. Many other disorders including those of the nervous system, heart, bones, joints, liver, and intestine exhibit the effects of apoptosis. Needless to say, there are also genes whose function it is to keep apoptosis in check!

Clock Genes

In 1729, French astronomer d'Ortous de Mairan noted that a sun-loving plant could open and close, following a day and night rhythm. Over years, and especially recently, internal rhythms have been recognized in fungi, bacteria, frogs, fruit flies, and other organisms. Elegant studies in toads have revealed "clocks" that function in each cell and even demonstrable during early embryo development. These developmental "clocks" signal the timing of key mechanisms that control growth and specialization of cells into tissues and organs. In many organisms, the molecular clocks are mainly located within the nervous system. The pineal gland of birds, reptiles, and fish have light-sensitive cells with pacemaker properties, which direct the rhythmic production of hormones. We probably have clock genes in the front portion of the area of the brain called the hypothalamus. These cells rhythmically send out signals that control sleep, certain behaviors, mating, or, of course, hibernation in animals.

Clock genes represent a beautiful example of the need for environmental action and interaction, because light-sensitive cells are necessary to send

---

2. The term apoptosis was coined from an old Greek word that described the falling off of leaves from trees or petals from flowers.

signals to help regulate the master clock genes. Interestingly, horseshoe crabs have clock sensors on their tails, whereas swallows have them just within their skulls. Fruit flies have clock genes in their legs, wings, and hair bristles. Therefore, it was not terribly surprising that when biologists at Cornell University Medical College in New York shone a bright light on the backs of human knees, they remarkably reset the master biological clock in the human brain! The mechanism by which light signals from behind the knee are detected and transmitted to the master clock cells in the brain remains to be discovered.

Biological rhythms we commonly recognize include the flux of body temperature and levels of the hormone melatonin. The body's temperature rises throughout a day, peaks in the early evening, and begins to decline around 7 to 8 o'clock in the evening, falling to it lowest point at about 5 a.m. Melatonin levels begin to increase around 10 p.m., inducing a state of sleepiness, with the level dropping off during the day. When this flux of melatonin secretion is reversed because of a mutation of a gene(s) on chromosome 17, the result is a birth defect syndrome (Smith-Magenis) with sleep inversion (Chapter 24).

Cyclical hormone production is also under control of some master body clock mechanism since both the age when menses starts and when menopause begins are strongly influenced by genes. Similar influences exist for uterine fibroids (benign tumors) and for the common disorder of endometriosis (cells from the uterine lining growing and causing problems outside of the uterus in the pelvic area).

Meanwhile, a human clock gene has been identified, and mutations demonstrated, that affect specific daily rhythms. This gene and others like it may have mutations that influence consequences such as jet lag and various sleep disorders, including the familial advanced sleep phase syndrome characterized by an intrinsically short sleep cycle and chronic primary insomnia. The partners of day or night people may now finally have an explanation, and once again, genes are implicated. Even sleepwalking is thought to be transmitted as an autosomal dominant trait due to a mutation or variation in a gene on chromosome 20.

In fact, a gene found lacking in some mice causes insomnia. Such mice need twice as long as normal mice to fall asleep, and when they do, they sleep 30% less than their normal cousins.

Mutations found in two different genes associated with narcolepsy (a debilitating chronic sleep disorder) provide further clues to the genetic basis of sleep. Certain gene mutations in Doberman Pinschers cause them to have narcolepsy, and a mutation in another related gene causes a condition in mice that is remarkably similar to human narcolepsy. Understanding the genetic basis of sleep will undoubtedly lead to the discovery of new medications for narcolepsy and other sleep disorders. Who would have thought that when we go to sleep, our parents, through their DNA, still influence our bedtimes?

On Dictating Left from Right

Yes, here we go again. Establishing left from right, or laterality, is coded in your genes Your heart is on your left side, your liver on your right, and your spleen on your left. In the male, the left testis is lower than the right, while the left breast in the female is often larger than the right. The origins of left–right axis are indeed within the control of genes dedicated to the body's symmetric or asymmetric development. For example, a cascade of noncardiac genes dictate the looping of the embryonic tube that becomes the heart, even before 26 days following conception. Mutations within such a controlling gene may result in a failure of positioning, resulting, for example, in a right-sided heart, a left-sided liver, and a right-sided spleen. This disorder is called situs inversus (*see* Chapter 24). Both recessive and dominant genes causing failure to establish normal left–right asymmetry during embryonic development are known. Not infrequently in these situations, defective formation may occur, with a child being born with a structural heart defect.

Brain asymmetry favoring right-handedness and control of speech in the left side of the brain is probably also dictated by genes yet to be discovered.

The Power of Silence

Earlier I referred to members of the gene orchestra—gene silencers—DNA sequences that reduce or prevent a gene from functioning. The most impressive is on the long arm of the X chromosome, where a controlling gene (*XIST*) is located at a spot called the inactivation center. Within days after conception of a female, signals from one randomly chosen X-inactivation center silence most of the genes on that chromosome. Due to this random process, about half the cells in a female have an active maternally derived X, the other half having the paternal functioning X. Females need only one X to survive, whereas males cannot live without an X. In kangaroos, the process is not random—the X chromosome from the male is silenced.

When a translocation of an X chromosome occurs, the unaffected X may be silenced, leading to the possible occurrence of an X-linked disease (seen almost always in males) in females.

Imprinted Genes

We inherit our genes in pairs—at least on our 22 paired, **non-sex** chromosomes. Each pair occupies the same "geographic" location on the paired chromosomes, as would be seen on either side of a rung on a ladder. Generally, the pair of genes is thought to function equally. We now know, however, that for a number of genetic disorders, one of the gene pair becomes silent (inactivated). If the silenced gene is of maternal origin, only the paternal gene is functionally active, and vice versa, in a process called imprinting.

Imprinting occurs before fertilization, and is passed into all of our cells and through eggs or sperm, but it is also reversible.

Two disorders in particular serve to illustrate this phenomenon of imprinting. Both result from a mutation or abnormality at the same spot (although different genes) on the long arm of chromosome 15. Prader-Willi syndrome (short stature, obesity, learning disorder) and Angelman syndrome (severe retardation, absent speech, seizures, and other features) may both arise, for example, from a tiny deletion (or structural abnormality) on chromosome 15. For Prader-Willi syndrome, the deletion is invariably on the father's chromosome, whereas it is the mother's number 15 that is deleted when a child has Angelman syndrome (*see* Chapter 21).

Besides the deletion described, other mutations or structural rearrangements of the genes in this imprinted region of chromosome 15 may occur, causing either Prader-Willi or Angelman syndrome, depending on the parent-of-origin. Deletions account for 70% of these two syndromes. Another mechanism with the same parental sex influences accounts for 20% of these cases. You are likely to be surprised that such a process occurs.

Either at the time the egg (or sperm) is formed or one step later, a pair of chromosome 15s might fail to separate. This would leave the egg or sperm with two chromosome 15s from one parent, which meet the one 15 from the other. An offspring with three chromosome15 (called Trisomy 15, characterized by multiple birth defects) could result (almost all such pregnancies end in miscarriage), or one chromosome 15 could immediately be lost. The remaining two chromosome 15s could be from one parent (called Uniparental Disomy), and either the Prader-Willi or Angelman syndrome would be the consequence, depending on the parental origin of the two chromosome 15s.

Now you must be wondering what could happen if there were a gene with a mutation on a chromosome, which because of the process just described, ends up in duplicate in an offspring. If, for example, it is chromosome 7 and the mutation is in the cystic fibrosis gene, this recessive disorder will occur, although the other parent is **not** a carrier! This mechanism accounts for less than 1% of those with cystic fibrosis.

Imprinting regions occur elsewhere, other than with chromosome 15, and some rare birth defect syndromes and certain cancers may occur as a consequence.

Who would have thought that a parental stamp could be anything but one of approval!

CONSERVED GENES

It comes as a surprise to some that many of our genes are conserved over generations. Because of their critical function for life, even primitive organisms have remained in the genomes of many other species. One of my earliest teachers in medical school, Nobel Laureate Professor Sydney Brenner, chose the 1-millimeter worm (*C. elegans*) to study fundamental biological processes. This worm grows from embryo to full size (1 millimeter) in 3 days and is entirely transparent. Not only are the precise number of cells known in each of its organs, but its complete set of genes has been sequenced. Would you believe that today we know these very same or similar genes in this lowly worm that we share, when mutated, result in scores of genetic diseases that affect us? Examples include the genes involved in cystic fibrosis, colon cancer, deafness, muscular dystrophy, Long QT syndrome, and on and on.

Much the same can be said for other species, including chimpanzees (with whom we share 98.5% of our genes), mice, and fruit flies. In fact, it is sobering to realize that the fruit fly[3] has just over half the number of genes we have.

THE FUTURE

So-called "next-generation sequencing" is based on the tremendous advances in genetic biotechnology that now enables rapid sequencing of our entire genome. The cost of the Human Genome Project to elucidate the entire human genome approximated $3 billion. The incredible biotechnical advances now point to the possibility of having a complete gene analysis for close to $1,000 in

---

3. *Drosophila melanogaster*

the next 5 years. Thus far, dozens of individuals, including some celebrities as well as one of the discoverers of DNA (Dr. James Watson) have had their genomes sequenced. However, data that emerge from analysis of a single individual's genome containing 3 billion bits of data present major challenges in interpretation. Although discovery of precise gene mutations or recognition of those who might be carriers of certain genetic disorders might not pose great difficulty, computational genetics (bioinformatics) will be necessary to figure out an individual's likely risk for developing many different and usually complex diseases. The ability to achieve accurate risk prediction from such analyses remains controversial at present, given the limited opportunity for meaningful interventions, should certain high-risk predictions obtain. Conclusions about risk might also be followed by studies that examine gene expression, which might in turn lead to an understanding of how genes function and open avenues to therapeutic intervention, including the development of new drugs. Certainly, such interventions are likely to be more successful than pure gene therapy in the near term.

In this, the golden era of genetics, we can certainly look forward to continuing resolution of our genomes and a better understanding of the cause of genetic disease and the opportunities that this progress will engender in the prevention and treatment of such ailments.

HOW GENES ARE TRANSMITTED

Each one of us was created by a matching set of genes contributed by our parents. Often a particular feature such as a chin dimple points to the parent who contributed that particular gene. If you have fair skin and suffer badly in the sun, it may be a characteristic of only one side of your family. These variations are mostly the result of inheriting single genes. More commonly, inheritance of multiple genes interacting with environmental factors result in recognizable family traits such as short or tall stature or remarkable intelligence. There are some famous cases, such as the Darwin family, who produced outstanding scientists for five generations. On the other hand, genius often springs from completely average families of no particular intellectual distinction, as was the case for Newton, Keats, and Einstein.

Certain genes convey advantage in fertility or survival, but defects within single genes are mostly disadvantageous. Understanding precisely how defects in single genes are transmitted is critically important, especially if there are opportunities to avoid or prevent serious genetic diseases.

HARMFUL GENES FROM ONE PARENT

We inherit matching genes in pairs, one from each parent. One of these genes may have a stronger effect than its mate and is called a **dominant** gene. If a defect exists in this dominant gene, then the contributing parent is likely to have a genetic disorder as a consequence and have a 50% likelihood of transmitting the defective gene to each of his or her offspring (*see* Figs. 6.1 & 6.2). The resulting dominantly inherited genetic disorder may result from the defective protein produced, its dysfunction, or its absence.

Single dominant genes may therefore cause variable traits, such as large and unusually shaped ears, and when mutated, serious/fatal genetic disorders

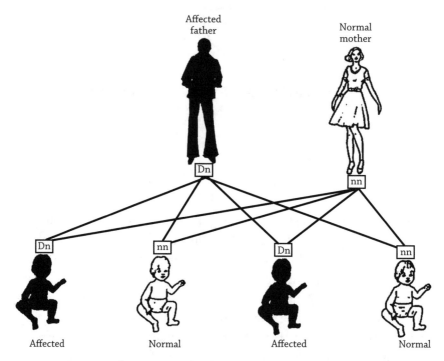

FIGURE 6.1 Dominant inheritance One affected parent (in this case, the father) has a defective gene (*D*) that dominates its normal counterpart (*n*). Each child has a 50–50 chance of inheriting the defective gene from the affected parent and thus of having the disease.

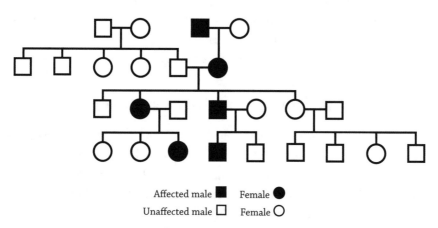

Affected male ■   Female ●
Unaffected male □   Female ○

FIGURE 6.2 A typical family tree involving dominant inheritance—as seen, for example, in Huntington disease, heart disease caused by hypercholesterolemia, and hundreds of other disorders.

(such as Huntington disease). Thus far, almost 20,000 genetic disorders or traits have been catalogued[1] as caused by a single gene. More than half are dominantly inherited, about 36% are recessively inherited, and less than 10% are linked to the X chromosome. About four-fifths of these transmitted gene defects are associated with genetic disorders.

Characteristics of Dominant Inheritance

Certain general "rules" govern this form of inheritance, in which the gene in question is located on a regular, or autosomal, chromosome, rather than on one of the two sex chromosomes.

1. Any child of an affected person has a 50% risk of inheriting the gene from that parent.
2. Males and females are equally affected and equally likely to pass on the harmful gene.
3. Family members who have not inherited the harmful gene do not have the disorder and do not transmit it.
4. The disorder appears in every generation (if not a new mutation), with no skipping, but may not be detected easily.

Considerable variation may be seen in the expression of a dominant genetic disorder within a family. Some affected members may have severe involvement, whereas others may appear not to have any obvious disease, only to bear a seriously affected offspring. Explanations of this phenomenon in terms of a "skipped generation" have often been provided by families. More often, however, incomplete examination or subtle signs that are missed is the better explanation for this apparent lack of **penetrance**.

A single defective gene transmitted through the family may have several effects. For example, in Marfan syndrome (a dominantly inherited disorder in which the elastic fibers of the body's connective tissues are defective and weak), blood vessels, bone, and eye defects may all occur. However, one affected individual may simply have very tall stature, long fingers, and one or two other bony defects, whereas his or her offspring with the identical gene defect may suffer from a dislocation of the lens of the eye and even rupture of a major

---

1. In Online Mendelian Inheritance in Man (OMIM).

blood vessel such as the aorta. Reasons for this variability are unknown but may in large part reflect the type of mutation, the function of the other inherited normal matching gene, or modifying effects of other genes.

Different mutations in the same gene may cause remarkably different disorders. One superb example is the *RET* gene in which a mutation can result in developmental failure of nerve control centers (ganglia) that serve the colon. The result is a failure of colonic function to allow passage of stool effectively, causing a bowel obstruction (called Hirschsprung disease). A different mutation in the same gene can cause thyroid, adrenal, and other cancers in hormone-producing organs (for a disorder called multiple endocrine neoplasia types 2A and 2B).

Given the complexity of how our bodies are structured, it is not surprising that certain dominantly inherited disorders may arise from defects in different genes. Two good examples are illustrative. Profound deafness from birth may result from mutations or variations in one of a few hundred different genes. Indeed, dominant, recessive, and sex-linked genes (see below) may all result in congenital deafness. About 1 in 10 persons carry a mutation in one of these deafness genes. A second example is the adult form of a kidney disorder characterized by progressive and slow development of cysts within the kidneys, causing high blood pressure and kidney failure. Thus far, at least three different dominant genes may cause the same adult form of polycystic kidney disease (*see* Chapter 18).

If a dominant genetic disorder is common, then two affected individuals may easily meet and subsequently have children. If a child receives the defective gene from both parents, the "double dose" is likely to cause a much more serious or fatal form of the disorder affecting each parent. The resulting disorder could be that severe that death would occur in the womb or in the first days, weeks, or months of life. A common disorder (affecting 1 in 500 people) called familial hypercholesterolemia, results in early heart disease and is due to mutations in a dominant gene. A "double dose" in the offspring of a couple who both have this disorder could result, if untreated, in heart attacks before the age of puberty.

Gene Mutations

Inherited gene defects are transmitted via the eggs and sperm. Hence, virtually all the body's cells will contain the same gene defect (called germline mutations) because the gene change exists in the reproductive cells passing from generation to generation. Mutations may, however, arise spontaneously in some sperm in the testes or in some eggs in the ovaries and thereafter can be transmitted randomly. When a disorder caused by a mutation in a single gene (dominant or sex-linked) occurs in an individual whose parents have been definitively shown not to harbor the culprit gene (usually in their blood DNA), and paternity has been confirmed, the conclusion is that the new mutation originated in the ovaries or testes. Previously, proof unfortunately came when such couples had a second affected child, despite having been told that with their negative tests, their risks of having a second affected child were not increased. Now we know that in these cases the ovaries and testes house a mixture of eggs and sperm with a normal or mutated gene (called germline mosaicism). An increasing number of single-gene disorders are recognized in which germline mosaicism may occur (see Appendix 2). For example, as many as 15% of mothers who have had a son with Duchenne or Becker muscular dystrophy and who show no evidence of a mutation in the muscular dystrophy gene are germline mosaics.

Mostly we do not know the cause of mutations. Irradiation either from X-rays, atomic energy, or from the atmosphere can cause mutations. Various chemical products may do the same. We do know that for a handful of genetic disorders, mutations in the sperm of older fathers occurs more frequently (examples include Marfan syndrome and achondroplastic dwarfism).

Occasionally, a mutation may occur in a single cell when the undifferentiated embryo is still literally a ball of cells. That precursor cell may be the origin, for example, of a patch of skin, a limb, a digit, and so forth. The result may therefore be a segmental, patchy, or localized birth defect. This so-called "somatic mutation" may occur in various genetic disorders, including neurofibromatosis type 1 (*see* Chapter 20).

Current estimates indicate that a new mutation in a given gene occurs about once in every million as that gene is passed from parent to child. This would mean that a surprising 8% to 10% of all newborns may carry a new mutation. Thankfully, most of these mutations are silent, probably because of the normal status of the matching gene from the other parent. However, a significant number of people with a genetic disorder that affects neither their parents nor any other family member have a brand new mutation. This is the case in about one-half of those with neurofibromatosis type 1 (*see* Chapter 20), two-thirds of those with tuberous sclerosis complex (*see* Chapter 20), and about one-third with Duchenne muscular dystrophy (*see* Chapter 13), and similarly for hemophilia.

The various types or mutations are described in Chapter 5. It is evident that a change even in a single base within a gene can lead to lifelong disease or death (e.g., sickle cell disease). Gene deletion or duplication mutations that are not visible under the microscope may cause recognizable disorders (called microdeletion or microduplication syndromes). Each of these disorders may arise from a new mutation or be transmitted (as a dominant) by one parent to half the offspring. Features may vary from one person to another. In addition to the Prader-Willi and Angelman syndromes discussed in Chapter 21, dozens of other microdeletion/microduplication syndromes are now known. Typical signs include mental retardation, speech and language delay, autistic behavior, minor or unusual facial features or anomalies, various birth defects, short stature, small head, and seizures. For each of the examples given, there is considerable variability, probably reflecting the additional deletion of one or more contiguous genes.

Another type of mutation resulting from instability ("stuttering") in specific genes is discussed later in this chapter, and disease onset and severity will both be considered.

HARMFUL GENES FROM BOTH PARENTS

Each of us carries a number of harmful "mutated" genes. Because our genes are inherited in pairs (one from each parent), when one is defective and no disease results, the other has sufficient protein product to keep the body stable and without evidence of any disorder. This is the case with all the chromosomes, with the exception of the sex chromosomes, discussed shortly. Defective genes that have no obvious (or very little) effect on the body are termed **recessive**. Measurement of the product of the normally functioning gene would usually show about half the function or, if an enzyme, half the activity. Hence, a person who carries a defective gene for the degenerative brain disorder called Tay-Sachs disease is likely to have half the activity of the produced enzyme (hexosaminidase A) and can be diagnosed by measuring this enzyme activity. A carrier of a recessive disorder would have a 50% likelihood of transmitting that defective gene to each of his or her offspring. A child who receives only this single defective gene would also be a carrier and also show no evidence of any disorder. Only if two individuals who are **both** carriers of the same defective recessive gene, both transmit their flawed genes will there be a 25% risk of having an affected child. As shown in Figures 6.3 and 6.4, there is also a 25% chance that two carriers would have a child who is neither affected nor

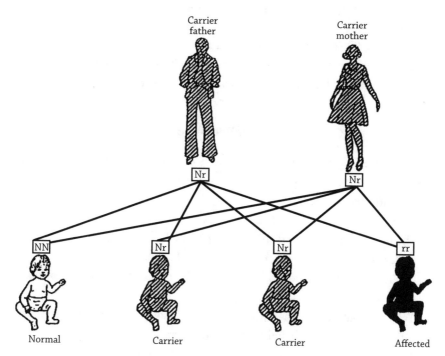

FIGURE 6.3 Recessive inheritance Both parents are usually healthy, but each may carry a defective recessive gene (r), which generally causes no problem when paired with its normal counterpart (N). Disease results when a person receives two of these recessive genes. When both parents are carriers, each child has a 25% chance of inheriting a "double dose" of the defective gene, a 50% chance of being an unaffected carrier, and a 25% chance of being neither a carrier nor affected.

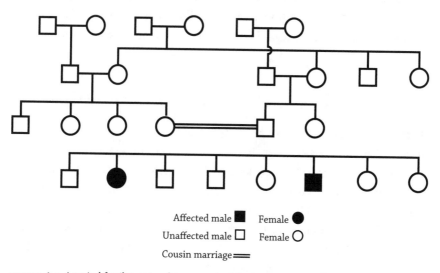

FIGURE 6.4 A typical family tree involving recessive inheritance—as seen, for example, in cystic fibrosis. Note that there were no affected individuals in the early generations. It is not unusual to find cousin marriages in the family history of individuals with recessively inherited disorders.

a carrier. The likelihood that two individuals carrying the same defective gene have children together is increased dramatically if they belong to the same ethnic group (*see* Chapter 15) or are related (e.g., first cousins; uncle–niece).

Characteristics of Recessive Inheritance

Specific criteria govern recessive inheritance in which an individual receives the same harmful gene located on a non-sex chromosome from both unaffected (although carrier) parents.

1. The parents of an affected child may be related.
2. Males and females are equally likely to be affected.
3. On average, once one child has the disorder in question, the risk of recurrence is 25%.
4. Typically, but not invariably, the disorder is not present in the parents or other relatives, but only in brothers and sisters.

Not infrequently, the mutation in the gene in question is different in the one parent than in the other. In such circumstances, the disorder may still manifest in their offspring but may be somewhat different than expected. A perfect example is found in the cystic fibrosis gene (*see* Chapter 14). A person with two severe mutations will have cystic fibrosis, whereas the presence in a male of one severe mutation and one mild mutation may only result in congenital bilateral absence of the vas deferens[2] and no systemic signs of cystic fibrosis.

HARMFUL GENES FROM MOTHERS TO THEIR SONS

A female who has a defective gene on one of her X chromosomes will pass it along to half her male children and half her female children (*see* Fig. 6.5). The daughter who receives the defective **X-linked** gene also receives a matching gene (usually normal) from the father. Such a daughter is then a carrier retaining about half the function of the two genes in combination.

A key example among the hundreds of X-linked disorders is the bleeding disorder called hemophilia (*see* Fig. 6.6). This condition results from an inherited dysfunction of one factor that enables blood to clot normally. If a female

---

2. The tube in each groin that carries the sperm from each testis to the penis.

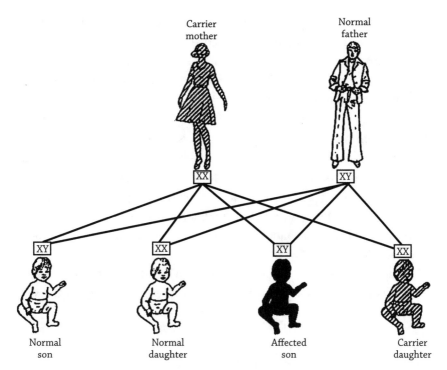

FIGURE 6.5 Sex-linked (X-linked) inheritance. Here, the defective gene (X) is carried on one X chromosome of the mother, who is in most cases healthy. Disease occurs when the X chromosome containing the defective gene is transmitted to a male. The odds of being affected are 50-50 for each male child, and 50 percent of the daughters will be carriers.

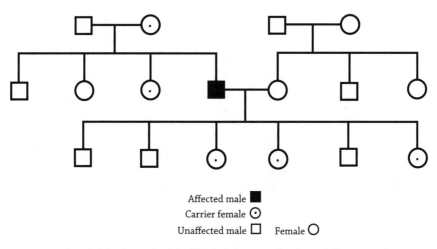

FIGURE 6.6 A typical family tree involving X-linked disease, such as hemophilia or muscular dystrophy.

passes along the hemophilia gene to a male child, then he will actually be affected by the disease. Because the defective gene she carries is on only one of her two chromosomes, there is a 50% chance that her male child will receive the normal one and not be affected (*see* Fig. 6.5). If the male child inherits the defective X chromosome and then marries a woman who is a non-carrier and later has daughters, then all of them will receive the X chromosome with the defective gene and become obligatory carriers of this disorder (*see* Fig. 6.7). Their brothers, because they receive their father's normal male (Y) chromosome, will neither be carriers nor have the disease. Of course, when an affected male impregnates a female carrier, the probabilities are quite different (*see* Fig. 6.8). Incidentally, the most common condition transmitted on the X chromosome is red-green color blindness: about 8% of White males (less in other races) are affected.

Hemophilia is one of the oldest recognized genetic disorders. There are records noting the disorder in the Talmud dating back to before the sixth

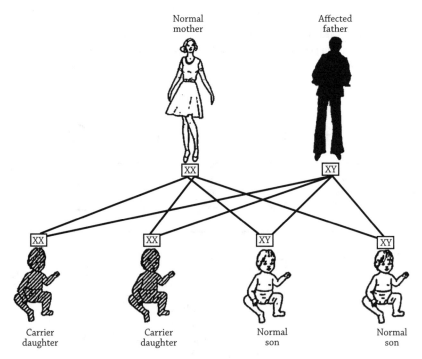

FIGURE 6.7 Sex-linked (X-linked) inheritance. Here, the defective gene (X) appears only on the father's X chromosome. He has the disease (such as hemophilia). He passes his X chromosome to all his daughters, who become carriers, but none of his sons are affected.

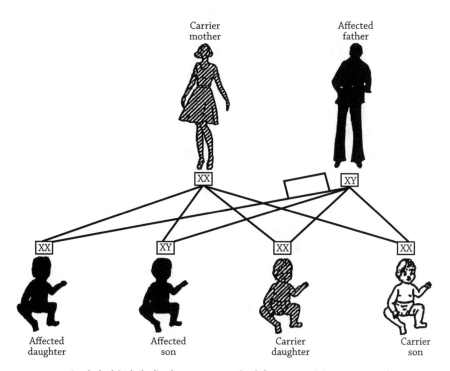

FIGURE 6.8 Sex-linked (X-linked) inheritance Here, the defective gene (*X*) is present on the X chromosome of the father as well as on one of the mother's X chromosomes. The father has the disease (such as hemophilia), and the mother is a carrier. There is a 25% chance that a daughter will be affected and a 50% chance that a son will have the disease.

century C.E. The rabbis at the time exempted from circumcision a male child whose brother had bled heavily following this ritual. These exemptions extended to the nephews of a woman who had a male who bled excessively after circumcision. In their wisdom, this exemption was *not* allowed for the father's son born to other women.

The British royal family provides a typical family "pedigree" for sex-linked disease. Queen Victoria was a carrier of hemophilia, as was her daughter Princess Beatrice. Two of the princess's sons had hemophilia and one daughter (Queen Ena)[3] was a carrier. Queen Ena, in turn, had two sons who were also affected. And on and on.

---

3. New gene sequencing technologies were used to analyze historical specimens from the Romanov branch of the Royal family to show that they had severe hemophilia (*see* Chapter 16).

There is a devastating disorder caused by a mutation in a particular gene (*MECP2*) near the tip of the long arm of an X chromosome. A mutation in this gene causes the X-linked disorder called Rett syndrome.[4] This startling disorder occurs almost exclusively in females, almost all the affected males having died in the womb. Typically, pregnancies are not complicated and prenatal and early development appear normal. However, somewhere between ages 6 and 18 months the affected children usually begin to lose the milestones they had achieved (sitting, walking, talking) and steadily become spastic, lack proper balance, are extremely irascible, and develop autistic behaviors. Typical features include sudden outbursts of crying or screaming and characteristic purposeless wringing or flapping of hands and arms. Growth of the brain slows and a small head (microcephaly) becomes apparent. At least 50% develop seizures. After a few devastating years, the neurological deterioration ceases and the affected females may then survive for many decades with profound disability. The few males who are born alive mostly manifest profound neurological deficits with severe mental retardation and seizures. In recent years, some seriously retarded males have also been recognized as having the Rett syndrome gene mutation.

Another potentially serious disorder, which like Rett syndrome is transmitted as a sex-linked dominant disorder, appearing almost exclusively in females, again results from a mutation in a gene not far from the Rett syndrome gene on the X chromosome. Incontinentia pigmenti is a rare disorder presenting at or soon after birth with a blistering rash that slowly resolves, leaving whorls of pigment on the trunk and limbs. At least one-third of affected females have neurological consequences that may even resemble cerebral palsy, with or without seizures. Other findings include hair, teeth, and nail abnormalities. Blindness may occur as a consequence of detached retinas. The mutation in this disorder is primarily a gene deletion.

Symptoms and Signs in Carriers

A woman who is a carrier of the gene for an X-linked disease rarely has a similar harmful gene on the other X chromosome. But even with this single dose of the mutated gene, it would not be remarkable for her to show some manifestation of the disorder in question. If it is the Duchenne form of muscular dystrophy, she

---

4. Named after Andreas Rett, an Austrian neurologist.

may well have symptoms of weakness when walking, which may become increasingly obvious as she tires during the day. Or, she may have weakness walking up stairs or running even though her calf muscles seem well-developed. Of greater importance is the realization that as many as 84% of mothers who carry a gene mutation for Duchenne muscular dystrophy have some form of heart involvement. These signs may take the form of changes on the electrocardiogram, a tendency to rhythm disturbances of the heart with a potential for serious consequences, cardiac enlargement, and possible heart failure. Hence, once again, it is important to know your genes in this regard and immediately seek a consultation with a cardiologist to arrange for annual surveillance and appropriate pre-emptive prevention and treatment. If you are a carrier, this knowledge and action could save your life.

In the Fragile X syndrome (*see* Chapter 10) almost 50% of women who carry the dynamic mutation manifest cognitive abnormalities and, not infrequently, premature ovarian failure resulting in infertility. Female carriers of hemophilia may also not have entirely normal blood-clotting ability. Mothers who are carriers of a white blood cell defect that leads to chronic granulomatous disease (a condition in which the offspring are especially subject to serious infections) can also be shown to have decreased functional ability of their white blood cells to kill bacteria. Another example is mothers of certain albino children who may show some pigmentary changes in their own eyes.

Rarely a female actually has an X-linked recessive disease. In such cases, she would have had to be the daughter of an affected father and a mother who is a carrier, and she would have to inherit an abnormal gene from each of them.

Characteristics of X-Linked Recessive Inheritance

Five main criteria help determine whether a disorder is transmitted as an X-linked condition.

1. The disorder is passed from an affected man **through all** his daughters to, on average, half **their** sons.
2. The disorder is never transmitted from father to son.
3. The disorder may be passed through carrier females eventually to affected males who are all related to one another through these females.
4. Female carriers may show signs of the disorder.
5. The incidence of the disorder is much higher in males than in females.

HARMFUL GENES FROM MOTHERS TO THEIR CHILDREN

Situated within the fluid (cytoplasm) bathing the nucleus in every cell are several hundred small bodies called mitochondria, also made up of DNA. Curiously, the DNA is circular but also codes for certain protein subunits, called enzymes. At fertilization of an egg, the sperm nucleus enters, but the mitochondria are enzymatically destroyed. Hence, the genes contained within the mitochondria are maternal in origin and are transmitted by the mother to all of her children, regardless of their sex (*see* Chapter 22 for a fuller discussion; *see* Fig. 6.9).

A brand new defect (a sporadic mutation) may occur in a mitochondrial gene. One condition rarely recognized, and caused by a sporadic mutation in a mitochondrial gene, is characterized by a feeling of fatigue and exhaustion even during normal play or daily activity, worsening with age. Some complain as early as age 5 years of a feeling of exhaustion and nausea and feeling that their jaw muscles are too tired to chew. All of this exercise intolerance may sometimes be accompanied by weakness or by muscle cramps during exercise.

There are also many mitochondrial genes in the nucleus of every cell.[5] These nuclear genes are transmitted in the same way as other single genes

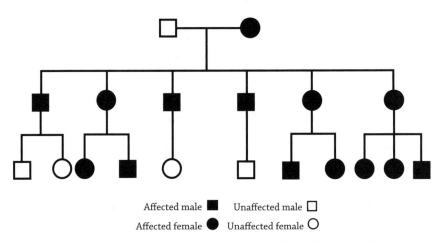

Affected male ■   Unaffected male □
Affected female ●   Unaffected female ○

FIGURE 6.9 Mitochondrial inheritance. The affected mother passes her mitochondrial mutation to all her children, but her affected sons do not transmit the mitochondrial disorder.

---

5. Mature red cells have no nucleus.

discussed earlier. There is, however, a direct relationship with the cytoplasmic mitochondrial genes that assist in the maintenance of their integrity. Similar disorders may occur as a consequence of mutations in either mitochondrial or nuclear mitochondrial genes and may not be easily distinguishable clinically.

The characteristic pattern of mitochondrial inheritance has been used not only in forensic cases to identify remains, even from long-buried bones, but also in notorious cases. Examples include the identification of "the disappeared children" of Argentina abducted during their military dictatorship and recognition from the bones of nine people that confirmed the fate of the Russian royal family at the time of the Bolshevik revolution.

Characteristics of Maternal Inheritance

Mitochondrial inheritance (also called maternal, extranuclear, or cytoplasmic inheritance) involves the transmission of a mother's genes to each of her children. The prime criteria are:

1. Women who harbor a mitochondrial mutation in all cells (called homoplasmic) will transmit it to **all** offspring and of both sexes (*see also* Chapter 22).
2. Women who are heteroplasmic (meaning that not all the mitochondria carry the mutation) for a mitochondrial point mutation or duplication will pass them on to all of their children. The number of mutant mitochondria will vary in their children, making the risk and severity of disease highly variable.
3. Affected and carrier males do not transmit the mutation to any of their children.

In families in which there is a recognizable mitochondrial disorder (not nuclear mitochondria) with demonstrable maternal inheritance, a variable spectrum of disease is expected as a consequence of the varying fraction of mutant mitochondria in different tissues.

GENES FROM FATHER TO SON

Genes on the Y chromosome are only transmitted to the sons, and fortunately there seem to be none that cause death or serious disability. Y-linked (or Holandric) inheritance passes a set of genes located on the long arm of the Y,

Zebra male finches learn to sing elaborate songs from their fathers. There isn't any good evidence, however, that this occurs in humans.

which all function in the production of sperm. Deletions of one or more of these genes result in no sperm (azoospermia) or few sperm (oligospermia). Deletions in 5% to 18% of these sterile or infertile men have been reported. Even in these cases, recovery of a single sperm via a needle in the testis will frequently lead to successful pregnancy. This step is accomplished by inserting the sperm directly into a harvested egg—a process called intracytoplasmic sperm injection—and implanting the fertilized egg into the hormonally prepared uterus. The gene for hairy ears is also located on the Y chromosome.

AGE OF ONSET AND SEVERITY OF A GENETIC DISORDER

One would think that the presence of a defective gene that causes a serious genetic disorder would be obvious at birth. In fact, the time of onset of serious to fatal genetic disorders varies from the earliest days following conception in the womb, all the way through to the late 70s or 80s. Many factors influence the expression, penetrance, age of onset, and severity of a genetic disorder. Where a gene is so vital to the structure and function of a cell or organ, a mutation may prove lethal within days or weeks of conception. A somewhat less severe mutation might lead to fetal death at some time during pregnancy. Witness the case of a severe form of brittle bone disease (osteogenesis imperfecta) in which a child may be born with almost all bones fractured.

In contrast, some mutations for the same disorder may lead to few obvious signs, which may only become detectable in middle age.

Of the more than 1600 mutations in the cystic fibrosis gene recognized thus far, one is the most common (called the ΔF508 mutation). When both members of a couple contribute this mutation to their offspring, the more severe form of cystic fibrosis (see Chapter 14) occurs. Some rarer mutations may be associated with such mild cystic fibrosis as to not raise the question of a diagnosis until middle or even old age. Such individuals may in fact present with chronic bronchitis, problems with the pancreas (pancreatitis), or gallstones. Others may be spared the more grave involvement of the lungs with chronic infection.

Other mutations, especially in disorders affecting the nervous system and the muscles, may exert their effect conditioned by the sex of the parent transmitting the culprit gene. For example, in the neurodegenerative Huntington's disease, an affected father passing the gene mutation to his son results in an earlier onset than he had for that disorder. Huntington disease could manifest even as early as age 3 years (*see* Chapter 12), although the average age of onset of detectable symptoms and signs is age 37 years.

In the dominantly inherited myotonic muscular dystrophy (the most common form of adult muscular dystrophy), in an affected mother who transmits the defective gene to an affected offspring (the risk is 50%), frequently severe manifestations will be present at birth. Hence, pregnant mothers who know they have this disorder should know about the implications of this gene. They should ensure that they deliver in a tertiary care medical center with sophisticated facilities for newborn intensive care and be certain that a pediatric newborn specialist (neonatologist) is present at the birth. Moreover, because of the increased personal risk to herself for obstetrical as well as anesthetic complications, high-risk specialists in obstetrics (perinatologists) should be sought for the best care. Again, knowledge of the potential hazards of this defective gene will secure the health and could save the life of both mother and child. The phenomenon of sex-influenced effects on the offspring of affected men or women results from a process called imprinting (*see* Chapters 5 and 21).

The mutations that are typical in more than 20 inherited neuromuscular disorders are characterized by a stuttering type of defect in the bases that constitute the gene (*see* Chapter 5)—in the chain of letters making up a gene. Not infrequently, in normal genes, there could be runs of three letters (called triplet repeats). For example, there could be triplet repeats of CAG for 10 to 30 copies normally. However, in Huntington disease, there are an increased number of triplet repeats mostly ranging between 40 and 121. Similarly, an increased run of triplets (different numbers for different diseases) may be seen—for example, in myotonic muscular dystrophy, Friedreich's ataxia, various types of spinocerebellar ataxia, spinal bulbar palsy, and the fragile X syndrome (*see* Appendix 3).

A safe but not absolute generalization is that the higher the number of triplet repeats (note that some are CAG, others are CGG, etc.), the more severe the disease and the earlier its onset. Indeed, for all of these disorders, there is the phenomenon of **anticipation**. This means that over the generations there is a progressively earlier age of onset of the disorder in those who have inherited the dynamic triplet repeat mutation (*see* Appendix 4 and Chapters 10 and 12).

DNA FINGERPRINTS

There are more than 3 billion bits of DNA information from which individual patterns, mutations, or markers can be used for identification. Moreover, for forensic use, the DNA within tiny specks of blood, for example, can be expanded infinitely, as an aid to identification of an individual. The so-called "DNA fingerprinting techniques" (not actually fingerprints, but much better) can reach billions to one odds—a standard no court requires. Moreover, a distinguishing feature of this method makes positive identification virtually certain, compared with other methods that serve only to exclude persons under investigation.

Incest

Intercourse between brothers and sisters, fathers and daughters, or mothers and sons constitutes incest and is not only illegal but considered taboo in most societies. The reported studies of incest all note a devastating increase in the occurrence of serious birth defects, mental retardation, or both when offspring result. Such unions would be expected to result in about a fivefold increase in the birth of defective offspring. A 1982 Canadian report on 29 children born of incestuous unions showed that most had severe abnormalities, low birth weight, mental retardation, or medical problems. Four (13.8%) had specific recessively inherited defects.

The advent of precise DNA analysis now provides remarkable accuracy in the determination of paternity and even maternity. Many legal cases of claimed incest by a father with his daughter have been successfully prosecuted based on definitive DNA evidence. Demonstrated in these cases is the appearance of a unique pattern of genes in the offspring that could only have derived from the male committing incest. Degrees of certainty in these cases mostly exceed 99%.

Cases of questioned maternity have arisen mostly through immigration services where claims of maternity by someone applying for immigration status have had to be addressed. Once again, proof of maternity in such cases has been achieved in the 99% to 100% region of certainty.

Rape and Murder

The uniqueness of an individual's set of genes provides a telltale DNA set of "fingerprints." Cells containing DNA from any site can yield identifiable DNA.

Such sites successfully mined for DNA in criminal cases have included blood specks, semen stains, hair roots, nasal mucus, skin cells (e.g., from scrapings under the nails of a victim), cells from saliva (e.g., taken from a bite site or from the mouth found under a licked stamp), or skin from a touched envelope or instrument of murder. A 25-year-old vaginal swab taken for semen was successfully used in a criminal prosecution. Many convictions of murderers and other felons through DNA identification have been achieved. Also noteworthy and desperately sad is the discovery of innocence and false incarceration of individuals subsequently exonerated and freed by DNA evidence.

PRENATAL DIAGNOSIS

The anguish shared by parents following the birth of a child with a serious birth defect, genetic disorder, or mental retardation is profound and everlasting. The feelings engendered by this sadness are compounded by distress and anger upon realization that all could have been avoided or prevented and that a lifetime of suffering for a child, as well as the complex family burden, could have been averted. Such an opportunity is rare indeed. Prenatal genetic diagnosis is a rare exception.

To avoid or prevent birth defects, genetic disorders, or mental retardation, pregnancies should be **planned**. Such a plan presupposes careful consideration and knowledge of the family history and consultation with the obstetrician and, if necessary, a clinical geneticist (*see* Chapter 1). Armed with the knowledge of risks and informed about all the available options, parents have the freedom to choose their own approach. This chapter focuses on the critically important option of diagnosing a defect in the embryo or fetus in early pregnancy.

EARLY WARNING

We are all comforted by the knowledge that about 96 in every 100 babies are born without evidence of major birth defects. The 3% to 4% that represent each of our average risks and who are not born sound are the root cause of our anxieties during pregnancies. Virtually all of us take on these background risks and have our families. However, when there are indications of birth defects or genetic disorders in the family, or other risk indicators exist (*see* Chapters 2–6), genetic evaluation and counseling should be sought and prenatal diagnosis may be a considered option.

PRECONCEPTION PLANNING

It is the careful and judicious couple who seeks **preconception** counseling. Much grief can be avoided by couples who follow key recommendations, including folic acid supplements (*see* Chapter 25), adjustments of medications, and control of conditions such as epilepsy and diabetes (*see* Chapters 23 and 26). Clearly, once parents make a decision to have a pregnancy and elect prenatal diagnosis, the possibility of abortion of a defective fetus may need to be addressed. Those at known risk but opposed to terminating a pregnancy should explore all other options prior to conceiving so as to avoid even having to address the issue of abortion later. *Preconception planning* is the most important step parents can take to avoid having a child with a serious birth defect or genetic disorder. This critical step is the one most parents omit and spend a lifetime regretting.

INDICATIONS FOR PRENATAL GENETIC STUDIES

Prenatal genetic diagnosis is done to detect chromosome abnormalities, single-gene mutations, biochemical genetic disorders (which result from single-gene defects), and anatomical defects of the fetus.

Chromosome Defects

A couple would need to consider having prenatal chromosome studies to detect such abnormalities for any one of the reasons outlined in Table 7.1.

A brief look at these indications may be helpful. With advancing maternal age, there is an increased risk of having a child with one of five chromosome disorders, each characterized by the presence of an extra chromosome (see Chapter 2). The most common is Down syndrome (Trisomy 21), and the others are Trisomy 18, Trisomy 13, Klinefelter syndrome (XXY), and Triple X

Table 7.1 Reasons for Prenatal Diagnosis of a Chromosome Defect

1. Advanced maternal age
2. An abnormal maternal serum screening result
3. A previous child with a chromosome defect
4. One parent is a carrier of a structural chromosome rearrangement
5. A fetal abnormality detected on ultrasound study
6. Previous removal of an ovary (or sections of one or both ovaries)

(XXX chromosomes; *see* Chapters 2–4). Precisely why advancing maternal age is associated with an escalating risk of these disorders remains uncertain. Although the mechanism of sticky chromosomes (called nondisjunction) is understood (*see* Chapter 2), the initiating mechanisms remain obscure. The escalating risk with age may be tied to the body's natural protective mechanisms against harboring chromosomally defective offspring. For example, the body is remarkably efficient at naturally discontinuing (by miscarriage) the vast majority of chromosomally abnormal embryos and fetuses. One likely reason for the increasing rate of certain numerical chromosome defects among older women may be a progressive breakdown in the body's surveillance (possibly a flaw in the immune mechanism), which allows more chromosomally defective embryos to survive.

Prenatal genetic studies have been recommended routinely for women who become pregnant at age 35 years or older, but more recently the American College of Obstetricians and Gynecologists have backed the availability of such studies for all women. There is a steadily, although slowly, rising risk of chromosome abnormality beginning in the late 20s. The new recommendations emerged against a background realization that the procedural risk of fetal loss may be less than the likelihood of a chromosome defect. After all, some 80% of babies born with Down syndrome are delivered by mothers younger than age 35 years!

Maternal serum screening, as discussed later in this chapter, facilitates recognition of pregnancies at unexpected risk for fetal chromosome defects. These screening studies serve as a very common indication for prenatal genetic studies. Parents who have had a child with the common Trisomy 21 form of Down syndrome have a 1% to 2% risk of recurrence in a subsequent pregnancy when the mother is younger than age 35 years. If this has occurred after age 35 years, the risk of recurrence or another chromosome defect depends on the maternal age at the time of the future conception. At age 36 years, the risk of some type of chromosome abnormality approximates 1%; at age 40 years, it is about 2% to 3%; and at age 45 years, the risk ranges between 7% and 10%.

Women who have had a child with a chromosome defect, or who have had a miscarriage in which a chromosome defect was detected, may have increased risks of recurrence in a subsequent pregnancy. Those women who suffer through three or more miscarriages have a 3% to 8% likelihood that either she or her partner carries a chromosomal abnormality. Blood chromosome analysis of both partners is indicated in these circumstances to determine whether one or the other has or carries a chromosome abnormality. The risk that one partner carries a chromosome abnormality after two miscarriages is between 1% and 3%.

Another risk indicator for having offspring with Down syndrome exists in women who have had an ovary (or part of one or both ovaries) surgically removed or who were born without one ovary. A report from the Centers for Disease Control and Prevention noted a 9.6-fold increased risk of Down syndrome in the offspring of women with a "reduced ovarian complement." Although the mechanism is uncertain, the physiological state of the ovary is the focus of attention. The reported risk is clear enough to offer prenatal genetic studies.

Single-Gene Disorders

The chromosomal disorders just discussed are mostly associated with risks of recurrence below 15% and mostly in the region of 1%. In contrast, risks of occurrence or recurrence resulting from disorders caused by single-gene defects range (almost always) between 25% and 50%. In this high-risk group especially are parents who in the past, faced with such high risks and prior to the availability of prenatal diagnosis, decided against having a child or another child. Prenatal diagnosis now provides the reassurance that allows such parents to have as large a family as they wish. Specifically, prenatal diagnosis allows couples the opportunity to have unaffected children selectively, sparing the parents the agony of losing a child and, more important, sparing an affected child the pain and suffering of disease, serious deformity, or early death.

I discussed disorders caused by defects in single genes (dominant, recessive, X-linked, and mitochondrial) fully in Chapter 6, including their risks of recurrence. For prenatal diagnosis in any of these four categories of single-gene disorders, the first requirement is to identify precisely the gene mutation(s) in one or both parents or in a previously affected child. Only with fulfillment of that requirement can prenatal diagnosis proceed to a specific definitive conclusion. Indications for prenatal studies for single-gene disorders are for couples who have had a previously affected child or where one parent is affected or a known carrier or both are known carriers with recognized mutations. If a mutation has yet to be described or cannot be determined, tracking blocks of DNA containing the likely mutation (called DNA linkage analysis) in an informative family could provide prenatal diagnosis with certainties exceeding 99%. Such studies, however, require the cooperation of family members in the form of blood samples—for example, from parents, siblings, grandparents, great-grandparents, nieces. nephews, and cousins. Obviously not everyone has to participate, but the more key members who do, the greater the certainty of diagnosis, as long as there is clear evidence of who is and who is not affected among those family members. Given the variability of expression among certain, especially dominant single-gene diseases, DNA linkage analysis is sometimes difficult to accomplish.

Needless to say, because prenatal diagnosis of single-gene disorders represents complex challenges, couples are advised to seek a consultation with a clinical geneticist **prior to pregnancy.**

Single-gene disorders that manifest themselves through disturbed biochemical functions of cells are individually rare. Collectively, however, they occur about once in every 100 children born. Many of these cause severe mental retardation, seizures, stunting of growth, and early death. Prenatal diagnosis is achieved by cultivating the fetal cells, which are then subjected to analysis of the potentially defective, or absent, enzyme. The first prenatal diagnosis of a biochemical genetic disorder was made in the late 1960s. That disorder was Tay-Sachs disease (*see* Chapter 15).

An uncommon indication for prenatal studies is when carrier detection in one of the parents is either inconclusive or impossible. In such very specific cases, it may be possible to assess accurately the activity, or lack thereof, of a specific enzyme in the cultivated fetal cells.

Prenatal Studies for Physical Defects in the Fetus

About 2% of all newborns have a significant physical defect. Included in this group are cleft lip and palate, spina bifida, heart defects, hand or limb defects, and brain abnormalities. Prenatal detection of these defects mostly requires imaging by high- resolution ultrasound, primarily between 16 and 18 weeks of pregnancy. Such studies are not normally done unless there is a history in the family, a previous affected child, a report of an abnormal maternal serum screen (*see* following discussion on Screening in Early Pregnancy), or a suspicion of fetal growth restriction or abnormality on a routine ultrasound study.

SCREENING IN EARLY PREGNANCY

Among the most important advances following the introduction of prenatal diagnosis in the mid-1960s was the development of screening pregnant women's blood samples for two specific classes of fetal defects—neural tube and chromosome defects. These two represent the most common groups of serious birth defects in the Western world. Neural tube defects encompass disorders that result from a failure of closure in the embryo of the tube that forms the brain and spine. Failure of closure results in exposed brain (called anencephaly), whereas an opening along the spine exposing the spinal cord is termed spina bifida. Anencephaly is not associated with survival much beyond birth (with rare exceptions), whereas spina bifida will almost always cause a lifetime of serious problems (see Chapter 18).

The various chromosome defects, including Down syndrome (see Chapter 2), have mental retardation and multiple birth defects as their most serious potential consequences.

Before the advent of screening, about 95% of all babies born with neural tube defects and close to 80% born with Down syndrome were delivered without any advance warning of the fetal defect or recognition of any increased risk. The vast majority of other chromosome abnormalities also occurred without prior warning. Screening facilitated recognition of pregnancies with increased risks for these defects and represented an enormous advance.

> The prime purpose of screening is to identify pregnancies not otherwise known to be at risk for birth defects and then to provide precise diagnostic studies to secure the safest delivery or the option to discontinue the pregnancy.

Although maternal serum screening for neural tube defects has been possible since the early 1970s, it only became the expected standard of care in the United States in mid-1985. Even now, some Western countries do not provide screening for all their patients. Screening pregnancies to detect those at increased risk of chromosome defects has also been available for almost two decades.

Screening for chromosome defects is effectively accomplished between 11 and 13 weeks of pregnancy. Maternal blood samples are analyzed for the main pregnancy protein human chorionic gonadotropin (hCG) and a placental protein (PAPP-A). The levels obtained are entered into a statistical algorithm to which additional information is added (week of pregnancy, maternal age and weight, race, twins, etc). The result is compared to electronically stored databases from normal pregnancies, and the odds of a specific chromosomal abnormality affecting the fetus is computed. A precise prenatal diagnostic test is offered when the odds of a fetal chromosomal defect are considered greater

than the risk of pregnancy loss resulting from the prenatal diagnostic procedure. Most laboratories use risks greater than 1 in 270 or 1 in 250.

The detection rate of pregnancies in which the fetus has Down syndrome
ranges between 80% and 94%. Remember this is a screening, not a diagnostic
test. Maternal serum screening is also provided in the second trimester of
pregnancy, around 16 weeks. This is primarily aimed at detecting pregnancies
at risk of fetal neural tube defects (mainly spina bifida and anencephaly[1]).

Measurements are made of four blood constituents—alpha-fetoprotein
(AFP), human chorionic gonadotropin (hCG), unconjugated estriol (uE3),
and inhibin A (placental hormone). Measuring AFP enables the detection of
virtually all pregnancies where the fetus has anencephaly. Close to 95% of
pregnancies are detected where the fetus has spina bifida. These neural tube
defects are suspected when high levels of AFP leaks from the open defect into
the surrounding amniotic fluid and thence into the mother's blood circulation, where elevated levels are then found. Other defects that leak (e.g., via the
fetal kidneys or fetal skin) may also raise the maternal blood levels of AFP.

Because the level of AFP in the fetal blood is 150 to 200 times higher than it
is in mother's blood, even a small leak directly into the mother's blood may
raise the AFP level. Because the measurement of this protein is very accurate,
finding an elevation of AFP in mother's blood in the absence of a demonstrable fetal defect usually means a small breach in the integrity of the placental
interface between fetus and mother. Unexplained raised AFP levels signal
pregnancies at increased risk of premature labor, low birth weight, toxemia,
and other potential complications, highlighting the need for increased surveillance during the last 3 months of pregnancy and through labor and delivery.

A high-resolution ultrasound study of the fetus is recommended if an elevated maternal serum AFP is detected. Targeted (high-resolution) ultrasound
will reveal the diagnosis of anencephaly and close to 100% of spina bifida. The
possible exception is the tiny defect near the end of the spine. In morbidly
obese mothers (see Chapter 22), clear visualization of the fetal spine may
not be achieved. Other defects that may cause the elevated AFP may also
be detected at this time. Twins, triplets, and so forth, who each represent a

---

1. Spina bifida is a defect in the spine through which a portion of the spinal nerves could extrude,
forming a lump on the back and resulting in paralysis of the legs and possible lack of control of
the bladder and even the bowel. Anencephaly is an open skull with a deformed, poorly developed
brain that is not compatible with survival.

"factory" making AFP, will obviously raise maternal blood levels and be detected by the ultrasound study.

Parents faced with an abnormal maternal serum screen showing an elevated AFP level have the automatic recommendation of a high-resolution ultrasound study. Even in the face of a normal ultrasound report, I would encourage an amniocentesis. The aim would be to measure AFP in the amniotic fluid as well as an enzyme (acetylcholinesterase) that is secreted from exposed brain or nerve cells. The presence of this enzyme in a clear (non-blood-stained) amniotic fluid almost invariably points to a leak from the nervous system, such as that resulting from spina bifida. There are, in fact, a host of different disorders that may leak or cause elevations of AFP in amniotic fluid. Hence, again, even in the presence of a normal ultrasound report, an amniocentesis would be recommended and should include chromosome studies of the cultivated cells derived from the fluid. It should be noted that in about 5% of cases with spina bifida, the spinal lesion is covered by skin, does not leak, and will not be reflected by elevated levels of AFP[2] in either the amniotic fluid or the mother's blood. In such cases, high-resolution ultrasound would not ordinarily be done, except in cases where there is a family history of a neural tube defect, such as spina bifida or anencephaly, or because the mother has taken medication that may cause spina bifida (such as the anticonvulsant valproic acid; *see* Chapter 23).

In contrast, low levels of AFP and uE3 associated with temporarily higher levels of hCG and inhibin together indicate increased risks of Down syndrome or another chromosome defect. Risks of Down syndrome are calculated from complex formulas that account for the mother's age, weight, race, the week of pregnancy, presence or absence of diabetes, and the level of the various measured blood constituents. When such a risk exceeds 1 in 270, we recommend that an amniocentesis (*see* below) be done. By this method, between 80% and 90% of pregnancies in which the fetus has Down syndrome, as well as more than half of other chromosome abnormalities, will be detected. A host of other rarer fetal defects may be detected through screening.

Screening findings that lead to an amniocentesis for Down syndrome or chromosome defects and that conclude with normal chromosome and ultrasound results cannot be ignored. In close to two-thirds of such "unexplained" cases with increased odds for Down syndrome, late pregnancy

---

2. These cases include exposed bowel (called omphalocele or gastroschisis), skin defects, or a kidney disorder (such as a congenital nephrosis).

obstetrical complications may occur, and careful surveillance should once again be instituted. Because the hormones being measured are of placental origin, abnormal levels imply dysfunction in this organ or the fetus. Hence, abnormal screening results signal a disturbance in normal function as well as the possible presence of a fetal defect. That is precisely their value.

Fortunately, the vast majority of abnormal serum screening results are not associated with a fetal defect or an adverse outcome to pregnancy. Consequently, considerable anxiety may be engendered when an abnormal result is obtained. Remember, however, that without screening, up to 80% of pregnancies with fetal Down syndrome and up to 95% with spina bifida would go undetected. There are also advantages to detecting pregnancies at previously unknown obstetrical risk, encouraging much more careful surveillance that would not otherwise have occurred. Avoiding anxiety by not being screened does not remove a mother's chances—it removes her choices. Any anxiety generated "unnecessarily" during pregnancy is totally overshadowed following the birth of a child with one of these defects. The ensuing emotional chaos and economic family burden, coupled with the suffering of the child, weigh heavily in favor of maternal screening.

PRENATAL DIAGNOSIS

All couples wish to have a healthy child. Those couples who have an increased risk of bearing a child with a certain defect will most often seek ways to avoid or prevent such an outcome. Information couples should know about avoidance and prevention of birth defects, mental retardation, and genetic disorders is discussed in Chapter 1 and throughout this book. Preventive actions are best taken before pregnancy is initiated. To avoid having a child with a chromosome or gene defect, prenatal diagnosis with its option of selective abortion is available once pregnancy has begun. Unfortunately, fetal treatment remains a rare option. On average, more than 95% of prenatal genetic studies yield normal results.

Indeed, more children are born _because_ of the availability of prenatal diagnosis compared to the number of pregnancies otherwise terminated because of defects. Prenatal diagnosis is therefore a life-giving approach, as many more couples choose to have children in the face of high risks, given the assurance provided by prenatal diagnosis.

There are five methods used in prenatal genetic diagnosis and that are discussed in turn:

1. Preimplantation genetic diagnosis
2. Chorionic villus sampling (CVS)
3. Amniocentesis
4. Ultrasound
5. Non-invasive prenatal diagnosis

Preimplantation Genetic Diagnosis

Sometimes couples may be faced with high risk (25%–50%) that a future child would be born with a serious to fatal genetic disorder. An ideal solution would be to check the fertilized egg **before** it implants into the lining of the prepared womb. This procedure has been accomplished in a few thousand cases worldwide, and is called preimplantation genetic diagnosis (PGD).

Available Procedures

The entire process involves in vitro fertilization (IVF), in which a harvested egg produced after hormone stimulation of the mother is fertilized in a dish by contributed sperm. After fertilization, when the embryo is between 4 and 8 cells in size, it is possible through micromanipulation to extract 1 or 2 cells for analysis of a single gene or specific chromosome abnormality. Because each one of the cells possesses the entire genetic program of the future individual, removal of one or even two cells has not proved harmful to development of the embryo and fetus. This process of embryo biopsy of these individual cells (called blastomeres) has been followed by successful implantation and delivery of a healthy child in many pregnancies in highly specialized centers around the world. Many single-gene disorders have been diagnosed or excluded by PGD.

Preimplantation gene analysis proceeds only after the precise mutation has been determined in both parents (recessive disorders) or from one parent (dominant or X-linked disease). The discovery that chromosomal mosaicism (*see* Chapter 2) may already be present in an 8- to 16-cell embryo adds more concern. About 1 in 13 conceptions are not normal, and these embryos seldom implant or survive. If an abnormality is found, the fertilized egg is discarded. Hence, for those with an antipathy toward abortion, PGD might be a more palatable and important option.

Another approach to PGD is based on a basic biologic fact. When the usual 46 chromosomes in a cell (*see* Chapter 2), such as the one from which the ovary originates, splits in two to form the egg with 23 chromosomes, the remaining 23 crumple up into a tiny ball (termed the polar body) usually found within and at the periphery of the egg. Polar body biopsy of the egg enables assessment of the mother's (but not the father's) genome. Single-gene mutations detected by analyzing a single embryonic cell can yield an accurate diagnosis in 99% of cases. However, a misdiagnosis rate of up to 1% is known, leading some couples to confirm a (normal) result at about either 11 or 16 weeks by methods discussed below.

Couples undergoing IVF and PGD are likely to achieve a pregnancy about 40% of the time in very experienced centers. Pregnancy rates in less experienced centers may range upward from 26%. Note, however, that these figures don't translate to "take home baby rates," which will almost invariably be less than the best 40% figure. Although a number of eggs are often fertilized, transfer of no more than two into the uterus might be judicious. Couples who choose the IVF route (for PGD or infertility issues) frequently tell of the psychological stress, economic issues, and marital tensions. Logic might dictate that transferring three or more fertilized eggs significantly raises the chances one will implant. When all or some do, the dilemma to be faced is selective reduction (i.e., reducing the number of growing fetuses) or risk losing all. Choosing to go forward with triplets or quadruplets can invite potential catastrophes that are well-recorded. Premature delivery is an increasing likelihood with multiple births, and very tiny infants are at high risk of serious complications that include brain hemorrhage, strokes, chronic lung disease from ventilators, mental retardation, seizures, blindness, and other problems not related to the genetic disorder parents set out to avoid. Instead, they may end up with lifelong care of a severely handicapped child and later adult.

In addition to the many congenital or early onset, single-gene disorders detectable by PGD, diagnosis of adult-onset genetic disorders (including breast, ovarian, colon, and other cancers) have been performed (*see* Appendix 1). Once a culprit gene for any disease has been identified, PGD, chorionic-villus sampling (CVS), or amniocentesis can be used for diagnosis. Even detection of a mutation causing the hereditary early-onset form of Alzheimer's disease has been accomplished.

Among the more controversial innovations was the original successful approach by one of the pioneers, the late Dr. Yury Verlinsky, in Chicago.

He used PGD to select an HLA-matched embryo for a desperate couple who had a child with a rare fatal genetic disorder (Fanconi anemia). That selected embryo resulted in a successful pregnancy and a healthy child who, as a stem-cell donor, saved his sister's life! Cord blood or bone marrow can be used in these situations for more common disorders, such as the treatment for thalassemia (*see* Chapter 23).

Limitations

Beyond the economic constraints, and the need to seek a center of excellence performing preimplantation genetic analysis, is the recognition of some inherent limitations. Sampling a normal cell and not an abnormal one (because of chromosomal mosaicism) has led to missed diagnoses. Because extremely minute quantities of DNA are available from a single cell, chance contamination by extraneous DNA (from mother's cells or from sperm) can cause and has caused misdiagnosis. The process of analyzing DNA from a single cell requires that the minute amount present is amplified. However, failure to amplify may occur in between 5% and 15% of cases, resulting in an incorrect diagnosis. Although the diagnosis of cystic fibrosis and other disorders have been missed and the gender of the embryo mistaken, many precise diagnoses have been made, including Tay-Sachs disease, muscular dystrophy, and cystic fibrosis. Human error, by transfer of the wrong embryo, has resulted in failed diagnoses, as have some technical errors.[3] And sure enough, unprotected sex in a couple undergoing IVF has resulted in offspring with the disorder they were trying to avoid!

Pregnancies conceived after the rigorous efforts of PGD and IVF are precious indeed. Nevertheless, careful consideration should be given to confirming the normal result by amniocentesis at 16 weeks of pregnancy. Clearly, it is easy to comprehend that the majority of parents in such hard-won pregnancies might resist taking any further risk of fetal loss by having a confirmatory amniocentesis.

Given how frequently chromosome abnormalities occur in the embryo, it would make sense in couples having IVF to routinely check that an abnormal embryo is not transferred into the womb. Some experienced centers claim much improved rates of implantation, pregnancy, and good outcome. However, a

---

3. Use of incorrect and inappropriate probes and primers.

few randomized trials (with some flaws) have not confirmed such claims. The matter remains unsettled.

CHORIONIC VILLUS SAMPLING

Every couple with a significantly increased risk of having a child with a genetic defect and willing to have prenatal diagnosis would opt for the earliest possible stage of pregnancy for the tests to be performed. Indeed, diagnoses of chromosomal and single-gene disorders, although first described by the Chinese in the 1970s, entered the clinical arena in the early 1980s. Genetic diagnosis began to be routinely achievable between 10 and 12 weeks of pregnancy, thereby reducing stress, maintaining privacy, and facilitating termination before pregnancy became obvious. Moreover, maternal bonding with the fetus is much less likely to be a problem in the face of necessary pregnancy termination in the first 3 months of pregnancy, rather than between 16 and 20 weeks following amniocentesis.

Available Procedures

Very early prenatal diagnosis depends on sampling a tiny piece of the placenta, which is then used for chromosome or DNA analysis. The procedure is like amniocentesis, with introduction of a needle into the uterus under ultrasound guidance. A tiny piece of the branch-shaped tissue (chorionic villi) of the placenta in the area of attachment to the uterus is sampled (hence the procedure is called chorionic villus sampling [CVS]). Given good ultrasound visualization, CVS for twins (and even triplets) is also almost invariably successful.

The CVS tissue can be analyzed directly or the cells cultivated and then analyzed for chromosomes and genes. Direct examination for chromosomes, although achievable, is more reliable from cultivated cells. Because it is too early to obtain amniotic fluid safely between 10 and 12 weeks, ultrasound studies to detect spina bifida and similar defects should be done around 16 weeks of pregnancy.

There are very few instances in which CVS tissue cannot be obtained. Perhaps the most common situation is a malposition of the uterus. In such cases, and sometimes even for routine cases, some obstetricians choose to do the CVS procedure via the vagina and cervix. The presence of infection in the vagina adds risk and would need prior treatment.

Accuracy

Analysis of the tissue obtained during CVS for either chromosomes or genes is the same as that from cells cultivated from the amniotic fluid. Admixture of maternal cells is somewhat more likely to occur with CVS and potentially increases the possibility of a diagnostic pitfall. Moreover, because confined placental mosaicism may occur in 1% to 2% of placentas, sampling chromosomally abnormal cells by chance may lead to an erroneous diagnosis.

Risks

Major comparative studies between CVS performed in the 9- to 12-week period compared to amniocentesis between 14 and 20 weeks of pregnancy have mostly not revealed statistically significant differences for fetal loss. Some studies, however, have pointed to an increased fetal loss rate from CVS when compared to amniocentesis, with rates being around 2% compared to 0.5% to 1% for amniocentesis. Complications that could occur are similar to those noted for amniocentesis (*see* below).

In the early 1990s, concern arose about a reported cluster of four children born with limb and lower jaw abnormalities following CVS. Subsequently, major studies of more than 200,000 cases did not reveal a definitive association of such defects with offspring who had undergone the CVS procedure. The one recommendation that did emerge was to avoid CVS too early, suggesting 10 to 11 weeks as optimal.

Amniocentesis

The fetus floats within a cushion of fluid (amniotic fluid). Cells from fetal skin, intestinal and urinary tracts, lungs, as well as from the enveloping sac containing the fetus, are shed into the fluid. Most of these are dead cells, but a few are viable. A needle introduced through the abdomen and through the wall of the uterus into the fluid (a procedure called amniocentesis) allows for the aspiration of about 2 tablespoons of fluid. Cells are removed from this fluid sample, placed in sterile plastic containers, fed with sterile broth, and placed in warm, moist incubators. The modern enriched broth (culture medium) stimulates the growth of those cells that have adhered to the dish or glass cover slip. The cells slowly multiply, and about 7 to 10 days later, there are usually enough cells to analyze.

Amniocentesis is best (and safest) when done between the 15th and 16th menstrual weeks of pregnancy, when there are the largest number of viable cells, the uterus is easily accessible by an abdominal approach, and there is sufficient amniotic fluid to sample.

Procedure Risks

Introduction of a needle into the womb was first used in the early 1880s for the removal of excess fluid. Fetal evaluation by this method began in 1930, but modern prenatal studies as we know them today really began in the mid-1960s. Studies on earlier amniocenteses done between 12 and 14 weeks are more hazardous to the fetus than the indicated 15 to 16 weeks. The main risk is fetal loss. In highly experienced hands, the rate of loss approximates 1 in 1,000, with average rates ranging between 1 in 200 to 1 in 100. Clearly, then, the risk of the condition to be studied should exceed the potential rate of loss. Ultrasound guidance of the needle during amniocentesis is routine and clearly lessens the risks.

Amniocentesis for multiple pregnancy (twins, triplets, or more) is best done by an experienced obstetrician. In good hands, risks of fetal loss in twin pregnancies are about the same as for singletons. The need to consider amniocentesis for multiple pregnancy is not unusual, given that the frequency of nonidentical twins increases with advancing maternal age. The rate of nonidentical twinning is between 7 and 11 per 1,000 births, whereas for identical twins, the rate is 3 to 4 per 1,000 births. The widespread use of hormones to stimulate the production of ova (eggs) has resulted in a significant increase in the frequency of multiple pregnancy. Whereas identical twins are almost invariably affected by the same genetic disorder—although not necessarily equally—nonidentical twins are like siblings, and only one may be affected. It is therefore not rare to find that one nonidentical twin has Down syndrome. The option in such circumstances is continuing the pregnancy or having selective reduction of the affected twin. Removal of the affected nonidentical twin enables successful continuation of the pregnancy in about 95% of cases.

Life-threatening maternal risks are extraordinarily rare. There may have been two or three deaths in the world after millions of amniocenteses. Infection was the likely cause. Minor maternal problems occur in 2% to 3% of women and include transient vaginal bleeding or leakage of amniotic fluid and uterine cramps. Potential fetal risks other than loss include needle puncture and injury, infection, or placental separation, all of which are rare.

Women who have the Rh-negative blood group and who may be carrying an Rh-positive fetus should receive an immunoglobulin injection at the time of amniocentesis to prevent them becoming sensitized, leading to risks for a fetus in future pregnancies.

It is important for women to have a full discussion about their indications for study and the associated risks of amniocentesis prior to any procedure being done. Written consent is usually required.

Diagnostic Accuracy

Prenatal genetic studies rank among the highest in accuracy among laboratory tests.

Biochemical analyses are done on the cell-free amniotic fluid, and the free-floating cells and cultivated cells are used for the study of chromosomes, DNA, and enzymes. Accuracy rates are almost invariably in the 99% to 100% range. Analysis of the noncultivated cells using FISH (*see* Chapter 2) enables diagnosis of the most common serious chromosome anomalies within 24 to 48 hours. Although in good hands these results are accurate in about 99% of cases, confirmation from analysis of the cultivated cells is advised. Nevertheless, care should be taken in the selection of laboratories, with special reference to their experience and their ability to interpret results. Laboratory errors have certainly occurred but fortunately are very infrequent. One potential pitfall is the inadvertent analysis of maternal cells in the provided sample of amniotic fluid. On those very infrequent occasions where this occurs, a second amniocentesis study is recommended.

Ultrasound Imaging

The use of sound waves (sonar) to visualize both the external and internal features of the fetus has represented an enormous advance in fetal medicine. Routine ultrasound studies are not aimed at identifying fine fetal anatomical details. Rather, the focus is on the number of fetuses present; measurements to assess fetal age, size, and growth; and determination of the placental location with the aim of finding a safe spot to introduce the amniocentesis needle. Visualization of fine anatomical details, such as the inner spaces of the brain (ventricles) or the four chambers of the heart, requires high-resolution or targeted ultrasound performed by experienced obstetricians or radiologists. Despite the remarkable advances in fetal imaging, considerable limitations remain.

Although there may be high degrees of certainty excluding a particular defect, most ultrasonographers will stop short of providing absolute guarantees. Reservations are common when reference is made to cardiac defects and brain abnormalities.

Superb technical advances in fetal evaluation by ultrasound include 3-D and even 4-D imaging. Even without that much sophistication, ultrasonography is challenging the blood-screening approach to neural tube defect detection and may well replace it. However, not all ultrasonographers meet the required high standard of excellence. Although laboratory assays are accurate, interpretation of results can be bedeviled by incorrectly estimated weeks of pregnancy (by mother and by ultrasound), particularly when there is poor fetal growth (intra-uterine growth restriction [IUGR]) or a smaller head (which may occur in spina bifida and other genetic syndromes). If a significant fetal abnormality is seen by ultrasound, then serious consideration should be given to immediately doing a DNA micro-array analysis (Chapter 5) and chromosome study on amniotic fluid cells. The aim is to detect an unexpected numerical or structural chromosomal or molecular defect.

DIAGNOSTIC ERRORS

Despite an accuracy rate exceeding 99% for prenatal genetic studies, errors do and have occurred. Fetal sex determination has been incorrect a number of times, mainly because of admixed maternal cells in the amniotic fluid. Errors in biochemical diagnoses have occurred in laboratories that have not performed their biochemical analyses with the required care and rigorous standards. Errors in chromosome analysis, although very infrequent, probably constitute the majority of mistakes. Missed chromosomal mosaicism (*see* Chapter 2) and failure to detect a subtle structural rearrangement are the two most common errors. Given the complexity and the high technical skill required, the high degree of accuracy still achieved is remarkable.

PITFALLS AND PROBLEMS

Aberrant, but Normal

Chromosome analysis of cultivated amniotic fluid cells sometimes turns up one or more cells, derived from a single dish, that have a specific chromosome defect.

As long as no other such cells are found in any other dishes and sufficient numbers of cells are analyzed, this finding is referred to as **pseudo-mosaicism**, to which no clinical importance can be attached. It is likely that the origin of these abnormal cells may be placental or arise spontaneously upon cell division in the culture dish.

An Extra Fragment

About once in every 2,000 amniocentesis studies, an unexplained tiny extra chromosome fragment—technically called a **supernumerary marker**—is found in all or some of the fetal cells. A chromosome fragment may be directly inherited from one parent, who, if normal, provides inferential assurance that the offspring too will be normal. If neither parent possesses the fragment in question, then there is about a 14% risk that after birth there will be associated birth defects or mental retardation. New DNA technology using FISH and micro-arrays (*see* Chapters 2 and 5) now allow the precise identification of the origin of these fragments. Curiously, fragments derived from chromosome 15 occur most often. The clinical implications will depend on the chromosome origin of the fragment, its size, and the constituent genes in the fragment.

Disputed Paternity

From time to time, and much more frequently than many would believe, we are confronted with the **question of paternity**. Through use of DNA techniques and blood samples (or cheek scrapings for cells) from the mother and the child and two (or more) men, we are able to declare the identity of the father, with degrees of certainty usually between 99.9% to 100%. Despite the parental emotional pressures, amniocentesis to determine disputed paternity is inadvisable, the matter being best resolved after birth.

Multiple Pregnancy

As noted earlier, **twins or multiple pregnancies** occur where one may be detected prenatally as having a serious genetic disorder. In cases of nonidentical twins or multiples, selective reduction is possible by causing the cardiac arrest of the affected fetus, which is slowly absorbed, leaving only a tiny sac of tissue by the time delivery occurs. In the vast majority of such cases, the healthy twin has survived to bring joy to the parents.

Culture Failures

The growth of amniotic fluid cells in plastic containers using highly enriched culture medium rarely results in failure of cell growth. On the very unusual occasions where this does occur, a few common reasons are recognized. The sample may be very small (because of difficulty in aspirating sufficient fluid) and may, to boot, be very bloody. Amniotic fluid sent over vast distances may be subject to extreme heat or cold, and the few viable cells present may die. Careless laboratory technique or lack of proper sterile technique when the sample is drawn may result in infectious contamination of the sample, ruining any chance for cell growth. Samples in culture are kept in warm, moist incubators. Electrical failure or some other mechanical failure may cause a serious drop or elevation in temperature within the incubator, and the cells will almost always die. Major laboratories like ours are invariably wired directly to an emergency electrical generator to take care of such eventualities.

Some years ago, we and others discovered that the syringes or tubes into which amniotic fluid was placed contained chemical substances toxic to cells. Thankfully, these episodes have been few and far between and are rarely encountered today.

Diagnosis of the Unexpected

Prenatal studies performed for advanced maternal age or for an abnormal maternal serum screening result constitute the two most common reasons for amniocentesis. Although the search for Down syndrome and neural tube defects occupy central attention, an entirely unexpected defect may be discovered. I vividly recall the case in which we discovered that the fetus was an XYY male with all the implications (including involvement with the police, as discussed in Chapter 3).

Noninvasive Prenatal Diagnosis

It has been known for decades that fetal cells migrate via the placental interface into the mother's bloodstream. Decades of hard work to isolate these relatively few cells to detect fetal chromosome or gene disorders have thus far largely failed. This has mainly been due to the lack of a robust and reliable method to capture and analyze the relatively few circulating cells.[4] As a consequence, much effort has been expended to enrich these cell numbers to facilitate diagnostic studies. Unexpectedly, about a sixfold increase in the number of fetal cells in the maternal circulation was noted when the fetus had a chromosome abnormality such as Down syndrome. While enormous efforts continue to develop methods to efficiently isolate and analyze fetal cells in the maternal circulation, greater technological advances will be necessary before this noninvasive approach can be used for prenatal diagnosis.

Even before the discovery of the double-helical structure of DNA, demonstration of its presence in the bloodstream was achieved more than 60 years ago. Subsequently, significant amounts of cell-free circulating bits of DNA (called nucleic acids) were found in the bloodstream of cancer patients and later in pregnant women. The natural cycle of cells, with a limited lifespan that break down, serve as the origin of the circulating nucleic acids. In pregnancy, in addition to the break-up of fetal cells, there is likely to be a transfer directly of fetal nucleic acids into the maternal circulation.

The sheer volume of maternal circulating nucleic acids swamp the small volume of fetal nucleic acids, making it a serious challenge to achieve prenatal diagnosis.

Notwithstanding these difficulties, a few notable diagnostic successes have been achieved. Moreover, use of fetal RNA (*see* Chapter 5) instead of DNA has opened up additional avenues to recognize fetal-derived nucleic acids that contain a placental stamp of origin.

While major efforts continue to perfect noninvasive prenatal genetics diagnoses, the observation that there is quantitatively more fetal DNA in the circulation when a fetal chromosome abnormality is present opened a new research front. Subsequently, it has become clear that increased amounts of cell-free fetal DNA in the maternal bloodstream may herald the development of preeclamptic toxemia in pregnancy as well as preterm delivery.

It had also been known for years that women who had a pregnancy with a male offspring still had male cells in their bloodstream years later. Such cells have been found as long as 27 years after the last male pregnancy. Moreover, significant numbers of male cells—presumably fetal—have been found both in the blood and tissues of women with the auto-immune disorder scleroderma. Similarly, such cells have also been found in the thyroid glands of women with

---

4. Most studies report between 2 and 40 fetal cells per milliliter of maternal whole blood. New technologically sophisticated methods to analyze both the chromosome status and a single-gene mutation in one embryonic cell are in development and show promise.

auto-immune thyroid disorders. The theory is that some type of fetal graft versus maternal host disease has been caused by the invasion of persisting fetal "foreign" cells.

Thus far, use of cell-free fetal nucleic acids have found clinical use in the determination of fetal gender (for X-linked disorders) and for Rhesus D blood group determination. Much more work will be required to meet the 99% to 100% accuracy rate afforded by the other well-established prenatal diagnostic methods.

The Future Is Now

Analysis of genes now allows detection of mutations that have implications for genetic disorders that may manifest many decades after birth. One example is the uncommon, but serious, dominantly inherited brain–blood vessel disorder called CADASIL.[5] We were first to make a prenatal diagnosis of this disorder[6] in a pregnancy where the father had begun experiencing stroke-like symptoms and signs at age 27 years. Other examples include breast cancer, colon cancer, and degenerative brain diseases such as Huntington's disease. These issues are fully discussed in Chapters 8 and 13. Faced with a family history of one of these disorders and the ability to detect the mutation in your fetus or that of your partner, how and what would you decide? This will become an increasingly more common challenge.

In the foreseeable future—perhaps 10 years or so from now—routine sequencing of the entire fetal genome (already possible) will be available. Current huge costs can be expected to rapidly drop with further technical refinements. Much time, however, will be necessary to assure that interpretation of results is accurate and that there is no confusion between mutation and normal variation. Meanwhile, we are fortunate to have had the enormous technical developments in prenatal diagnosis that now assures parents that they can selectively have unaffected offspring in the face of serious risk.

---

5. Cerebral Autosomal Dominant Arteriopathy with Subcortical Infarcts and Leukoencephalopathy.

6. Milunsky A, Konialis C, Shim SH, Maher TA, Spengos K, Ito M, & Pangalos C. (2005) The prenatal diagnosis of CADASIL. *Prenatal Diagnosis* 25: 1057.

8

WHEN GOOD CELLS GO WRONG

It was hot and humid. The fan of an air conditioner clanged noisily from its poorly fitting perch on the wall adjacent to our table in this small restaurant in Playa Del Carmen. I noticed a bead of sweat chasing another down the worried brow of our dinner companion, Richard. We had met Richard and Susan at a Mayan resort at Mayakoba, Mexico, and were having dinner when the conversation turned to books and publishing. When they discovered that I had only recently published **Your Genetic Destiny**, *I noticed a momentary awkwardness. They knew I was a physician but did not know that I was a clinical geneticist. The reasons for the awkwardness became immediately apparent as the story spilled out.*

Richard's mother's non-identical twin sister had died from breast cancer diagnosed at age 39 years. A first cousin once removed and her daughter who both lived out of state were thought to also have and have had breast cancer, respectively. There were no other forms of cancer in the family (see the family pedigree in Chapter 1).

Susan related that in her 40s she had been diagnosed with colon cancer after a single "lump" was found in her colon following an evaluation for anemia. She was sure no polyps were found. Subsequently, cancer of one fallopian tube (the connecting channel from ovary to the uterus traversed by released eggs on their hopeful way to fertilization) was detected by a CAT scan as a follow-up for her colon cancer. Major surgery to remove both tumors had thus far been successful and she had remained cancer-free for the past 8 years. Susan's father and a paternal uncle had both had colon cancer, diagnosed too late, resulting in an early untimely death of both. Susan's paternal grandmother apparently also died from colon cancer. No other family member had ovarian or any other cancer.

The inevitable questions tumbled out without hesitation. "Am I at any risk of developing cancer?" asked Richard. "Are there DNA tests to determine whether I have a gene mutation that could affect me and even be transmitted to my son or daughter?" Susan wanted to know if it was possible that she had inherited a colon cancer gene from her father and maternal grandmother and whether a DNA test was available to determine if she had inherited a colon cancer gene that could also be transmitted to either her son or daughter.

I recommended that they see a clinical geneticist when they returned home and suggested testing for specific genes. A few months later, I received an e-mail from Richard. They had followed my recommendations, had family members tested, and were astounded by the results.

Richard found that he harbored a mutation in one of the common breast cancer genes (BRCA1), as did his unaffected mother, who was 83 years old and in good health. Her deceased twin sister's son also proved positive for the same mutation that his mother must have had. Moreover, Richard's daughter, Cheryl, inherited his BRCA1 gene mutation. His son declined testing.

Susan was found to have a gene mutation in one of four common hereditary nonpolyposis colon cancer genes. Her sister, who was still in good health, was found to have the same gene mutation. Her brother proved negative. Susan's paternal first cousin, the son of the affected uncle, was also found to have the same mutation and was also in good health.

Richard expressed his appreciation for this chance meeting in Mexico that resulted in the discovery of two mutant genes in the two families. Lifelong surveillance had now been instituted and would also, by making them aware of risks and taking pre-emptive action, certainly save the lives of those with the mutation if a cancer reared its ugly head.

The pattern of inheritance for the *BRCA1* mutation in Richard's family is autosomal dominant. This means that every family member who carries the culprit gene mutation has a 50% likelihood of transmitting it to his or her offspring. The early onset of breast cancer in Richard's maternal aunt at age 39 years invariably points to a genetic form of this malignancy. As a general clinical rule, cancers that are diagnosed prior to age 50 years are regarded as genetic in origin until proved otherwise. Richard's mother, as the non-identical twin, and a carrier of the *BRCA1* mutation, has an 80% to 85% lifetime risk of developing breast cancer.

This risk applies to Richard's daughter and any other female carrier of this mutation. Richard and his male first cousin face less than a 6% risk of developing breast cancer and an estimated 8% risk of developing prostate cancer by age 70 years, which is about threefold higher than the general male population. Cheryl, faced with future high risks of breast or ovarian cancer and after much agonizing, made the extremely difficult decision to have an elective bilateral mastectomy and removal of her ovaries (oophorectomy). The fact that many women have opted for bilateral mastectomy in these circumstances does not in any way diminish the personal anguish. Patients who have shared with me their personal angst describe their feelings of loss of femininity and sexuality with changes in their body image. Analysis of 23 published studies fortunately points to the fact that most women do, in fact, recover with much reduced worries and with few experiencing serious depression.[1] A feeling of regret is uncommon and invariably trumped by the great relief engendered by the dissipation of anxiety caused by the high risk of cancer. In the United States about 1 in 5 BRCA1/2 mutation carriers who have not had cancer opt for prophylactic mastectomies.

There is indeed compelling published evidence to support her decision for surgery at the optimal recommended time between ages 35 and 40 years. The best data point to a reduction of breast cancer risk by about 90% in women with a mutation in either of the two common breast cancer genes (*BRCA1* and *BRCA2*) who chose bilateral mastectomy. This obviously means that continuing lifetime surveillance remains important given the 1% or 2% possibility of breast cancer still developing in residual cells left after mastectomy, either on the chest wall or in the extended breast tissue toward the armpits.

Similarly, an 80% to 96% risk reduction in ovarian cancer is achievable following bilateral oophorectomy. Surgery will remove not only the ovaries but the fallopian tubes as well. Once again, however, a residual risk of 1% to 2% of ovarian cancer in the subjacent tissue remains, even following surgery, and requires lifetime surveillance.

Testing for the *BRCA1* or *BRCA2* mutations in Richard's grandchildren or other children in the family is not recommended at least until their

1. Cochrane Database

late 20s. Fortunately, Richard and Susan's daughter had completed her family. However, their son had not. If he proves positive for the *BRCA1* mutation, he would have a 50% risk of transmitting it to any future offspring. He and his partner would have the choice of preimplantation genetic diagnosis (PGD; *see* Chapter 7). This test involves in vitro fertilization (IVF) with fertilization of a harvested egg and mutation analysis of a single cell when the fertilized egg has reached at least a size of eight cells. Their option then would be to discard the fertilized egg if affected and to implant an unaffected one in his partner's womb. Alternatively, prenatal diagnosis is available at about 11 weeks of a normally established pregnancy via chorionic villus sampling (CVS) or via amniocentesis around 15 weeks of pregnancy (*see* Chapter 7). Discovery of a gene mutation would present the option of pregnancy termination.

It is noteworthy that Richard's mother has never developed cancer despite having the *BRCA1* mutation and is healthy at 83 years of age. This may be a hopeful sign for the family and may result from the type of mutation or from modifying genes, promoting what geneticists call a lack of penetrance.

BREAST AND OVARIAN CANCER

More than 190,000 women are diagnosed with breast cancer each year in the United States, and more than 40,000 succumb each year. Worldwide the figures are in excess of a million diagnosed and more than 500,000 deaths each year. About 90% of all breast cancers are not directly inherited. In 2006, the National Cancer Institute reported that there were more than 2.5 million women alive in the United States with a history of breast cancer. The prevalence of *BRCA1* mutations in the general population approximates 1 in 500 to 1 in 1,000, while the *BRCA2* mutation frequency occurs in about 1 in 1,000. Among those of Ashkenazi Jewish ancestry (Eastern Europe), about 1 in 40 women carry a mutation in one of these two genes. Three mutations (two in *BRCA1* and one in *BRCA2*) account for about 90% of carriers. Among people of Dutch ancestry, three large mutations (described as deletions due to tiny missing bits of DNA within the gene) are well-known. Curiously, and probably as a consequence of a founder effect, a single specific mutation in *BRCA2* has been found in many Icelanders and present in 7.7% of women and 40% of men with breast cancer from Iceland. In fact, original estimates (and diagnoses) may well have missed the now known occurrence of deletions within the BRCA1 and BRCA2 gene mutations.

The incidence of ovarian cancer is highest in Europe, the United States, and Israel and lowest in Japan and developing countries. The average lifetime risk in developed countries approximates 1 in 70. Only 10% to 15% of women with ovarian cancer have a BRCA1 or BRCA2 mutation. Those with a BRCA1 mutation have a 39% to 46% lifetime risk of developing ovarian cancer, whereas the risk in BRCA2 carriers is 12% to 20%. For the majority of women, increased risks are associated with a number of factors, including having had no children, early onset of menses, and late menopause. A reduced risk is associated with a history of oral contraceptive use, pregnancy, and breast feeding.

The BRCA1 and BRCA2 genes are termed tumor suppressors. We all possess these genes and now know that their action is to control cell growth. When there is a mutation in either one of these genes, their function is diminished or lost, and cells grow without control and form a tumor. There are also multiple other genes that operate along the pathways that control cell growth and, when mutated, result in uncontrolled cell growth, called cancer. Fortunately these other genes account for very few breast or ovarian cancers and are not routinely tested.

Even when there is a family history of multiple affected individuals, DNA analysis may not reveal a specific mutation in either BRCA1 or BRCA2. This could be due to a failure of detection by the method used, a mutation in an entirely different gene, or even no direct genetic factors. Although hundreds of mutations have been discovered in both BRCA1 and BRCA2 genes, it is not uncommon for an alteration in one or the other of these genes to be found and be uninterpretable or inconclusive. Determination of whether this alteration is ominous will require testing of other family members. The aim is to discover if the alteration is present or absent in the affected members compared to the unaffected. This step will often, but unfortunately not always, resolve the question of significance.

Women with very dense breasts have a fourfold to fivefold greater risk of breast cancer than women of the same age and BMI whose breast tissues are not dense. Moreover, a variation in a particular gene (called ZNF365) has been recognized to be associated with both breast density and breast cancer risk.

Clearly the family history of breast and/or ovarian cancer and ethnicity are critically important to the assessment of risk. Especially important is a history of breast cancer in a male. Every male with a diagnosis of breast cancer is strongly urged to have a DNA study and if found to be mutation-positive, to recommend that his parents and grandparents and siblings and other family members be tested. Testing the grandparents facilitates discovery of which side the mutation originated, enabling communication and timely diagnostic studies of more distant family members.

The occurrence of breast cancer in one breast and then the contralateral breast, or both at the same time, invariably spells a dominantly inherited form of malignancy. Such an occurrence should immediately alert the family about their risks and the wisdom of seeking genetic counseling.

Surveillance

Current recommendations for early detection of breast cancer in those who carry a BRCA1 or BRCA2 mutation include:

- Monthly breast self-examination beginning in early adulthood
- Annual or semi-annual clinical breast examination beginning at age 25 years
- Annual mammography beginning at age 25 years

For those with mutations in either of these two genes, the National Cancer Center Network has recommended breast MRI, which has been found to have a much higher detection rate than mammography alone. The use of both modalities is likely to achieve a detection rate exceeding 90%.

For men with one of these mutations, monthly self-examination, semi-annual clinical breast examination, and an annual mammogram are recommended, if marked breast development is present.

Women not known to carry a BRCA1 or BRCA2 gene mutation are likely aware of a 2009 controversy about the age at which mammography screening should begin. All experts agree on age 50 years. Well-known is the fact that for women in their 40s, more than 1,900 must be screened for 10 years to prevent a single death from breast cancer. Moreover, there are about 60% more false-positive results and unnecessary biopsies in this age group. Mammograms are imperfect and miss about 10% to 15% of cancers. Women in their 40s should carefully consider their options and decide whether they wish to be more safe than sorry.

Surveillance for ovarian cancer is unfortunately much less effective. Standard recommendations for women with a known mutation include:

- Annual or semi-annual pelvic examination beginning at age 25 years
- Annual or semi-annual transvaginal ultrasound examination at age 35 years

- Annual blood sample for analysis of CA-125 concentration also beginning at age 25 years, and graphically tracking the level year by year to determine the rate of any elevation

A University of California study focused on 1,939 families with 97 males with breast cancer. The authors reported that males who had a *BRCA2* mutation had a 6.8% risk of developing breast cancer, whereas those men with a *BRCA1* mutation had a 1.2% estimated risk of developing breast cancer by the age of 70.

Men with mutations in either *BRCA1* or *BRCA2* should have annual digital rectal examinations and prostate-specific antigen (PSA) testing beginning at age 40 years. At present, screening for pancreatic cancer in individuals with a mutation in *BRCA2* is not effective. Men or women with a mutation in *BRCA2* have a slightly increased risk of developing a skin cancer called melanoma. This malignancy may affect not only skin but also the pigment cells of the eye. Recommendations for surveillance include annual examinations of both the skin and the eyes by specialists.

Avoidance of hormone replacement therapy, even at menopause, is probably a wise step. Certain oral contraceptives are not contra-indicated for women with a mutation in either *BRCA1* or *BRCA2*. Researchers in Seattle have reported a link between migraine headaches and breast cancer. They found a 26% reduction in breast cancer among premenopausal and postmenopausal women who suffered from migraines. The association of female hormones and migraine is well-known. This may eventually explain the observation, but other factors, such as nonsteroidal anti-inflammatory drugs used for treatment, need further study.

Another option for preventing breast cancer in women who have inherited a mutation in *BRCA1* or *BRCA2* is the use of medications such as Tamoxifen or Raloxifene (partial estrogen antagonists). This effect applies only to tumors that are estrogen-sensitive (so-called "estrogen receptor positive"). Various studies have reported a 41% to 62% reduction in the risk of breast cancer in these women. Just as for some other drugs (certain anticoagulants, some anti-depressants), a particular enzyme[2] may break up Tamoxifen too quickly or too slowly (called a fast or slow metabolizer). The result could be insufficient Tamoxifen when processed too fast and excessive amounts that accumulate if processed too slow. A simple genetic test of the enzyme-related gene (*CYP2D6*)

2. The liver enzyme cytochrome P450 2D6.

should help determine the best Tamoxifen dosage. Well-designed clinical trials are still necessary to determine the use of this test. Note, however, that this treatment may cause increased rates of uterine cancer and blood clotting (including pulmonary embolism) that could prove fatal.

BREAST CANCER IN OTHER GENETIC DISORDERS

As mentioned, other genes are involved in causing breast cancer. A number of rare genetic disorders[3] resulting from entirely different genes may convey risks of breast cancer as part of the specific disorder. Almost all are characterized by cancers in multiple different organs.

While the most important risk factor for breast cancer in males is an inherited mutation in *BRCA1* or *BRCA2*, other disorders probably with a disturbance in the body's hormones (especially estrogen) are also associated with breast cancer. A study by the U.S. Veteran's Affairs Team at the National Cancer Institute examined the medical records of some 642 males with breast cancer whose records they culled from more than 4.5 million men between the ages of 18 and 100 years. They noted significant risks with a condition called Klinefelter syndrome (tall men with a female body build, prominent breasts, and small testes who have an extra female [X] chromosome, discussed in Chapter 3), those who were obese, and those who had a history of testicular infection.

The fact that Richard's and Susan's families both harbored serious cancers is startling but not uncommon. The mode of inheritance reflected in Susan's family tree is again consistent with autosomal dominant inheritance. Therefore, Susan's two children have a 50% risk of inheriting her colon cancer mutation (called *MLH1*). This is one of five genes[4] that

---

3. Li-Fraumeni syndrome; ataxia telangiectasia; Cowden syndrome; Bloom syndrome; hereditary diffuse gastric cancer; *CHEK2* gene mutations; Peutz-Jeghers syndrome; Xeroderma Pigmentosum; Werner syndrome.
4. Five genes are currently known to be causally related to HNPCC—namely, *MLH1*, *MSH2*, *MSH6*, *PMS2*, and EPCAM. A major multicenter international comparative genome study of 289 human disease genes found 177 genes with similar DNA sequences (called orthologs) in the fruit fly (*Drosophila melanogaster*) and the tiny worm (*C. elegans*). Orthologs for these four colon cancer and other cancer genes (but not breast cancer) were detected in *Drosophila*.

when mutated may result in hereditary non-polyposis colorectal cancer (HNPCC). Clearly this mutation had been transmitted from Susan's grandmother to her father from whom she had inherited this unwelcome burden.

Susan, in her mid-40s, was at the average age for HNPCC and ovarian (including Fallopian tube) cancer to be discovered. Susan had an 80% lifetime risk of developing colon cancer and a 9% to 12% risk of developing ovarian cancer. Unfortunately, mutations in the HNPCC genes also convey risks for other cancers. Susan's risk of developing cancer in the uterus in her lifetime ranges between 20% and 60%; in the stomach, between 11% and 19%; and single digit risks for her urinary tract, small bowel, bile duct, brain, and nervous system.

Susan had the recommended surgery, which entailed total removal of the colon (colectomy) with connection of the small bowel to the remaining portion of the rectum (ileorectal anastomosis). Resection of only a segment or part of the colon is not recommended because of the high likelihood of cancers developing again in any remaining colon. Susan also underwent surgery to remove both the uterus and ovaries, a step others would consider as a preventive maneuver, especially after childbearing has been completed. Obviously, lifetime surveillance, even after all this radical surgery, is recommended given the smaller risks of other cancers as noted above. Because early detection of these other cancers is difficult, individuals at risk should pay close attention to their health and not delay indicated consultations. Incidentally, smoking increases the risk of colorectal cancer in individuals who have inherited a HNPCC gene mutation.

It should already be obvious from the earlier discussion that testing of Susan's children, her siblings, and other family members on her father's side of the family is necessary for this specific mutation Susan inherited. Although testing of children for primarily late-onset genetic disorders is not recommended, HNPCC has been diagnosed at surprisingly young ages, and hence screening or testing should be considered even before the age of 18 years.

COLON CANCER

In the United States in 2009 there was an estimated 147,000 new cases of colon cancer and nearly 50,000 deaths. Although the lifetime population risk for developing colorectal cancer is about 1 in 19 (5.4%), less than 5% result from the inheritance of a single mutated gene. HNPCC (also known as Lynch syndrome in honor of Dr. Henry Lynch) accounts for about 3% of all colorectal cancers.

Individuals with HNPCC may have a single lump or just a few polyps in the colon. Their lifetime risk is 70% to 80% for developing this cancer. This cancer is almost always inherited from one parent, and only rarely is there a new mutation accounting for this disease. Among those of Ashkenazi Jewish ancestry and with a family history of colon cancer, one particular mutation (A636P) is found in the *MSH2* gene in 7% diagnosed at 40 years or earlier.

If you inherited a mutation in one of the HNPCC genes, a schedule of annual colonoscopies is recommended, beginning between the ages of 20 and 25 years, or 10 years before the earliest age of diagnosis in an affected family member. Knowing that you have one of these gene mutations enables you to set up a colonoscopy schedule for a procedure that is likely to save your life. Moreover, close attention to your health with reference to the small but definite increased potential for developing cancer in the other organs is also important.

It is critically important, once a mutation has been identified, for that person to contact and inform siblings, parents, and (where appropriate) adult children of the need to seek a medical consultation and DNA testing. Just imagine if you developed colon cancer and a relative failed to let you know to be tested and treated in time; how you would feel? Sadly, I have repeatedly seen many families with various serious genetic disorders who, despite advice, have not contacted family members only to learn later about a family loss. Unfortunately, the family dynamics I have witnessed indicate how common it is for members to lose contact or, worse, not to be talking to each other—especially when a serious genetic issue arises.

These necessary communications may not be easy. Issues beyond estranged and alienated families complicate the needed transfer of information. The affected individual may not fully understand the complex information received (sometimes poorly communicated by a professional). The personal stress may be paralyzing, leading to inaction. Guilt about having passed on the disease mutation may dominate. Survivor-like guilt may be felt after testing negative, but communication is still necessary. A strong disinclination, perhaps tinctured by previous family stress, to be the bearer of "bad" news may interfere with necessary contact. Waiting for the "right time" may be another reason to postpone intrafamilial communication.

Regardless of the personal, psychological, familial, or other obstacles, those who harbor a potentially life-threatening mutation must communicate with family members at risk. This is a moral imperative. Physicians, clinical geneticists, and genetic counselors also have the duty to warn and instruct at-risk vulnerable family members. Successful litigation has found physicians negligent in not having communicated high risks of colon[5] and medullary thyroid[6] cancers to family members.

Prenatal diagnosis or preimplantation genetic diagnosis (*see* Chapter 7) for a mutation in one of the HNPCC genes remains rare for this highly treatable disorder. Nevertheless, these avenues remain open to couples still in their childbearing years and knowledgeable about their 50% risks of transmission to offspring. One mother expressed the view to me that she would rather avoid having a child with this mutation. Since she was 32 years old and single, who, she asked,would care for her child if she succumbed to one of these cancers?

In the event DNA testing does not reveal a mutation in one of the HNPCC genes in an individual with colon cancer **and** a family history, further consultation with a clinical geneticist is recommended, given that there are some other rarer genetic disorders in which colon cancer can occur.[7]

Eric remembered the day clearly. He had been sitting in the biology and molecular genetics honors class during the last semester prior to graduating with a Bachelor of Science degree. The lecture was discussing single-gene inheritance when Eric's mind wandered as he began to think of his extended family. His mother, who had developed colon cancer, was diagnosed at the age of 35 years. She had died within a year of the diagnosis, the cancer having spread by the time she had surgery. His maternal grandfather had died in his 40s from an "abdominal tumor." Apparently, real details were not available. Recently, he had learned that one of his first cousins, still in his 20s, had his entire colon surgically removed.

---

5. Safer v. Estate of Pack (1996).
6. Pate v. Threlkel (1995).
7. Familial adenomatous polyposis; juvenile polyposis syndrome; Peutz-Jeghers syndrome; PTEN hamartomatous syndromes; breast/ovarian cancer; hereditary diffuse gastric cancer.

Overwhelmed by the anxious realization of the potential importance of his family history, he left the class and immediately called his father. It took 10 days to get an appointment for a colonoscopy. During this time of waiting, he contacted his cousin who lived on the West Coast. He learned that the colectomy had been done when colonoscopy had revealed the presence of thousands of polyps throughout his cousin's colon. No DNA studies were available at the time.

Eric's colonoscopy revealed an entirely normal colon, relieving him of the persistent anxiety that had enveloped his every living moment while waiting for his colonoscopy. His sister, however, only 2 years younger, was less fortunate. Colonoscopy revealed many polyps. Subsequent DNA studies of the gene (called APC) for the condition termed familial adenomatous polyposis (FAP) revealed a mutation. Other family members of Eric's maternal side of the family were informed, many were tested, and some were found to harbor the culprit mutation. Eric's sister also had the recommended total colectomy.

Eric's sudden recognition of the importance of his family history, while sitting in a biology class, saved his sister's life. The period between the teens and the late 20s, which some regard as the period of infallibility, is only infrequently attended by awareness of the genetic importance of the family history. Despite the considerable educational level of Eric's own and extended family, no member had been referred for genetic counseling. They would have learned that anyone with this dominantly inherited disorder had a 50% risk of transmitting it to each of their children. Also, routine mutation analysis of the *APC* gene would relieve at least 50% of any further anxieties about FAP, while the others could save their lives and secure their health by elective colectomy.

When Eric's sister came for genetic counseling, she learned that close attention to her physical health would be necessary throughout her lifetime. While occasional polyps may occur in the stomach, the risk for them developing cancer in the duodenum (the portion of the small bowel connected to the stomach) ranges between 4% and 12% in a life-time, a far cry from the virtually 100% risk of cancer if she had not had her colon removed. The need to remain watchful is also underscored by the small (usually 1%–2%) risk of cancers occurring in other organs.[8]

For safety's sake, visual examination (endoscopy) is recommended every 2 to 3 years, even after colectomy. Visualization of the duodenum is also wise every 1 to 3 years.

COLON POLYPS AND CANCER

Thankfully, FAP is relatively rare, occurring in about 1 in 31,000 to 1 in 35,000 individuals. Although on average a diagnosis of FAP is made around age 39 years, polyps have been found as early as age 7 years. In some cases, there may only be a few dozen polyps (usually called attenuated FAP). Also, in some families, syndromic names have been given when FAP has been associated with certain typical other findings such as benign lumps in bones or brain tumors.[9]

Curiously, when the retina (the back of the eye) is examined in FAP, flat pigmented spots are often seen[10] and fortunately cause no problems. However, I have seen patients with this finding in both eyes that immediately alerted the need to test both the patient and the family for FAP. In other words, this concurrent eye finding serves to alert the physician to check for FAP. Remarkably, in about 17% of those with FAP, unerupted teeth, absence of one or more teeth, extra teeth, or dental cysts may occur.

A founder effect is probably the explanation for the observation that about 6% of individuals of Ashkenazi Jewish ancestry carry a particular mutation[11] in the *APC* gene.

When dozens of polyps are found and no mutation in the *APC* gene is discovered, consideration is given to a recessively inherited type of multiple polyp disorder caused by a different gene (*MYH*). In such cases, the mutation has

---

8. Pancreas, thyroid, brain, liver, and bile ducts. Benign fibrous tumors that may occur in the abdomen or elsewhere may cause a nuisance or an aggravation in about 5% of those with FAP.
9. called Gardner and Turcot syndromes, respectively.
10. called hypertrophy of the retinal pigment epithelium.
11. I1307K.

been transmitted from both parents with a one in four risk that each child inherited a copy from each parent and would be affected. This is an even rarer disorder than FAP.[12]

In couples planning childbearing in whom a mutation has been defined, prenatal diagnosis or preimplantation genetic diagnosis remains an option (*see* Chapter 7).

Esmeralda rushed home to telephone her husband and her father in the Philippines. Esmeralda and her husband, Hilario, had been trying to conceive for 2 years, and she had just had an ultrasound study that showed she was carrying twins. Her husband, who was of Hawaiian ancestry, could also hardly contain his excitement.

Pregnancy continued uneventfully and delivery by Cesarean section was electively done because of the fetal positions in the womb at term. Two beautiful babies emerged, a boy and a girl. Hilario's parents, who lived nearby, joined the celebrations, as did Esmeralda's father. Her mother had died of some type of cancer when Esmeralda was still a toddler.

The twins developed well, gained weight, and provided enormous joy to the parents. At the 6-week check-up, the family doctor noticed that the female twin, Juan, had "crossed-eyes" (strabismus). The same observation was recorded in the doctor's notes at 3 months and again at 6 months. Shortly thereafter, and upon recommendation by their family doctor, they sought a consultation with an eye specialist to consider if and when surgical correction of the one eye was appropriate. To their horror, at the back of the crossed eye, a small whitish tumor was found (called a retinoblastoma.)

This malignant tumor required immediate treatment, and chemotherapy and radiation therapy followed. The treatment was successful, and her sight in that eye was preserved.

Prolonged and difficult communications with health-care providers in the Philippines eventually revealed that Esmeralda's mother had suffered some type of cancer that had spread to her brain. DNA testing of the retinoblastoma gene (RBl) revealed a mutation in the affected twin but not in her co-twin, mother, or father.

---

12. A rare condition caused by a deletion in the long arm of chromosome 5 is associated with colonic polyps, intellectual impairment, and unusual facial features.

Unexplained strabismus at age 3 months is an indication for a referral to an ophthalmologist. The family doctor discussed the subject but failed to actually refer the twin for a consultation. Strabismus is the second most common sign indicating a retinoblastoma, the first and most common one being a white appearance behind the pupil. Fortunately, treatment was successful, but continued surveillance would be necessary for many years with special reference to examination of the unaffected eye. Moreover, a significantly higher lifetime risk exists for developing a later onset cancer, more particularly of bone and soft tissues (sarcoma), leukemia, lymphoma, or even melanomas, especially among those who have received radiation therapy.

In the fullness of time, this twin has a 50% risk of transmitting the retinoblastoma gene mutation to each of her children. Prenatal diagnosis or preimplantation genetic diagnosis would of course be available given the known gene mutation.

RETINOBLASTOMA

This eye tumor occurs in 1 in 15,000 to 1 in 20,000 live births and may be evident shortly after birth, indicating initial growth during fetal development. About 60% of those affected have involvement of only one eye. When a mutation is found in the retinoblastoma gene on one chromosome (13), we now know that an alteration also is present in the gene on the other chromosome 13 in the cells that initiate the tumor. In about 5% of children with unilateral or bilateral eye tumors, a tiny deletion or structural rearrangement is found in the long arm of chromosome 13. In such cases where neighboring genes may be deleted, other associated consequences include possible mental retardation and other birth defects. These may include microcephaly (small head), genital, urinary tract, ear, and other anomalies.

Once again, similar to breast cancer, bilateral involvement invariably spells a genetic origin and immediately implies the need for family testing. Babies born with a 50% risk of developing retinoblastoma (having one affected parent) need to have their eyes examined soon after birth under light anesthesia and then monthly for a year and then quarterly for 3 years, even under anesthesia when necessary. Early diagnosis has at least a 90% chance of saving life and sight.

As a result of the genetic defect or the consequences of chemotherapy or radiation therapy, there is a three- to sixfold overall increased risk of other malignancies. Clearly, added lifelong surveillance of already handicapped children and adults is necessary.

OTHER CANCERS

Invasive cancers can occur in any organ or tissue. Thankfully, most are uncommon or rare and the vast majority not inherited directly. Nevertheless, the cell chemistry in normal and tumor cells is almost totally dependent on gene action or inaction.

Genes and their products restrict and control cell growth. Such genes (called tumor suppressors), when mutated, result in uncontrolled cell growth called cancer. Not unexpectedly, these control genes exerting their influence from the earliest stages of embryo development, if mutated, can also be involved in the creation of birth defects.

Indeed, there is an association between birth defects and the subsequent development of certain cancers. In a Canadian study, some 90,400 children with and without birth defects were followed for 18 years. The risk of developing cancer during the first year of life was almost sixfold higher in children with birth defects. The risk was specifically higher for developing leukemia, tumors of the nervous system (central and sympathetic), and soft tissue tumors (sarcomas). Children with Down syndrome carry an almost 20-fold increased risk of leukemia but have a much lower than normal rate of developing solid tumors. This may be due to a gene on chromosome 21 (of which there are three in Down syndrome; *see* Chapter 2) that functions to "starve" potential or developing tumors of their blood supply. Children without birth defects but born with certain genetic disorders due to mutated genes may also be at risk for developing childhood malignancies.[13]

There are a number of genetic disorders in which tumors may occur in association with learning disorders and mental retardation[14] These conditions frequently involve brain, heart, face, and skin. Remarkably, the gene *PTEN*, when

---

13. Including leukemia, lymphomas, brain tumors, neuroblastoma, Wilm's tumor, hepatoblastoma, rhabdomyosarcoma, Ewing sarcoma, and retinoblastoma.
14. Including Costello syndrome, cardio-facio-cutaneous syndrome, neurofibromatosis type 1, tuberous sclerosis, and others.

mutated, is known to cause certain intestinal and other cancers and separately has been found in association with autism and macrocephaly (large head).

Parents with certain genetic disorders with a propensity of developing cancer (such as familial adenomatous polyposis), and whose children have a high (≥50%) risk of developing cancer, sometimes request testing of a very young child. Worried and upset and enormously anxious and sad themselves, they face a mix of emotions that include anger, denial, blame, and guilt. In trying to exert some control, parents may insist on the child or children being tested to see if they have inherited the culprit gene mutation. The guideline we most follow is to test children only if there is clearly recognizable benefit to the child and some important intervention/surveillance (such as colonoscopy) can be initiated. This is usually not the case, with the exception of rarer instances of risk such as thyroid cancer, where immediate testing (even before age 1 year) is performed since surgical removal of the thyroid gland, even in a toddler, would be recommended. A clash between the parents' wishes and the guidelines to do no harm may occasionally generate powerful but not helpful disagreements. Sophisticated and experienced clinical geneticists and counselors are often needed in these extremely difficult circumstances.

Severe chronic stress as a proximate cause of cancer is supported by some epidemiological evidence. In the Dutch Famine of 1944 during World War II, survivors whose food rations were reduced by 70% were later found to have a statistically significant increase in breast cancer rates. Holocaust survivors, compared with European émigrés before and during the war, reportedly have an increased rate of breast and colon cancer. Moreover, in the Israeli study[15] of 300,000 in these two cohorts, the risk of all-site cancer was especially increased in those who suffered at a younger age. The known anticancer effects of calorie restriction appear to have been overwhelmed by the extreme stress.

There are many different types of cancer. After heart disease, cancer is the next most lethal disease in the United States with more than 560,000 deaths annually. There are about 1.5 million new cancer cases each year, and about 1 in 5 will succumb from this scourge in a lifetime. My aim here is to focus on a few well-known examples with some clear life-saving messages. A short discussion on the genetic aspects of three common cancers serves to illustrate additional important advice and useful insights to prevention.

---

15. Kernan-Boker L and colleagues. (2009) Cancer incidence in Israeli Jewish survivors of World War ll. *Journal of the National Cancer Institute*. 101: 1489.

Melanoma

Malignant melanoma is a skin cancer responsible for the vast majority of deaths from all types of skin cancer. Melanoma is the fifth most common cancer among men and the sixth among women in the United States. The frequency of melanoma has risen dramatically over the past 80 years—especially in the United States, the United Kingdom, Australia, and New Zealand. The increase has been attributed largely to escalating sun exposure, particularly in white-skinned individuals. People with red hair and fair skin and freckles, as well as people with multiple moles, have significantly increased risks for developing melanoma (and skin cancer in general). Note, however, that wherever the pigment cell is (melanocyte) that makes melanin, melanoma may occur (e.g., the eyes, the intestine).

A significant family history of melanoma has been reported in up to 7% of cases. One important report estimated the risk of melanoma rising to 6.9% by age 80 years in male first-degree relatives (parents, siblings, and children) and 6.1 % in females, and 10.8% and 9.5% in males and females, respectively, for relatives of cases diagnosed before age 50 years.

Two well-known genes[16] that control cell growth (called tumor-suppressor genes) when possessed of a mutation account for less than 5% of cases of melanoma. In such families, dominant inheritance leads to a 50% risk of transmission. There is both evidence and likelihood that additional genes still to be identified also contribute to tumor susceptibility. Mutations in either of these two genes are found in at least 40% of families with three or more affected members. Melanoma may also occur in families in whom retinoblastoma has occurred, in male carriers of a mutation in the breast cancer gene (*BRCA2*), and in association with other cancers or genetic disorders.[17] Appendix 1 lists family cancer syndromes for which preimplantation genetic diagnosis has been done. In some families with melanoma, there is also an increased frequency of pancreatic cancer.

After little change in the treatment approach to melanoma over the past 30 years, in 2010 there was a paradigm shift to genetically based therapy. At least 60% of those with melanoma have gene mutations in their tumor(s) that encode a cancer-promoting mutated protein called B-RAF. The Plexxikon biotechnology company developed a drug (called PLX4032) that selectively

---

16. CDKN2A and CDK4.
17. Pancreatic cancer, Xeroderma pigmentosum, Werner syndrome, and neurofibromatosis.

blocked the mutated B-RAF protein. Early results have been promising, if not startling, in that tumors disappeared entirely in two patients and shrank by 30% in 24 of 32 others. A large trial of treatment involving 700 patients is ongoing. There is much room for hope given the experience with this approach. Successful examples include blocking mutated proteins in breast cancer with Herceptin, in chronic myeloid leukemia with Gleevec, and non-small-cell lung cancer with Tarceva.

Once again, you should know your family history. For the most part, mutation analysis in non-familial cases is not routinely recommended, since careful surveillance would be the key preventive step to be taken together with avoidance of sun exposure, especially of the intermittent type (sunny holidays). Skin cover and protective lotions (between 30 and 50 sun protective factor) are additional important steps.

Pancreatic Cancer

The American Cancer Society estimated that more than 43,000 Americans were diagnosed with pancreatic cancer in 2010. The high mortality associated with this cancer is due to the silent nature of the disease process that results in signs of the disease (abdominal pain, weight loss, and jaundice) only late. Endoscopic ultrasound remains the single best diagnostic tool at this time.

The first report of pancreatic cancer occurring in a family was described in 1973, in which four of six siblings were affected. Since then, many more families have been reported, but fortunately a genetic basis only occurs in 5% to 10% of affected individuals. Clearly, environmental factors such as smoking play an important role in the genesis of pancreatic cancer. There are susceptibility genes for pancreatic cancer, already discovered in the Japanese, which may act in concert with environmental carcinogens, such as smoking. Obesity, too, is associated with an increased risk of pancreatic cancer and a poorer prognosis. Those with blood group O seem to have a lower risk of pancreatic cancer than people with groups A or B.

There are a number of cancer-associated genetic syndromes in which pancreatic cancer may also occur. In the hereditary breast and ovarian cancer syndrome caused by mutations in the *BRCA1* and *BRCA2* genes discussed earlier, pancreatic cancer may occur especially, but not only, from mutations in the BRCA2 gene. The probability of a mutation in *BRCA2* increases to between 6%

and 12% in patients with pancreatic cancer who have a first-degree relative (e.g., sons, daughters, or siblings of an affected individual). Among 145 Ashkenazi Jewish individuals, with pancreatic cancer, 1 of 3 founder mutations[18] in the BRCA1/2 genes were determined in 5.5% in a major study. There is an approximate 7% lifetime risk of developing pancreatic cancer for Ashkenazi Jews with this mutation. Thus far, in general, the most common known genetic mutations associated with pancreatic cancer occur in the *BRCA2* genes. Very significant risks of developing pancreatic cancer exist in individuals who have familial atypical multiple mole melanoma. In certain intestinal polyposis syndromes (such as familial adenomatous polyposis and the disorder called Peutz-Jeghers syndrome[19], pancreatic cancer is a significant risk. This is also the case for the hereditary non-polyposis colon cancer syndrome. The rare hereditary type of pancreatitis (an inflammatory disorder of the pancreas) is also associated with a much greater risk of pancreatic cancer.

Prostate Cancer

Internationally, prostate cancer is the second most common cancer diagnosed among men (lung cancer is first) and is the sixth most common cause of cancer death among men. In North America, the most common cancer in men is of the prostate.

Major studies have found that between 13% and 15% of those with prostate cancer had an affected first-degree relative (father or brother). The greater the number of affected relatives, the higher the risk of developing prostate cancer. This was especially the case when prostate cancer occurred early, such as prior to age 55 years. About 2% of men with early onset prostate cancer have been found with a mutation in the breast/ovarian cancer *BRCA2* gene.

African-American men have the highest reported frequency of prostate cancer in the United States; significantly lower rates are found among Asian-Americans, Pacific Islanders, and Alaskan natives, as well as Hispanic men.

For the most part, there seem to be at least a dozen or more susceptibility genes that increase the risk of prostate cancer, possibly in combination with environmental factors such as excess fat in the diet.

---

18. Specifically 6174delT in BRCA2; 185 delAG and 5382 ins C in BRCA1.
19. This dominantly inherited disease with polyps in the intestine is recognized by pigmented spots on the lips and in the mouth. Besides pancreatic cancer, cancers of the uterus, lung, and breast may occur.

Besides breast/ovarian cancer families, prostate cancer may also occur in association with other cancer genetic syndromes, including hereditary non-polyposis colon cancer and familial adenomatous polyposis.

Surveillance is especially important for individuals with a family history. Annual digital rectal examinations and biopsies (when necessary) are important. The frequently used prostate-specific antigen blood test is still used but has fallen into disrepute in recent years; however, it can still be helpful.

Remarkable genetic technological advances (such as next generation gene sequencing) have accelerated the pace of discovery in cancer genomics. Hundreds of genes within tumors are now analyzable and compared with similar tumors in others and with the body's normal gene complement. Understanding the pathways of mutated gene dysfunction will follow and open avenues to rational treatments, sparing individuals of invasive and painful treatments instead of just about destroying a person while trying to demolish a tumor. There is now good reason for a hopeful future.

MATTERS OF THE HEART

It had been a scorcher, with temperatures hovering around 95°F and humidity to match. The whole family had decided to picnic at a beautiful lake an hour's drive away from home. The six grown children, some with children of their own, and their parents all met at the lake and had been enjoying a spectacular but hot day at the lake beach. About two o'clock in the afternoon, the mother and her two bachelor sons decided to have a swim in the surprisingly cold lake water. All were good swimmers as they set out to cross the narrow expanse of the lake where they had camped.

When the boys (who raced to reach the opposite shore) turned around, they suddenly realized that their mother was nowhere to be seen. A frantic search aided by the lifeguard on duty was fruitless. Only after police divers had arrived did they recover the mother's body from a deep section of the lake.[1] The grief-stricken family returned home, distraught and bewildered by this tragedy that had befallen them all. The mandated autopsy revealed no discernable cause of death.

Two years later, Maryanne, one of the daughters, went to the local library and was in the process of checking out a book when she suddenly had a cardiac arrest at the desk. The librarian vaulted over the desk and immediately began CPR and successfully resuscitated Maryanne while a colleague called for an ambulance. In one of those twists of fate, it turned out that the librarian had previously been an emergency medicine technician and was an expert at resuscitation.

---

1. Francesco A. Pia Ph.D. decades ago noted that drowning is mostly silent, without splashing, yelling, waving, or calls for help. He named this the Instinctive Drowning Response used by people to avoid actual or perceived suffocation in the water.

During transport to the hospital, the EMTs had connected an electrocardiogram that was electronically linked to the hospital. A characteristic pattern showing an increased interval between the Q and T waves was observed while in transit. However, on entry to the hospital, that particular diagnostic pattern was no longer evident, the electrocardiogram reflecting a normal tracing.

The next day, Maryanne felt well. After her overnight electronic monitoring had revealed perfectly normal heart rhythm and an echocardiogram had also indicated an entirely normal heart structure, she was discharged, having been in hospital barely 24 hours.

Five years later, Maryanne received an urgent call from the middle school that her daughter Adelle attended. Adelle had apparently fainted but had recovered spontaneously. The worried Maryanne nevertheless took Adelle to her pediatrician, who could find no physical reason to explain Adelle's fainting episode. He did, however, know about the cardiac arrest Maryanne had suffered years before, and this alert physician then sat Maryanne down to take a detailed family history. He learned that a niece had also had a few fainting episodes in school for which a cause had never been established. He also learned of Maryanne's mother's drowning and the subsequent sudden death of one of Maryanne's uncles as well as the sudden death of her maternal grandfather that had been ascribed to a heart attack. Subsequently, Maryanne also discovered that her living grand-uncle had for many years an implanted cardiac defibrillator (ICD) that her late mother knew about.

The newly minted pediatrician immediately considered the condition called the Long QT syndrome and was aware of DNA analysis that could potentially make a definitive diagnosis. He obtained blood samples, and some 6 weeks later, the molecular results showed that Maryanne and Adelle both had the identical mutation in the first Long QT syndrome gene (LQTI). Both Adelle and Maryanne were placed on beta-blocker medication and referred to a cardiologist. Later, we tested all Maryanne's siblings, nieces, nephews, maternal aunts, uncles, and cousins for this one specific mutation. Four of the nine tested (three adults and one child) were found to harbor the culprit mutation. A beta-blocker was prescribed for the child, at least for the next few years, and two of the three adults elected to have an ICD. Maryanne subsequently experienced a profound heart rhythm disturbance, which would have proved fatal had she not had an ICD.

Once again, the importance of the family history was not recognized and resulted in a catastrophe. Maryanne's mother was of course aware of her brother's sudden death and that of her own father. Apparently she had also been told about her uncle's ICD. With the exception of the latter information, Maryanne and her five siblings were fully aware of the sudden deaths in the family. Even after their mother drowned, none of the college-educated siblings considered the family history as representing a potential genetic condition, and none sought genetic evaluation or counseling. In a way, it was fortuitous that Adelle fainted in school as it resulted in the discovery of the Long QT syndrome gene mutation segregating in the family. An unexplained fainting episode should prompt an immediate consultation with a cardiologist, and at least an electrocardiogram. That event led to multiple family members' lives being saved, thanks to the well-informed pediatrician.

Obviously in retrospect, Maryanne's mother suffered a fatal heart rhythm disturbance (probably a ventricular arrhythmia) caused by her Long QT syndrome.[2] The arrhythmia was almost certainly precipitated by swimming in cold water—a typical and well-known trigger in this condition. Other well-known triggers that may set off a profound if not fatal cardiac arrhythmia include physical exertion, emotional stress, and, hard to believe, the sudden ring of a telephone or alarm clock.

An arrhythmia during sleep is not uncommon. Fainting is a typical presentation in the Long QT syndrome and reflects a sudden but transient arrhythmia that may even be punctuated by a brief seizure. Unfortunately, in about 10% to 20% of cases, sudden death is the first and only indication of the syndrome.

The tell-tale widening of the interval between the Q and T waves on the electrocardiogram frequently, but not always, helps clinch the diagnosis clinically. However, the electrocardiogram may be normal or, as occurred with Maryanne, may be transiently abnormal and then revert to normal. The gold standard for making a diagnosis is DNA mutation analysis of one of the associated genes.

This is a dominantly inherited disorder with an affected individual having a 50% risk of transmitting the condition to each of his or her

---

2. Also called the Romano-Ward syndrome

children. We reported on 8 infants with the Long QT syndrome ages 1 day to 1 year. Prenatal diagnosis and preimplantation diagnosis is achievable.

There is a rarer recessive form of the Long QT syndrome in which the child is born deaf. A mutation in a Long QT syndrome gene in this form is inherited equally from both parents who have a 25% risk in each pregnancy of having a child with this disorder. There are also those with a variation in a Long QT syndrome gene in whom a drug-induced arrhythmia may occur. Examples of drugs that prolong the Q-T interval and hence predispose to an arrhythmia in an individual at risk include certain antibiotics, antihistamines, anti-arrhythmic drugs, antipsychotics, and antidepressants.

THE LONG QT SYNDROME

This is not a rare condition, probably affecting about 1 in 3,000 individuals. Mutations thus far have been discovered in at least 12 different genes, all of which exert control on the movement of ions (such as sodium, potassium, calcium) as they move through channels between and through heart muscle cells.[3] Faulty gene action is the result of a mutation that interferes with the electrical impulses controlling heart rhythm and contraction, leading to a chaotic arrhythmia, which, if not treated immediately, may cause sudden death.

Most families exhibit a serious disinclination to agree to (or request) an autopsy on a loved one. This is unfortunate because a precise diagnosis with family implications of risks is not infrequently missed. If permission for autopsy is withheld, and sudden death has occurred in a young to middle-aged family member, I would urge that a sample of liver be obtained (by needle or tiny incision) for subsequent DNA studies if needed. The tissue should be frozen immediately in a sterile plastic tube without any preservative. Remember, the lives of other family members are at stake.

Although the mainstay of treatment is beta-blockers, for some Long QT types they do not work. Moreover, they provide no guarantees, whereas ICDs provide a much greater sense of security. Unfortunately, as with all treatments, there may be certain complications. In the process of implanting the ICD lead, there is a small risk of perforating the lung, a major blood vessel, or even the heart. Infection is possible and extraction of the lead could tear vital tissues.

---

3. The Long QT syndrome is just one of the hereditary so-called "channelopathies."

In young active individuals especially, an inappropriate, unexpected shock from the generator in the chest may occur. ICD devices may malfunction or even fail. The frequency of all complications and risks combined ranges between 7% and 13%, figures that are otherwise dwarfed by the high lifetime risk of death without treatment or an ICD. Moreover, given the risk that the lead may break, all contact sports should be avoided. Affected individuals are therefore advised to seek consultations with experienced cardiologists.

The recent demonstration of a permanent ICD placed directly under the skin of the chest alongside the sternum (breast bone) holds much promise. This development is expected to lead to much fewer complications, a hope that is still to be confirmed in larger clinical trials.

As always, relatives should be informed and advised to have genetic counseling and testing if a family member has a diagnosis of the Long QT syndrome. Affected individuals should also be advised to avoid competitive sports or heavy exertion and emotional stress (such as amusement park rides or scary movies). It is important to remember that most affected people live entirely normal lifestyles.

Rarer than the Long QT syndrome is the Short QT syndrome, which also predisposes to potentially fatal abnormalities of heart rhythm. Both Long and Short QT syndromes are dominantly inherited and transmitted. Episodes of sustained palpitations, fainting, a family history of premature sudden death, and rhythm disturbances—especially from the lower chambers of the heart (ventricles)—point to a possible diagnosis of this Short QT syndrome. Similar gene mutations to Long QT syndrome are determinable by DNA mutation analysis. Beyond the sheer structural anatomy of the nerves and muscles of and to the heart is the physiological mechanism that conveys the "electrical" impulses that make our hearts beat for a lifetime. The "current" that flows from tiny "power stations" (nodes) within the heart and from the brain is generated via channels traversed by sodium, potassium, and calcium ions. The products of multiple genes control both structure and function. A mutation in any key gene may interfere with the "electrical" transmission of impulses, resulting in serious or fatal heart rhythm disorders.

In addition to the Long and Short QT syndromes, other rarer disorders with known gene mutations are recognized[4] that may also cause serious to

---

4. These include Brugada syndrome, catecholaminergic polymorphic ventricular tachycardia, sick sinus node syndrome, atrial fibrillation, and dilated cardiomyopathy.

fatal arrhythmias. Sudden cardiac arrest (annually more than 400,000 in the United States and more than 50,000 in Canada) occurs most commonly because of coronary heart disease. Sudden death in a relative not known to have heart disease should make next of kin request an autopsy for their own sakes. In 10% to 20% of all sudden cardiac deaths, no structural abnormality is found. Failure to find an obvious cause should promptly lead to an appointment with a cardiologist. This is the action that saves lives!

As noted earlier, various drugs can lead to an acquired Long QT syndrome in genetically susceptible individuals. One 71-year-old Canadian woman had a cardiac arrest necessitating resuscitation and cardioversion with a defibrillator. She had a history of prolonged constipation and resorted to consuming large amounts of licorice for its laxative effects. This led to a dramatic fall in her potassium levels and the cardiac arrest!

You have to be careful what you eat, if you want not to miss a beat!

Jim Fixx, the athlete who is credited with initiating the worldwide jogging craze in the early 1970s, collapsed and died of a heart attack on July 20, 1984, while jogging in Vermont. For the 15 years prior to his death, he had been running about 80 miles per week. He was aware of a family history of early death from heart disease. Friends reported that Mr. Fixx had complained of exhaustion and tightness in his throat (angina) while running. A physician friend tried to persuade him to have a stress test. He refused. A former wife mentioned that he avoided doctors and appeared to deny the risk he ought to have acknowledged from his family history. It is noteworthy that 17 years earlier he was a two-pack-a-day smoker and overweight (220 pounds). He took up jogging and slowly saw his weight drop to 159 pounds. At autopsy two major coronary arteries were completely blocked. For the rest, he was in "fine, excellent shape!" Sadly, Jim Fixx failed to recognize the significance of his family history or to heed multiple signals indicating his need for attention and refused to see a physician.

It is extremely disturbing to realize that a marathon runner can suddenly drop dead from a heart attack while running. You might have imagined that with such extraordinary fitness and a lean, wiry build, no fat would dare accumulate in the coronary arteries of such an athlete. While genes rule supreme, environmental insults like smoking and excess weight gain don't help. There is unfortunately a long history of marathon (and other) runners suffering a cardiac arrest and dying during the race. Many well-published examples of such catastrophes are known from Boston to Berlin and London to Seattle, among others.

The blockage in Jim Fixx's coronary arteries resulted from fatty deposits in either the lining and/or in the wall of the arteries. These deposits either reached a critical size (together with adherent clots) or a fatty plaque ruptured under the stress of his running. Given his family history, it would have been wise for him to have known the level of his total cholesterol, low-density lipoprotein (LDL) cholesterol, high-density (HDL) cholesterol, triglycerides, and apolipoprotein B. Markedly elevated levels of triglycerides and cholesterol are recognized in a condition called familial combined hyperlipidemia (FCH). This turns out to be the most common genetic cause of high-circulating fat levels (hyperlipidemia), affecting about 1 in 100 people. Familial combined hyperlipidemia contributes to more than 20% of coronary artery disease in males under age 60 years. In some families, the transmission of FCH seems to follow a dominant pattern, with an affected person having a 50% likelihood of transmitting this trait. However, more recently, more complex genetics have been invoked and it is more likely that multiple genes are involved.

With his history, Jim Fixx might also have had familial hypercholesterolemia (FH), which affects about 1 in 500 people and accounts for about 40% of premature heart attacks. High levels of triglycerides can occur independently, making it difficult to easily categorize these disorders. Hence, it becomes even more important to know your family history and be alert to symptoms and signs that could indicate a cardiac threat. Avoidance and prevention are more easily accomplished than a cure.

CORONARY HEART DISEASE

Knowledge of these statistics concerning heart disease and stroke should make everyone stop and think about their family history, their own medical status, and the lifestyle they pursue. In 2006, only 57% of women surveyed by the American Heart Association knew that heart disease was the leading cause of death among women.

Indeed data from the Centers for Disease Control and Prevention revealed that 1 in 2.6 women die from coronary artery disease (CAD) contrasted with 1 in 4.6 from cancer. Not only do more women than men with CAD die, but a greater proportion die of sudden cardiac arrest before their arrival at a hospital! The failure of women to recognize their increased risks may be at the root of the problem, but a host of often synergistic risk factors conspire against their better survival. Awareness of and attention to these risk factors could help secure their health and save their lives.

Some of the easily preventable, avoidable, and treatable well-known risks include obesity (*see* Chapter 27), smoking, hypertension, elevated cholesterol and/or triglyceride levels, and lack of exercise. Early detection, treatment, and control of diabetes (*see* Chapter 26) are vitally important. Less well-known risk factors include elevated levels of C-reactive protein (CRP),[5] presence of an auto- immune disease (such as rheumatoid arthritis or systemic lupus erythematosis), estrogen deficiency, irregular menses in premenopausal women, and polycystic ovary syndrome.

However, coronary artery disease is not new. Computed tomography X-ray scans of Egyptian mummies have revealed tell-tale evidence. Meanwhile, about 80 million American adults (1 in 3) have one or more types of cardiovascular disease. In 2006, an estimated 16,800,000 had CAD, and almost 8 million had heart attacks. The lifetime risk of developing CAD after age 40 years was estimated as 49% for men and 32% for women. Coronary artery disease caused about one in every five deaths in the United States in 2005 and was recognized as the largest single killer of American males and females, ahead of cancer and stroke. Estimates were that every 25 seconds an American would suffer a coronary event and about every minute someone would die from one.

Virtually all coronary heart disease results from either susceptibility genes interacting with environmental factors or from defective single genes. Situated on the short arm of chromosome 9 is a gene variation, possession of which increases the risk of CAD. About one in four of the population carries this variation on both chromosomes 9, doubling the risk of early onset heart disease, when compared to persons without these variations. Moreover, this

---

5. In addition to the deposition of cholesterol and other fats in the lining of heart, brain, and other arteries, inflammation compounds the problem. CRP is a marker of inflammation that has been shown to predict risk of heart attacks, strokes, sudden cardiac death, and peripheral arterial disease. CRP is a stronger predictor of cardiovascular complications than cholesterol.

molecular signature on chromosome 9 also increases the risk of stroke, peripheral artery disease (e.g., in the legs), abdominal aortic aneurysm, and surprisingly, intracranial aneurysm. Those with a family history of early onset heart disease can determine their chromosome 9 status and take pre-emptive actions (*see* below) to avoid cardiovascular complications.

In the common so-called "multifactorial (genes and environment) CAD," control of the known risk factors is paramount. Attention to risk factors that are known to reduce the incidence of CAD include stopping smoking; control of diabetes and hypertension; exercise; reducing cholesterol to normal levels by dietary discipline and the use of a statin medication; weight loss; reduction, if elevated, of the level in the blood of the amino acid homocysteine (by taking folic acid supplements daily); and eating a diet with daily fruit and vegetables, with alcohol only in moderation. Cigarette smoking is recognized as the most important preventable cause of premature death and disability being responsible for between 17% to 30% of all deaths resulting from cardiovascular disease. Note, too, that cigar smoking significantly increases mortality as well. Worldwide estimates indicate that about half a billion of the world's current population will eventually die from tobacco-related illness between ages 35 and 69 years. Even among nonsmokers living with smokers, there is a 20% to 30% increased risk of death from CAD.

The incidence of fatal heart attacks among smokers averages about 70% higher than in nonsmokers. While there is a dose relation (the more cigarettes, the worse the prognosis), smoking as few as one to four cigarettes per day increases the risk. Women who both smoke and use an oral contraceptive have a 13-fold increase in risk of fatal CAD compared to those who take the pill but do not smoke. Smokers also have about a five times higher risk than nonsmokers of having a stroke. A poor circulation, amputation, or even rupture of the aorta all occur with much higher frequency among smokers. The good news is that stopping smoking reduces the risk of CAD markedly within 3 to 4 years after quitting.

A predisposition to clot may also add additional risk. Two genes in particular (Factor V Leiden and Prothrombin) in which a mutation may occur predispose an individual to an increased risk of blood clotting (*see* Chapter 17). Among Caucasians, between 3% and 5% harbor a mutation in the Factor V Leiden gene, and about 2% have a mutation in the Prothrombin gene. DNA analysis of these two genes is indicated when someone has had clots forming in the legs (deep vein thrombosis), clots shooting into the lungs (pulmonary embolism), or early age strokes.

The crowd were on their feet, cheering, shouting, and generally making a deafening noise. The score was equal in this neck-and-neck tussle between longtime high school adversaries in the regional basketball league. The pace was fast, furious, and physical. Tyrone, playing at center, had just scored and had taken but a few steps back toward his team when he collapsed. His teammates and a medic rushed to him as he lay facedown on the court. Administered CPR continued even as he was lifted onto a trolley and into an ambulance. Tyrone, however, had suffered an instantaneous sudden cardiac death. He was 16 years old.

Subsequent inquiry revealed that he had no health complaints. His grieving mother said that he had mentioned that he would have to train harder since he did not feel as fit as he should be.

Tyrone's mother's family had no history of heart disease or sudden unexplained death. Tyrone's father was "not in the picture," and nothing was known about his whereabouts.

Sudden death in a teenager not caused by an accident or violence mostly points to a cardiac disorder or a brain hemorrhage. Autopsy showed a markedly enlarged left ventricle consistent with a diagnosis of hypertrophic cardiomyopathy (HCM). Tyrone's sudden death must have resulted from an acute onset heart rhythm abnormality (arrhythmia)[6] resulting in a failure of the left ventricle to pump blood to brain and body. Tyrone may well have been asymptomatic, but his mention of needing to train harder may have reflected his awareness of shortness of breath with exertion, an early and important warning sign. Apparently he did not complain of other signs such as palpitations or dizziness, and he had no history of fainting. I would recommend an electrocardiogram for all high-schoolers intending to play competitive sports.

Tyrone's death spawned fear and anxiety in his three siblings. He died at a time when no DNA testing was available, and hence no specific mutation analysis could be offered to his siblings. For HCM (at the time) and many other genetic disorders where specific genes have not yet been identified or are not available for testing, banking DNA from an affected

6. Probably ventricular tachycardia or fibrillation

individual (even obtained hours after death) can prove extremely valuable, even many years later when gene analysis for the disorder in question becomes available.

Since it was uncertain whether Tyrone was the first in his family to have HCM, his siblings, all younger, underwent a careful physical examination and had an electrocardiogram and an echocardiogram, all of which revealed no abnormality. However, at the time, that provided no consolation because the age of onset of HCM is variable. The family was therefore advised to keep in touch with a clinical geneticist at least annually to determine if and when diagnostic gene analysis would become available. The family moved out of state and all further contact was lost.

Meanwhile, at least 17 different genes were discovered in which mutations occurred that resulted in HCM. Mutation analysis of these genes is now routinely available, and more than 600 different mutations have been reported.

CARDIOMYOPATHY

Hypertrophic cardiomyopathy accounts for about one-third of sudden cardiac deaths among athletes in the United States. Hypertrophic cardiomyopathy occurs in one to two per thousand individuals and is dominantly inherited or transmitted. This means that the affected individual has a 50% risk of transmitting the mutation in one of the genes to each of his or her offspring.

There are, in fact, many different rarer causes of disorders of the heart muscle (cardiomyopathies). In one such condition, called Noonan syndrome, 20% to 30% have HCM. This syndrome is characterized by short stature, a broad or webbed neck, a shield-shaped chest, a variable degree of developmental delay, frequently undescended testes, and a characteristic facial appearance with down-slanting eyes (palpebral fissures). Congenital heart defects are also frequently present. Five different genes account for this syndrome[7] and are available for routine analysis. Arrhythmogenic right ventricular cardiomyopathy is another heart muscle disorder that occurs in 1 in 1,000 to 1 in 3,000 people. The concerns, complications, and consequences are similar to HCM, as are the treatment and prevention strategies. The mode of inheritance is

---

7. Specifically PTPN11, RAF1, SOS1, KRAS, and SHOC2.

dominant and gene analyses currently yield mutations in about 50% of cases. Many other genetic muscular and neurological disorders may involve heart muscle.[8]

Determining the significance of a family history when HCM is suspected requires that attention be directed to any relatives who have had heart failure, sudden death, arrhythmias, unexplained strokes, or a heart transplant. Certainly, individuals with HCM are at markedly increased risk of an arrhythmia (particularly atrial fibrillation) that could result in a clot forming in the upper left chamber of the heart (left atrium). This clot could be ejected via the left ventricle as a projectile directly into the brain, causing a major stroke. A family history should prompt a consultation, preferably with a cardiologist, to determine the presence of HCM. If the evaluation is inconclusive, DNA studies of a possible affected family member (if cooperative) would be valuable. Absent that opportunity, annual evaluations would be important. Dr. Norman Cousins, writing in the *Saturday Review* more than 30 years ago, made the point that wisdom was the ability to anticipate and, I would add, to take preemptive action.

An unexpected problem concerning HCM and that recently came to light, highlights an area of medicine that receives scant regulation. A young man repeatedly provided sperm donations to a tissue bank. Ultimately, 22 children were conceived from his sperm. In addition, he had two of his own children. Only after the child of a recipient was diagnosed with HCM was attention paid to the donor. DNA mutation studies of all the conceived children eventually revealed that nine were identified as having HCM. One died at age 2 years from progressive and unrelenting heart failure, while two experienced serious heart enlargement at age 15 years. The donor is at high risk of cardiac failure, including sudden death. The team from the Minneapolis Heart Institute Foundation reporting on this case recommended consideration of a detailed electrocardiogram on every donor, which, of course, would be done in tandem with other genetic and infectious disease tests. To secure their health, individuals with HCM are advised to avoid competitive sports and to have only moderate physical activity. There should be no weightlifting or sudden bursts of activity such as sprinting. Medications used include beta-blockers and other

---

8. These include Friedreich's ataxia, myotonic muscular dystrophy, Duchenne or Becker muscular dystrophy, Limb-Girdle muscular dystrophy, amyloidosis, mitochondrial cardiomyopathy, and many others.

anti-arrhythmic drugs. In the event heart failure supervenes, heart transplantation becomes an important option.

A sense of well-being enveloped John as he ended his 3-mile jog around the neighborhood. He had made this an early morning habit since he had moved his family to a suburban location 6 years ago. Now 36 years old, he felt he was in excellent shape, fit, and happy with his wife and two young children. He had, however, noticed that he seemed more out of breath at the end of the run than he used to be. He mentioned this in passing to his wife, who happened to be a nurse. That was how John found himself in the cardiologist's office having a heart check-up, an electrocardiogram, and an echocardiogram.[9]

To his utter amazement, the cardiologist explained that he had been born with two rather than three leaflets that constituted his aortic valve (called bicuspid aortic valve [BAV]). As a consequence, John's valve had begun to leak, resulting in his left ventricle having to pump harder and slowly enlarge. Left alone, his doctor explained, two important complications could ensue. John could develop heart failure, but worse still, infection could settle on the surface of the valves, causing serious illness and even strokes as a consequence of tiny pieces of infected material breaking off the valve's surface and ending up in the brain.

When questioned about his family history. John described his late father having had an aneurysm (ballooning or marked dilatation) of his aorta, which had ruptured and from which he died at the age of 60 years. He did not specifically know whether his father had BAV. He was unaware of whether any other family member had any type of cardiovascular disease.

Not long after this consultation, John had an aortic valve replacement and at least 10 years later has been well, in good shape, and still jogging.

Major problems were averted because of the attention and watchfulness of his wife. Her knowledge and pre-emptive action in insisting and arranging his appointment with a cardiologist was critical for John's continued health. Any family history of aortic aneurysm occurring in individuals who are not old (60 isn't old!) should raise questions about the cause.

9. Heart imaging by ultrasound.

BAVs are highly heritable and probably via a dominant mode of transmission. This might mean a 50% risk of transmission by an affected person to his or her children. However, thus far no culprit genes have been clearly implicated in the vast majority of individuals with BAV.

John was advised to have an annual cardiology check-up because the basic defect causing the aortic valve problem frequently also involves the wall of the aorta. Hence, an annual echocardiogram would help keep an eye on the size of the aorta. Should the aorta begin to bulge, surgical intervention would be recommended to avoid rupture.

BICUSPID AORTIC VALVE

Bicuspid aortic valve affects 1 in 50 to 1 in 100 of the population and represents the most common congenital cardiac malformation. Complications of or associations with BAV include aortic valve narrowing (aortic stenosis), leakage (regurgitation as experienced by John), valve infection (infective endocarditis), and bulging (called aneurysm) or rupture of the aorta or an artery in the brain. A study of patients with BAV in Los Angeles showed that 1 in 10 had an aneurysm in the head. It would therefore be wise to have imaging of the brain arteries (by MRA).[10] Early detection of an aneurysm would allow pre-emptive surgery to clip or tie off the bulge before rupture, thereby saving a life! Since only 20% of those with BAV maintain normal valve function throughout their lives, careful attention should be given to those in whom a diagnosis has been made.

Interestingly for what is probably a disorder of connective tissue collagen, BAV is found surprisingly frequently in a condition called Turner's syndrome (see Chapter 3), in which it occurs in about 16%, while sharp narrowing or constriction of the aorta (called coarctation) occurs in about 11% of those with this sex-chromosome disorder.

Disorders caused by the interaction of multiple genes and environmental factors account for about 80% of deaths worldwide. Coronary heart disease and heart attacks account for about 40% of these deaths. Much is now known

---

10. Magnetic Resonance Arteriography.

about the avoidance, prevention, and treatment of heart disease, but public health authorities have failed in educating the public and inculcating key information beginning in early school education.

Since exhortations don't accomplish much, strong government incentives (funding) and disincentives (no funding) should be in place in all schools. The ever-increasing risk of premature heart disease is self-evident given the obesity epidemic. Childhood obesity is associated with a shorter lifespan. We owe it to our children and grandchildren to foster a healthier diet and lifestyle with much less heart disease.

10

CONSEQUENCES OF FAILURE TO DIAGNOSE

I got to know James and Mary when I was consulted by their lawyer, who asked for my opinion in their case against Mary's obstetrician and her children's pediatrician.

This Irish Catholic couple had five children. Their first son, John, had marked speech delay and was eventually diagnosed as mentally retarded. Their second child was a daughter, Lynn, who was perfectly fine. Their third child, Jeremy, also had major speech difficulties and was also diagnosed as mentally retarded. Their fourth child, Peter, was born barely 10 months after their third child. He, too, had marked speech delay, was late in walking (20 months), was subject to severe tantrums, was hyperactive, flapped his hands frequently, and was thought to have autistic behavior. Their fifth child, Rose, seemed generally okay but had considerable learning difficulties, especially in mathematics.

Mary had left school in the 10ᵗʰ grade, and James worked in construction. Mary had two brothers with mental retardation of "unknown cause"and who lived in Ireland. One of her two sisters had no children since "her periods stopped when she was 32." Mary's one maternal uncle, also in Ireland, was thought to have developed Parkinson's disease when he was 52. James had only one sibling, a brother, who also had mild mental retardation, cause unknown.

James and Mary moved to a larger home to accommodate their growing children and, in the process, had to change pediatricians. Their new pediatrician examined Peter first, as he appeared to be the source of considerable management difficulty at home. He noted that Peter's head was rather large (in the 90th percentile), that he had large, prominent ears, a prominent forehead and jaw with a long face, and obvious intellectual deficits, which included poor speech and autistic behavior. He immediately suspected a diagnosis of the Fragile X syndrome, and the DNA studies he ordered quickly confirmed the diagnosis. Over the ensuing weeks, he examined John, Jeremy, and Rose and ordered DNA tests on all, including their mother Mary. Not unexpectedly, John and Jeremy were also diagnosed as having the Fragile X syndrome, and both Rose and Mary were found to harbor the same gene mutation.

The lawsuit was occasioned by the realization that their first pediatrician had not evaluated either John or Jeremy by doing appropriate genetic tests, including Fragile X DNA analyses. They sued their obstetrician because she had not paid attention to the family history, which had included Mary's two brothers with mental retardation and a sister with premature menopause. They claimed that at the very least she should have ordered chromosome and Fragile X gene studies for Mary when she first came for prenatal care in her very first pregnancy. This would have revealed that Mary carried the Fragile X premutation (see discussion that follows) and that for any male offspring she carried, there would be a 50% risk of mental retardation, and for any female she carried, there would be a 50% risk of her being a carrier and possibly showing mild manifestations of the Fragile X syndrome. James and Mary maintained that they would have had no children given such risks since they had both been aware of the "miserable experience" the family had had on both sides with their respective mentally retarded brothers.

The standard of expected care from Mary's obstetrician when she was originally pregnant was to recognize Mary's potential risk, given her two brothers with mental retardation, albeit without known cause. It would have been expected that she would have ordered testing for chromosomes and Fragile X syndrome, at the very least. She would then have discovered that Mary carried the Fragile X syndrome premutation and would have had to offer Mary prenatal genetic studies to determine whether or not the fetus was affected. Mary would then have had the option to terminate the pregnancy, a choice she had previously made from a union she had had prior to meeting James. Another clue about the possible Fragile X syndrome in the family was Mary's sister with her premature menopause (called premature ovarian failure). About 20% of women who carry the Fragile X gene premutation experience premature ovarian failure or insufficiency. Her obstetrician's failure deprived Mary of the opportunity to selectively have unaffected children, using the assurance provided by prenatal diagnosis.

Mary's first pediatrician failed to recognize the clinical signs of Fragile X syndrome or to order the appropriate DNA test. He perpetrated this failure twice, the second time being his failure to diagnose the Fragile X syndrome in Jeremy. All of this, of course, resulted in no prenatal genetic studies for Mary's pregnancy with Peter, who was also born affected. In her pregnancy with Rose, DNA studies revealed a premutation state similar to Mary herself, leading her to continue that pregnancy.

On the advice of the clinical geneticist to whom she had been referred after Peter's birth, Mary informed her family in Ireland and passed on the advice for her uncle with "Parkinson's disease" to be tested for the Fragile X premutation. Sure enough, not long after, she received the news that he indeed was "an unaffected transmitting carrier" of the Fragile X syndrome and that his diagnosis had been changed to the Fragile X tremor-ataxia syndrome (FXTAS; discussed below).

THE FRAGILE X SYNDROME

The observations the pediatrician made when he examined Peter encompassed key signs of the Fragile X syndrome (*see* Table 10.1). Not every sign appears in every affected individual. Most males will have IQs between 30 and 50, with only about 15% having an IQ above 70. About 70% of affected females with the full mutation have an IQ of 85 or less. They frequently exhibit problems with executive function, attention deficit hyperactivity disorder, language delays, impulsivity, and problems in learning—especially in mathematics. About 25% of females with the full mutation have a normal IQ and no learning problems but do have frequent emotional problems such as anxiety. Autistic features are seen in about 30% of boys and 10% to 20% of girls. Psychosis has been reported in less than 10% of those with the full mutation. Families experience most problems in rearing children with the Fragile X syndrome because of their behavioral issues, including impulsivity, anxiety, mood instability, and aggression. Clearly, multidisciplinary care is required for the range of problems noted above.

Table 10.1 Common Features of the Fragile X Syndrome

Infancy and Childhood

Feeding problems and reflux

Low muscle tone

Recurrent ear infections

Delayed milestones (late walking and speech)

Behavioral problems—tantrums and hyperactivity with attention deficit disorder

Autistic features—poor eye contact, hand-flapping, hand-biting, tactile defensiveness (doesn't like being touched), perseverative speech, and poor impulse control

Mental retardation: IQ of 30–50

Typical facial features: long face, large head with prominent forehead, large ears, and prominent jaw

---

Puberty and Adolescence

Large testes (macro-orchidism)

Behavioral issues continued with shyness and gaze aversion

Strabismus (crossed eyes)

Lax joints and flat feet

Mitral valve prolapse

Soft smooth skin

Anxiety, depression, or mood disorder

Groin hernias

Seizures

A mutation in the Fragile X syndrome gene (*FMR1*) results in deficiency or absence of the expected protein. It is this protein that should otherwise normally function in brain development and the maintenance of interconnections. The actual mutation in the *FMR1* gene involves the single nucleotide bases (ACGT) discussed in Chapter 5. Throughout our genome, we have repetitive runs of three nucleotides in a row. Normally in the *FMR1* gene, we harbor less than 54 so-called "triplet repeats" made up of CGG runs. Individuals with 54 to 200 of these triplets are regarded as premutation carriers. Within this range, the higher the number of repeats, the more likely transmission will occur to offspring. In addition to premature ovarian insufficiency, both male and female premutation carriers may exhibit some psychological problems. Some boys with the premutation do exhibit attention deficit hyperactivity disorder, anxiety, and autistic features. Most have a normal IQ, but some do indeed exhibit IQs in the mental retardation range.

However, more important is the occurrence of FXTAS, in which tremor, lack of balance, and involvement of the peripheral nervous system (neuropathy) and the involuntary (autonomic) nervous system may be associated with cognitive decline in some older males and occasional females. FXTAS is seen more frequently with increasing age of premutation carriers, with 15% of males in their 50s exhibiting neurological features and 75% being symptomatic in their 80s. Among female premutation carriers, about 8% older than age 50 years develop FXTAS with symptoms less severe than their male counterparts. It also appears that premutation females have a significant frequency (50%) of hypothyroidism. Children with Fragile X syndrome have an increased frequency of seizures, tics and behavioral problems if their mothers have an auto-immune disease (eg hypothyroidism, type 1 diabetes, rheumatoid arthritis, or lupus erythematosis). The reason(s) remain speculative. Remarkably, multiple sclerosis has been reported in 2% to 3% of female premutation carriers, suggesting some type of auto-immune component resulting in this debilitating disorder.

Triplet repeat numbers in excess of 200 generally translate to the fully fledged Fragile X syndrome. These triplet repeat numbers may, however, expand into hundreds and even thousands. Not unexpectedly, the greater the number of triplets, the more severe the manifestations.

Estimates of the frequency of premutation carriers range between 1 in 113 and 1 in 259 females. About 1 in 4,000 Caucasian males have the Fragile X syndrome.

In less than 1% of cases, there may be a gene deletion or other type of mutation. A DNA switch close to the *FMR1* gene silences it, resulting in loss of the protein product. Functional failure of the gene results not only in premature ovarian failure but also in the typical FXTAS. The risk of FXTAS in premutation males increases with advancing age, approximating 17% between ages 50 and 59 years and rising to about 75% after the age of 80 years. For some reason, females appear to have a lower risk that has yet to be quantified. This latter disorder is not infrequently misdiagnosed as Parkinson's disease, given the associated tremor, loss of balance, and—later in some—loss of faculties. This was specifically the case in Mary's uncle, initially diagnosed incorrectly with Parkinson's disease. The Fragile X gene protein product finds expression in many tissues of the body. Although the precise way it exerts its malfunctioning mechanism is unknown, we do know that the physical and behavioral features described for Peter are typical.

Prenatal diagnosis is available for this disorder. However, prenatal diagnosis by chorion villus sampling (*see* Chapter 7), optimally performed at 11 weeks of pregnancy, is <u>not</u> as reliable as studies done on amniotic fluid cells sampled a few weeks later (15–16 weeks) and is not recommended. Preimplantation genetic diagnosis has been accomplished.

The Fragile X syndrome was discovered by that well-worn research technique—serendipity! A technician in the laboratory made an error in setting up the blood culture for chromosome analysis and mistakenly omitted an essential ingredient (folic acid) in the broth used to grow the cells. The astute geneticist (chance favors the prepared mind) noticed that near the end of the long arm of one of the X chromosomes, the end piece seemed to be hanging by a thin, fragile thread. For awhile, that was the test used to diagnose this condition, ultimately replaced by direct DNA analysis.

Treatment for this condition is symptomatic, including attention to special education, medication for behavioral problems, speech and language therapy, and treatment of seizures. Studies in the mouse model of the Fragile X syndrome have encouraged ongoing trials in humans using new therapeutic approaches.[1]

For this X-linked dominant disorder, premutation males, who mostly appear entirely normal, transmit their premutation (on their single X chromosome) to all their daughters but none of their sons, who inherit their Y chromosome. Their daughters are unaffected premutation carriers who have a 50% risk of transmitting what becomes a full mutation to their sons and daughters. The birth of a son with Fragile X syndrome and subsequent demonstration that his mother is a premutation carrier means that her father or mother is at significant risk of developing FXTAS, as noted above.

The Fragile X syndrome is categorized in a group of disorders (*see* Appendix 3) that share the dynamic mutation mechanism of expanding triplet repeats. In this and the other disorders in the group, a phenomenon called anticipation (*see* Chapter 12) occurs in which there is increasing severity of the disorder with transmission of the premutation through generations. Typically, a transmission from a grandfather who harbors a premutation to his daughter does not affect her, but when she in turn transmits it to her son, mental retardation results. Anticipation mostly occurs when less severely affected premutation carriers transmit the Fragile X mutation to their children. Thankfully, there are

---

1. Such as a glutamate receptor antagonist.

many families who do transmit the premutation for generations and do not experience anticipation.

Again, be well-informed about your family history, and for possible Fragile X syndrome, take special note of family members with mental retardation (on mother's or father's side), of premature menopause on mother's side, and of tremor and balance problems in older parents and grandparents on either side.

I supported James and Mary in their lawsuit against their two physicians who had neither diagnosed nor referred their first two sons for genetic evaluation, thereby depriving Mary and James of the opportunity to avoid a lifelong burden. The governing legal doctrine in such cases is described as "loss of chance," and to which I referred to in Chapter 8 in the context of colon and thyroid cancer. I subsequently heard that the case had been settled and that James had had a vasectomy.

Michael was 3 years old when his pediatrician mentioned to his mother that he was very loose-jointed, had flat feet, and had knock-knees. Small sensitive lumps on the side of his tongue and on his lips were noticed by his mother when he was about 5 years old. The pediatrician said they were probably a result of a virus and were likely to disappear spontaneously. They didn't. At age 7 years, tiny nodules appeared under his eyelids, which were ascribed to allergies. He fell off his bicycle when he was 13 years old and sustained an injury to his right hip that required surgery[2] When he was 17 years old, the nodules on his lips really bothered him, especially cosmetically, so he was taken to an oral surgeon, who excised the nodules. The pathology report stated that the nodule was a neurofibroma, and his pediatrician therefore diagnosed him as having the condition called neurofibromatosis (see Chapter 20), adding that he also had spinal curvature (scoliosis). It was also noticed that he had puffy-blubbery lips, and the nodules recurred on his tongue, lips, and mouth. Further efforts by a plastic surgeon to remove these nodules also failed. At this stage, his pediatrician for all those years decided that his build was Lincolnesque, with his tall, thin body; long arms; long face; and long fingers. He was referred to a geneticist, whose impression was that he probably had neurofibromatosis, largely based on the previous biopsy result.

---

2. For a slipped capital femoral epiphysis.

At age 18 years, his medical care was switched to a family doctor, who made no mention of any of the features just described. He was treated for significant abdominal pain, which was presumed to be due to milk (lactose) intolerance. During one of these visits, a physician-in-training who examined Michael discovered that he had a lump in his thyroid gland. Studies that were ordered revealed that radioactive iodine was not taken up by the thyroid lump, and surgical removal was recommended. For the first time, at age 20 years, a physician to whom he had been referred drew attention to the relation between the thyroid lump; the studded lesions affecting Michael's mouth, tongue, and lips; and his typical body build, raising the question of a condition called multiple endocrine neoplasia (MEN2B). He ordered a calcium hormone level (calcitonin), and an astronomically high level was revealed.

Michael then underwent surgery, at which time the diagnosis was confirmed that he had medullary thyroid cancer. Worse still, the cancer had spread to his lymph nodes, deep into his neck. He underwent further surgery for a block dissection and removal of all lymph nodes that could be found in his neck, but to no avail. Michael died a year later from metastatic thyroid cancer.

I was asked to render an opinion on the care rendered to Michael since childhood as part of a lawsuit against the many physicians who had examined him over all of those years.

The various types of MEN,[3] although rare, are well-known and should have been recognized in Michael, especially by the geneticist and the pathologist who examined the biopsy. The fact that the submitted tissue came from the tongue or lip should have immediately signaled that this was a neuroma classically associated with MEN2B. The pediatrician

---

3. Multiple endocrine neoplasia type 1 (caused by mutations in the *MEN1* gene) is also transmitted as an autosomal dominant disorder. About 90% of cases are inherited. In this disorder, endocrine glands (those that produce hormones) overgrow and overproduce hormones that cause problems. These overgrowths, called adenomas, cause secretory hyperfunction such as too much insulin, leading to extremely low blood sugar. The endocrine glands included are the pituitary, thyroid, adrenal, pancreatic islets, parathyroids, to mention the most important.

should have recognized his distinctive facial appearance with enlarged lips; long, thin body build; and the abdominal pains due to involvement of his intestinal tract. The detection by a physician-in-training of the lump in Michael's thyroid gland gives one further pause in considering the standard of medical care in that practice.

Fortunately, MEN type 2 is relatively rare (perhaps 1 in 30,000). About 50% of the time, it is inherited as a dominant gene, and half the time, it arises spontaneously. Interestingly, when a brand new mutation does occur in the MEN gene (called *RET*) it happens to be almost always on the chromosome inherited (without the mutation) from the father.

MULTIPLE ENDOCRINE NEOPLASIA

Although there are three subtypes of MEN type 2, I will only focus here on type 2B. However, each of these subtypes are characterized by medullary thyroid cancer—and that is the critical message. If there is a family history of thyroid cancer, the family should inquire whether it was medullary thyroid cancer.[4] For anyone with this type of thyroid cancer, a DNA analysis of the *RET* gene would be recommended because that analysis would identify a disease-causing mutation in about 95% of affected individuals.

You will immediately realize, of course, that for this autosomal dominant inherited disorder, there is a 50% risk that the affected individual will transmit to each of his or her children. Hence, the DNA test of the *RET* gene would be recommended forthwith if a mutation is detected in an affected parent. Identification of a disease-causing mutation, regardless of the age (even in the first month of life), might lead directly to surgical removal of the thyroid gland. Sophisticated genetic evaluation and counseling is recommended because some difference exists with reference to the likelihood of thyroid cancer according to the specific mutation discovered. For some with the highest risk, thyroidectomy within 1 month or certainly the first 6 to 12 months of life is recommended, whereas others will be candidates for this surgery by age 5 years and occasionally by age 10 years. Obviously, thyroid hormone supplements will be necessary for life.

---

4. There is also an increased risk for a rarer tumor called pheochromocytoma.

Among those who do not appear to have inherited a mutation in the *RET* gene, about 7% did inherit the mutation that resided in a gene housed in a father's testes or mother's ovaries. Although that parent is not affected, their gonad is constituted by a mixture of eggs or sperm, only some of which possess the mutation (called germline mosaicism) (*see* Chapter 5). The other possibility for individuals with medullary thyroid cancer and MEN2B is the spontaneous development of a mutation in the *RET* gene within the thyroid gland. DNA analysis of the removed thyroid tissue would then be important if that person had no family history of MEN2B.

For those who have had their thyroid glands removed in childhood and who obviously possess the RET gene mutation, prenatal diagnosis or preimplantation genetic diagnosis is an option when they begin to plan having children of their own. Those with a family history should inform all of their first-degree relatives of the risk they may face and the availability of DNA testing. Lifetime surveillance to detect any recurrence or other tumor is important and includes annual testing of the hormone calcitonin. In addition, thyroidectomy may include removal of the tiny parathyroid glands that normally nestle within and behind the thyroid gland itself. Usually efforts are made to simply transplant these tiny glands into the muscles of the neck, but their function should be monitored thereafter to be sure that a lack of function (hypoparathyroidism) does not develop.

There are well over 2,000 genetic syndromes representing disorders in which there are recognizable combinations of signs that facilitate diagnosis. Clinical geneticists are assisted in making syndromic diagnoses by the use of computer programs.[5] However, there is hardly a week that goes by without publication or recognition of another syndrome or association. Unfortunately, in Michael's case, recognition came too late to save his life. I learned later that his case had been settled.

---

5. The Oxford Medical Dysmorphology and Neurology databases and the Australian POSSUM database.

GENES GONE MISSING

Carol and Gene had met in college, graduated together, and married soon after. They decided to start a family as soon as possible, since they wanted to be "young parents and grandparents." Carol soon conceived and both they and their families were ecstatic. Pregnancy, labor, and delivery were uneventful. The baby, whom they named Errol, weighed 7 pounds at birth and was lively and "beautiful." Carol breastfed and commented on how long it took for Errol to complete a feed. He gained weight and "looked great." At his 3-month check-up, Carol commented to the pediatrician that he seemed floppy but was quickly reassured that there was a wide normal range of development and she should be patient. Two weeks after the visit to the pediatrician's office, Carol's grandmother from the West Coast came for a visit. She was known in the family as smart but blunt, never hesitating to speak her mind. Two days into her visit, she became the recipient of angry retorts when she repeatedly said that there was something wrong with Errol. She pointedly insisted that he was too floppy and that he did not kick very much. They were relieved to have her out of the house after her 1-week visit. Over the ensuing weeks as Errol approached 5 months of age, they noticed that they could not remotely prop him up even on pillows because he would simply keel over. At the 6-month visit to the pediatrician, it had become abundantly clear that Errol was nowhere near able to sit and clearly seemed to have either a neurological or muscle disorder.

Referral to a neurologist days later resulted in a clinical diagnosis of spinal muscular atrophy (SMA).[1]

---

1. Also known as Werdnig-Hoffman disease.

Carol and Gene were devastated. They sought a second opinion from a geneticist who was able to confirm the likely diagnosis from the clinical examination. The geneticist at the Yale-New Haven Hospital also obtained a tiny skin biopsy with the hope that additional studies may help achieve a molecular diagnosis.

Over the next 15 months, Errol grew weaker and moved less and less. He was never able to sit unsupported and mostly lay on his back with his beautiful, wide, round eyes and spectacular smile. He had begun to learn different words and it was clear that his intelligence was intact. Repeated episodes of pneumonia occurred, and during one such episode in hospital, Errol died. He was 21 months old.

This dreadful experience stilled the couple's desire to have a family, and they both buried themselves in their work, trying to forget the grievous hurt they had experienced.

I saw Carol and Gene in consultation some 11 years later. That's when they told me this history and came with the hope that there might be new advances in genetics that would allow them to have an unaffected child. In fact, in that very year, the culprit gene with its mutations causing SMA (the SMN gene[2]) had been discovered, and the ability to achieve a prenatal diagnosis had been established. However, for prenatal diagnosis to proceed at that time, it had been necessary to have DNA from the affected child to precisely determine the genetic defect in the SMN gene.

I remember their looks of anguish as they sat back in their chairs with their hopes and dreams crushed. Gene was visibly but momentarily angered when I then asked about the skin biopsy that had been done. He was remembering the pain Errol suffered when the local anesthetic via needle was administered for the skin biopsy and the child's cry without being able to move much. I explained that it was likely that cells had been grown from this tissue and may well have been stored frozen, even after these many years. Since I knew the geneticist at Yale, it was easy to inquire whether the cells still existed, housed in liquid nitrogen. I made the phone call with Carol and Gene in the office, only to discover that the geneticist had moved from Yale to Stanford and had taken much of her equipment and biological samples she had used for research. I promised to contact her and let Carol and Gene know the result of my enquiry.

---

2. Also called the survival motor neuron gene (*SMN*).

To their amazement, the geneticist, Dr. Uta Franke, was able to find Errol's frozen cells. She kindly thawed the cells, had them grow again in cell culture, and dispatched them to us for genetic studies. We were then able to precisely identify the gene defect Errol had and, in a second consultation, explain to Carol and Gene that prenatal diagnosis in a future pregnancy was achievable. I well recall the tears in their eyes and the warm hug from each. They returned about 6 months later, carrying a sample of amniotic fluid from her new pregnancy, then 16 weeks along in gestation. We grew the cells from the amniotic fluid sample and achieved a molecular diagnosis of an unaffected fetus. Gene called me when the baby girl, whom they named Erin, was born and kept in touch intermittently through the first year of her life with the good news of her normal development.

The emotional pain and deep sadness experienced by parents who care for their dying child is indescribable. It has been my sad duty to care for many such children and their parents, and I have not become inured by these experiences. I have attended their funerals and cried. Long ago, I recognized that caring for a child also includes a family, and that the duty does not cease the moment a child dies. Carol described the loss of Errol as her "heart being ripped out of her chest."

Gene described how he felt crushed and full of despair. Fortunately, their closeness enabled them to survive the overwhelming grief, move on with their lives, and ultimately achieve happiness again. Spinal muscular atrophy is an autosomal recessive disease, and they faced a 25% risk of having a second affected child. They decided, in the absence of available prenatal diagnosis at the time, to desist from any future pregnancy. They never gave up hope and eventually returned to benefit from the remarkable advances in human genetics.

The fact that there was no family history was typical for autosomal recessive disorders. Carol and Gene were not related either, but both had French-Canadian ancestors. In all likelihood, they shared a common ancestor in a generation long past. They were both carriers of a mutation in the *SMN* gene and unknowingly had a one in four risk of having an affected child in every pregnancy. At that time, there was no molecular prenatal diagnostic test or carrier test available.

An important lesson emerges from their experience, pointing to the importance of remaining in contact with a clinical geneticist or genetic counselor at least annually if testing of the gene for the genetic disorder in the family has not yet materialized. Carol and Gene's experience also points to another important message. If a genetic disorder in the family is likely to prove lethal, then every effort should be made to obtain a blood sample or tissue from which DNA could be extracted and stored. We have been banking DNA for many years with samples stored in the deep freeze. A blood sample or a tiny skin biopsy can be obtained from the affected person and DNA extracted and stored so as to be of benefit to the rest of the family when questions arise about carrier status, diagnosis, prenatal diagnosis, or preimplantation genetic diagnosis. We also receive blood samples from which we isolate the white blood cells, transform them with a virus that make the cells immortal (growing forever), and freeze those cell lines away, which can later be thawed and grown again as a continual source of DNA. In the unfortunate situation of an unexpected death, a tiny sample of liver can still be obtained (even without an autopsy) and frozen immediately without preservative. Ample DNA can be extracted and stored from that sample.

SPINAL MUSCULAR ATROPHY

Errol had the typical form of infantile SMA in which there is progressive muscle weakness caused by degeneration and loss of nerve cells in the spinal cord and eventually the brain stem. The onset of signs is variable and may even be obvious when an alert mother notices that toward the end of pregnancy the fetus does not kick. While onset in the first 6 months of age is most common, signs may appear between 6 and 18 months, later in childhood, and even in adulthood. Since the same *SMN* gene is at fault, the possibilities explaining the later onset are that the mutation from one parent is different from the other parent or there are other genes modifying the effects of the defective gene.

Now we know from studies in the United States and Germany that about 1 in 50 individuals carries a mutation in the *SMN* gene and that SMA occurs in about 1 in 10,000 live births. DNA tests are now routinely available to determine an individual's carrier status, preferably before pregnancy is initiated.

More than 95% of carriers have a tiny deletion[3] in the *SMN* gene. The few other carriers may have a different type of mutation not detectable by routine screening. In about 2% of those affected by SMA, test interpretations can become complicated. For example, two copies of the *SMN* gene might occur on a single chromosome in one parent, while testing shows that the other parent is not a carrier, and yet the child is affected. In these unusual cases, a brand new mutation occurred when the child was conceived. This appears to be the case in about 6% of parents of an affected child after the carrier tests have been done. In these unusual situations, further studies (called linkage analysis) including other family members may be indicated. Given the increased availability of routine carrier testing, any doubt about a result should lead to a consultation with a clinical geneticist or genetic counselor.

If both parents are recognized as carriers of a mutation (usually a deletion) in the *SMN* gene, then for future pregnancies, they have the option of prenatal diagnosis or preimplantation genetic diagnosis.

Unfortunately there is no cure for this disorder as yet and treatment is purely anticipatory and palliative. The inevitable deterioration in breathing is eventually managed by the offer of a tracheotomy or the use of a ventilator, according to the parents' wishes. These are very tough situations and excruciating for parents faced with decisions, including their wishes not to resuscitate the child to spare the suffering. Continuous feeding may be necessary through entry directly into the stomach (called a gastrostomy) via the abdominal wall.

Whenever someone is found to be a carrier of an *SMA* gene mutation, the standard recommendations are to offer testing to their parents and siblings to track the mutation and provide an opportunity for other relatives to avoid future and unnecessary grief. Time and experience have taught that failure to contact and inform all relatives at risk occurs with distressing frequency. Imagine, I always say to my patients, how would you feel if a child of yours could have avoided having their own child with a fatal genetic disorder, but for the lack of communication by a relative.

The appointment had been made by Jill's mother, not withstanding her age (21 years). Jill, her mother explained, had always been in a special education class and eventually dropped out of high school. Shortly after she was born, a diagnosis of a heart defect was made and showed a hole in the wall

---

3. exons 7 and 8 of the *SMN1* gene.

between the heart's lower two chambers (ventricles, called a ventricular septal defect). She also had a cleft palate and throughout infancy experienced difficulty feeding, often choking on her food. The cleft in her palate was repaired without incident. Apparently, when it was clear that the ventricular septal defect would not close spontaneously, she had cardiac surgery to close the hole between the left and right ventricles. Besides a bout of postoperative infection, she recovered without any additional complication. Jill took her first steps at 18 months and only began to use single words at age 2 years.

When still a toddler, Jill's father was murdered while involved with gang warfare. The social and economic stresses and pressures on Jill's mother during those early years were difficult, and short shrift was paid to Jill's development. The local physician interpreted her delays in speech acquisition as "environmental." Jill's erratic behavior in her elementary school years was characterized by attention deficit disorder and cognitive limitations and mostly attributed to a less-than-optimal home environment. The school assessed her as having a verbal IQ of 82 with a performance IQ at least a few points lower than that. Her mother related that one social worker thought that her behavior was consistent with a diagnosis of autism spectrum disorder. In her teens, she became overly anxious and extremely impulsive.

In fact, Jill's mother said that was the reason for the consultation. Jill was pregnant—again! Moreover, she had no idea which male had impregnated her. She had had a first child 2 years earlier and again had no idea which male was responsible. That child, then 2 years old, was apparently very much like Jill at that age. A cleft palate had been repaired. The child started walking around 18 months and had not yet acquired any speech. Feeding had also been problematic, and chronic ear infections had been a problem. Significant hearing loss was a result.

No other clues emerged from a detailed family history, although the history was limited on Jill's father's side.

On examination, Jill had an unusual facial appearance. She had droopy eyelids, wide-set eyes, low-set and unusual looking ears, and a long, flat mid-face. Her eyes were crossed (called strabismus) and she wore spectacles. The tip of her nose was bulbous with a dimple at the tip. She had short stature (4 feet 10 inches) and webbing between the second and third toes of both feet. Subsequent studies I ordered showed that she had a single kidney. Brain imaging (MRI) revealed mild loss of brain cells (atrophy)—more especially in the front of her brain (frontal lobes) and at the back (occipital lobes).

Laboratory studies revealed no obvious chromosome abnormality, but a FISH study (see Chapter 2) showed a tiny missing segment (deletion) in the long arm of chromosome 22.[4] This test enabled the precise diagnosis of the 22q11.2 deletion syndrome.[5]

Jill's mother proved negative, and her late father (who apparently was a bright but misguided individual) was likely also unaffected.

Jill's diagnosis was obvious even before genetic testing, given her typical facial appearance, history of a cleft palate and heart defect, together with the typical story of her delayed development, limited capacity, and behavioral features. The various physicians who examined her from infancy through childhood neither made the diagnosis nor referred her to a clinical geneticist. Remember, however, that more than 2,000 syndromes have been described, so physicians untrained in the clinical skill of what we call dysmorphology might not easily recognize an uncommon or rare syndrome. However, the combination of physical features and defects and subsequent speech, language, and intellectual deficits should have resulted in a referral for genetic evaluation and testing. However, virtually every physical, behavioral, or psychiatric finding in this deletion syndrome may occur as an isolated abnormality in an otherwise normal person. For example, congenital heart defects (a child born with a cardiac defect) occurs in 0.85% of all births and is the most common major birth defect.

Jill was the first affected person in her family. Only about 7% of affected individuals inherit the deletion from a parent. But once affected, there is a 50% risk of transmitting the deletion to each of the affected person's children. Not unexpectedly we subsequently found that Jill's first child was also affected, as was the child she delivered subsequently. She had presented too late in the pregnancy for prenatal studies, reflecting a

---

4. specifically 22q 11.2.

5. Also known as the Velo-Cardio-Facial Syndrome or DiGeorge syndrome or Shprintzen syndrome.

serious problem seen in cities throughout the United States. Some 20% to 40% of pregnant city-dwellers make their first visit to a physician or clinic after 20 weeks of pregnancy, thereby foreclosing opportunities for prenatal detection of serious fetal abnormalities for which they could have had an option to terminate a pregnancy.

CHROMOSOME 22 DELETION SYNDROME

This deletion syndrome occurs in about 1 in 4,000 individuals and is probably underdiagnosed because of the great variability of presenting signs. Even in families with the same deletion, there can be marked variation of the multiple possible signs, which is also the case between families. There are, in fact, a staggering number of signs emanating from involvement of virtually all body systems. Heart defects occur in 3 of 4 affected individuals and can be severe enough to eventually cause death despite efforts at surgical repair. Almost 7 of 10 affected individuals have problems with coordinating swallowing or having a cleft palate and/or cleft lip. While almost all have characteristic facial features, developmental delay or learning difficulties are seen in 70% to 90%. At least 3 of 4 experience some type of deficiency in their immune system, making them more susceptible to infection. About half the time, very low calcium levels are seen in the newborn where feeding problems, kidney abnormalities, and hearing loss may also be detected. There may also be growth hormone deficiency resulting in very short stature; auto-immune disorders causing, for example, arthritis or thyroid disorder; seizures; and bony abnormalities. There also appears to be an increased risk of malignancy involving organs such as the liver and kidneys.

Typically, review of the history of an affected adult reveals a pattern such as that seen in Jill, with structural abnormalities (such as heart and palate) followed by behavioral problems (attention deficit disorder or autistic features) followed in adulthood by psychiatric problems that include bipolar disorder (manic behavior and depression) or schizophrenia. The given explanation for the wide variability of signs in this disorder is the number of genes deleted at the chromosome 22q11.2 location and the presence of modifier genes from either parent that serve to influence the manifestations. The deletion wipes out a number of genes whose functions are then obviously lost. The size of the deletion may vary in families with differences in the number of genes deleted and, hence, the variability of signs in affected individuals. Complicating the issue even further is the finding of a deletion in the short arm of chromosome 10, which much less frequently causes a similar panoply of features in a similarly named syndrome. (In a very few cases, the deletion may have been missed because of being too small to detect by FISH or because there is a tiny mutation determinable only by sequencing the specific gene, which may not have been done.)

Treatment in this deletion syndrome is focused on the myriad symptoms and signs that originate from involvement of many organ systems. Structural defects of the heart, palate, and urinary/genital tracts are mostly surgically remedied. Treatment of low calcium levels is initiated as soon as diagnosed in the newborn or infant. Given increased susceptibility to infection, antibiotic treatment is usually initiated promptly. If growth hormone deficiency exists, a treatment schedule for long-term growth hormone therapy is initiated. Early intervention for speech, language, and intellectual delays should begin as early as age 1 year. Later, attention and intervention are necessary for manifestations of psychiatric illness.

In the approximately 7% of families in whom the deletion has been inherited from a parent, family members should be informed and FISH testing or microarray analysis (*see* Chapter 5) recommended. This would include the affected parent's siblings and parents and subsequently the nieces, nephews, and first cousins of proven affected members. All of these steps are best coordinated following genetic counseling by a genetic counselor or clinical geneticist. For all those found to be affected, in addition to initiation of appropriate treatment, future availability of prenatal diagnosis or preimplantation genetic diagnosis is emphasized.

For 7 years, Rita and Alex had ferried their son Joe to different hospitals to see developmental specialists and geneticists. Following an uneventful pregnancy, Joe had been born with a normal birth weight and no complications in the delivery or newborn period. He had gone home with his mother on day 3 of life and seemed to feed and suck well, although he seemed a little floppy. In retrospect, Rita acknowledged that compared to her other two children, Joe never looked her "smack in the eye" when she breast fed him. He accomplished walking a little late (18 months), but more importantly, no speech developed at all until he was 2 years old. Only then did he articulate a few relatively unintelligible words, and it slowly became clear from his lack of understanding simple directives that formal testing was needed, which concluded that he had moderate mental retardation.

Distraught by this realization, Rita and Alex took him to the best medical institutions in Boston, where a series of sophisticated genetic tests were done. No diagnosis emerged, and they remained bewildered that despite every effort, including many genetic tests, no cause had been recognized. Like so many other parents in the same situation, they wondered about what they each could have done to have caused Joe's significant cognitive impairments. They did recognize that he had a slightly unusual facial appearance with thin lips, straight eyebrows, and short philtrum (the skin between the nose and the central portion of the upper lip). He resembled no one in the family. Both his testes had not descended into his scrotum for which he had surgery for correction. He had always remained with low tone to his muscles. At age 3.5 years, autistic behavior became evident with hand-flapping, walking around in circles, and repeatedly making a high-pitched noise.

At age 7 years, he was referred to us at the Center for Human Genetics where he was seen by my son, Jeff. After a full history and examination, a blood sample was obtained and a chromosomal microarray test was initiated in our laboratories. The advent of this test was relatively recent and Joe had never had this analysis.

The result unexpectedly revealed a tiny duplication within the long arm of chromosome 7. Testing both parents with the same analysis to determine if this was simply a variation that had been inherited showed that neither parent had this duplication. At the same time, reports of other patients with this specific duplication had begun to appear and to be recognized as an unnamed microduplication syndrome.

Rita and Joe were staggered to realize that this was a spontaneous event that had not been inherited and would not be remediable. At least their worries that they had in some way caused Joe's delays were dispelled.

When no explanation can be found to explain a child's developmental delay, most parents will spend years shuttling between physicians and institutions seeking to learn the cause of their child's disability or birth defect. This parental search may be driven by various and sometimes compounding factors. Early on there is an urgent need to know with the hope that there might be a remedy, a cure, or an effective treatment or intervention. Concern about recurrence in a future pregnancy often ranks high in the reasons for the persistent search. Worries about their other children being carriers of a fatal flaw is yet another reason for a continued search. On occasion, parents are driven, sometimes by guilt, that either one or both of them did something that could have caused or contributed to their child's deficits. Some, for example, have told me about their taking illicit drugs or binge drinking, not realizing that pregnancy had begun. For the most part, but not always, those behavioral missteps have not been causally implicated.

Rita and Alex were no exception, and in their long journey they appeared for yet another consultation at a time when new genetic biotechnology became a clinical diagnostic reality. They learned that a tiny snippet incorporating a few genes in the long arm of chromosome 7 were duplicated in their son Joe. This was a new occurrence, the precise cause of which no one yet knows. A gene or genes in duplication interfere with gene function at a critical phase of brain and organ development in the embryo. Nothing they could have done in the past could have caused this duplication. The invariable step taken after the discovery of a duplication or a deletion is to test the parents and determine whether the child has inherited the precise structural chromosomal abnormality. Clearly, Joe did not inherit his specific duplication.

DELETIONS AND DUPLICATIONS

The newly acquired technical ability to effectively assess the number of single nucleotide bases (SNPs; *see* explanations in Chapter 5) made it possible to discover tiny and heretofore undetected duplications or deletions throughout our genomes. In 2007, the journal *Science* called this the discovery of the year. These submicroscopic structural chromosomal imbalances are now known as copy number variations (CNVs). Rapid application of the new technology has revealed that some 12% of our genome is **normally** involved in these various imbalances and almost certainly accounts to an important extent for the differences—physical and mental—that we see among us all. More detail about our genome through this technology has materialized in the past 5 years than in the last 50 years!

Assessment of CNVs enables determination of areas in our entire genome where there are too few or too many SNPs. Application of these new SNP microarrays (it's all done on a single chip) has been rapidly applied to the evaluation of children with birth defects or developmental delay. Not unexpectedly, this has resulted in the emergence of a host of newly recognized disorders and syndromes. Depending on the chromosome location of the microdeletion or microduplication, and which genes are involved, the recognition of a range of characteristic findings have been found that include many different birth defects, mental retardation, autism, limb abnormalities, unusual facial features, skeletal defects, epilepsy, genital abnormalities, low muscle tone, and growth delay.

An important limitation of the SNP microarray approach is the failure to detect a chromosome defect that does not involve any imbalance. As described in Chapters 4 and 5, translocations that are balanced would not be detectable by the SNP microarray. Similarly, a chromosomal inversion would be missed. The presence of either of these structural abnormalities have the potential for causing birth defects or mental retardation in future children. Hence, where appropriate and indicated because of family history, pregnancy history, or known or possible structural chromosome abnormalities, both parents should have a routine chromosome study prior to a new pregnancy. Fortunately, new technical advances are resolving this limitation, and balanced chromosome rearrangements will soon become determinable by microarrays.

The discovery that Joe had a newly recognized duplication in one of his chromosome 7[6] is particularly startling. This very location is the site of a very well-known disorder that results from a microdeletion that occurs at precisely the same spot, called William's syndrome. It turns out that among the variable number of genes that are deleted in William's syndrome is the elastin gene that codes for the elastic fibrous component in all of our organs and tissues. Consequently, just above the aortic valve, there may be narrowing (called aortic stenosis) or narrowing in the blood vessel going to the lungs (pulmonary stenosis). Facial appearance is distinctive, the voice may be hoarse, and there may be hernias, loose-jointedness, and soft, lax skin. Almost all have some degree of mental retardation, but a few have average intelligence. Their unique personalities are characterized by excessive friendliness, general anxiety, and attention deficit disorder. Short stature and other findings related to malfunction of glands that produce hormones may also occur.

The experience of Rita and Alex serves to inform those seeking an explanation for the cause of their child's unexplained developmental delay to request

6. More precisely, at 7q11.23

a chromosomal microarray analysis. This test has provided a detection rate in such cases of 10% to 20%. While no remedy for Joe's deficits is available, Rita and Alex are not at increased risk of having another similarly affected child.[7] Moreover, their other children can be reassured that they do not harbor the microduplication discovered some 7 years after Joe's birth.

One other important matter needs mention. When literally identical blocks of SNPs (therefore genes) are found at the very same locations on pairs of chromosomes (each one of a pair from one parent), suspicion is immediate that the child (most often studied) was conceived by a first-degree relative (a brother or father). Microarray studies in such cases are likely being done to evaluate disabilities or birth defects, which are frequent in children born of incestuous unions.

---

7. Germline mosaicism (*see* Chapter 2) has not been described yet for CNVs. Because this mechanism is possible, notwithstanding a low risk, prenatal diagnostic studies would be prudent in any future pregnancy.

EARLIER AND MORE SEVERE
GENETIC DISORDERS

They had fallen in love when they were both sophomores in college and had been inseparable since. Howard and June celebrated their graduation and their marriage simultaneously at a spectacular family function. They decided to wait for about 3 years before starting a family, allowing themselves time to develop careers and earn some money. Both were live-wires and were invariably the liveliest personalities at parties.

Some 3 years later, while they were both doing well at work, friends noticed that Howard seemed more irascible and not that easy to get along with anymore. Once an avid tennis player, he no longer accepted invitations to play. He commented to June that he felt clumsy. She, in turn, had noticed outbursts of temper that he had not previously exhibited.

At that time, they were under considerable stress, given the realization that Howard's father (whose forebears "came to America on the Mayflower," he would proudly proclaim) was steadily losing his faculties. Initially, he was diagnosed by his family doctor as having presenile dementia. Howard and June insisted that he consult a neurologist and it was not long after that a precise diagnosis of Huntington disease was made by DNA testing. Howard's paternal grandfather was thought to have had some type of dementia but had died suddenly from a heart attack. His father's younger brother had also shown signs of mental deterioration and had refused to be tested.

Since Howard and Jane were planning to start a family, they appropriately sought genetic counseling. They learned that Howard had a 50% risk of inheriting the Huntington gene mutation. It was explained to Howard that DNA testing could be predictive in determining whether he harbored the mutation his father had and would therefore be destined to eventually also lose his faculties as part of a slow-developing dementia. Howard promptly refused any testing and made it clear to June that he did not want to know.

As luck would have it, June found that she was already pregnant at the time and, as she reported later, was "stressed out of her wits." She realized, after the genetic counseling, that if they found that the fetus was affected, Howard would know that he was destined to disintegrate slowly just as his father was in the process of doing.

At 16 weeks of pregnancy, June decided to have prenatal studies and determine whether the fetus was affected and not to tell Howard if there was bad news. Her obstetrician drew a sample of amniotic fluid[1] and was dismayed to learn that commercial laboratories refused to accept the sample without appropriate prenatal genetic counseling. I received the obstetrician's call, who said that he had in his hands an amniotic fluid sample and was desperate to find a reliable laboratory that would accept a sample for prenatal DNA diagnosis for Huntington disease. He explained the situation and had me also speak to June on the telephone. Through her sobs, she made it clear that she could never rest again if she had a child who was destined to develop this degenerative neurological disorder and that she fully understood the mode of inheritance from her genetic counseling session she and her husband had before discovering her pregnancy.

I accepted the sample and we performed the required analysis in our laboratories. Fate was a passenger, and we found that the fetus was affected. I let the obstetrician know the information and subsequently learned that June had terminated the pregnancy, telling Howard that she had a miscarriage!

About 6 months later, I received a call from June who promptly told of her excitement and anxiety about her new pregnancy. She had consulted with a genetic counselor in the state in which she lived and was ready again to have a prenatal diagnostic study. This time, at 11 weeks of pregnancy, a tiny pinch of the developing placenta was biopsied (by chorion villus sampling),[2] and we received a sample for the Huntington disease DNA test. I vividly recall her joyful scream at hearing the good news that the fetus did not

---

1. The procedure called amniocentesis (see Chapter 7)
2. See Chapter 7.

166 YOUR GENES, YOUR HEALTH

have the Huntington disease mutation. Some 6 months later, June called to say how happy she and Howard were at the birth of their beautiful daughter. She had not told Howard about her prenatal genetic study.

What are you thinking now, having just read about June's dilemma and her actions? Was she a false and deceitful wife? Or was she an extremely sensitive and concerned partner who, although desperately wanting to have a child, wanted to protect the potential pain her husband would suffer upon knowing he had a fatal flaw? Was it justifiable for her to make an effort to avoid bringing a child into the world who, if affected, would suffer the consequences of earlier onset Huntington disease (note that this disease has been reported in a child younger than age 3 years).[3] Was she right to keep secret her knowledge that he had inherited the lethal gene? What type of marriage did this partnership represent that led June to take the actions she did? Should she have forgone the powerful maternal urge and, together with Howard, chosen adoption? Would he not then have had his anxiety precipitated by an act that all but suggested he was already affected? Was June's act purely selfish or was it courageous? After all, in the final analysis, she presented them with the joy they could both share for at least some years. Should she have avoided the abortion issue entirely and opted for artificial insemination by donor? Without her husband's consent, a whole series of thorny and unwanted issues could materialize later without warning.

Should June simply have taken every possible precaution not to become pregnant? Should she have told her husband about her intention to have a test and that she would not tell him the result? Her reactions and actions after obtaining a result would have provided as clear a message as simple speech. Was June's act purely out of love so that they could together, for as long as possible, enjoy their own child together, albeit with her knowing that Howard would steadily deteriorate over a 10- to 18-year period, during which time he would lose all his faculties and be totally dependent on her?

---

3. Milunsky JM, Maher T A, Loose BA, Darras BT, & Ito M. (2003) XL PCR for the Detection of Large Trinucleotide Expansions in juvenile Huntington's disease. *Clin Genet* 64: 70–73.

June was also not oblivious to the stress and chaos that she had witnessed in her in-law's family as Howard's father and his uncle progressively demented. She thought that Howard and his sister in particular had psychologically suffered in that family environment—a situation that she desperately wanted to avoid. She had also read a great deal about Huntington disease and fully recognized the phenomenon of anticipation in which the disease would begin earlier and earlier in the generations with increasing severity, especially when paternally inherited (see Appendix 4 for other disorders in which anticipation occurs).

And what would you have done if you had been in my shoes, with my responsibilities? Would you have told the obstetrician to throw away the amniotic fluid sample, which had been obtained with some risk to both fetus and mother? The issues were challenging and riddled with ethical complexities. The decision to accept the sample when no one else would was required immediately and would be irrevocable, as the amniotic fluid cells would die if not placed in cell culture within a day or two. My thoughts that dictated the action to accept the sample for study were clear. June had taken a significant personal risk, including the potential small (less than 1 in 200) risk of losing the fetus because of the amniocentesis procedure. Being neither policeman, nor judge, nor jury, I did not see my role as one that prevented her from achieving an outcome with a 50% likelihood of a normal child. Moreover, women have the legal right to determine what they do with their own bodies, including in pregnancy. Although on the face of it, some would find it distasteful, disturbing, or simply sad that Howard would be kept in the dark about June's actions, all would agree that he would be protected from grievous hurt by learning of his unwanted genetic burden and the grim consequences that he had witnessed in his father and which would devastate his future.

HUNTINGTON DISEASE

It was a virtual certainty that Howard's paternal grandfather had Huntington's disease. This condition is yet another in the group in which expansions of triplet repeats occur (*see* Appendix 3 and Chapters 5, 10, and 13). For this disorder, 36 or more CAG triplet repeats in the Huntington gene are involved. Once again, the greater the number of repeats, the earlier the onset and severity of the disease (the phenomenon called anticipation; *see* Appendix 4). We all have variable numbers of triplet repeats up to 35 in our two Huntington disease genes on our pair of chromosome 4 (yes, we all have this pair of genes, but it is only when there is a triplet expansion mutation, representing the key defect in one of these two genes, that this degenerative brain disorder occurs). For those who have 36 to 39 CAG repeats, Huntington disease may not develop, but those individuals may be at risk personally or for transmitting an expanding defect. The disease will invariably manifest for those who have 40 or more CAG repeats in one of their Huntington disease genes.

Howard's personality change and his recognition of clumsiness were typical signs that presage the appearance of full-blown disease. Signs of this disease become obvious in those affected mostly between ages 35 and 44 years. June had noticed that her father-in-law had frequent twitches, was not well-coordinated, and was frequently irritable and depressed. Over time, he had difficulty in walking; developed writhing, clumsy movements; and had difficulty swallowing and speaking clearly. (I remember one patient, who had a staggering gait, told me that he had been arrested once because a policeman thought he was intoxicated.) Sometimes, at least early on, psychiatric features are dominant and include depression, delusions, and hallucinations, as well as aberrant behavior. In the late stages of this neurodegenerative brain disorder, the original signs are compounded by difficulties in walking, inability to speak or swallow, and finally incontinence and inability to care for oneself.

June was also aware not only of how common depression was in this disorder but also the increased rate of suicide, a matter which further motivated her actions. She was also petrified by the realization that even very young children may manifest signs of Huntington disease (between 5% and 10% of all Huntington disease cases present before the age of 21). Moreover, in the very young affected child, seizures and severe mental deterioration with difficulty in walking and talking are typical.

The decision to be or not to be tested that Howard faced falls into the category of pre-symptomatic or predictive testing. Guidelines promulgated by the World Federation of Neurology Research Group on Huntington Chorea and the International Huntington Association largely govern the genetic counseling approach to predictive testing—especially, but not only, for Huntington disease. These guidelines are that important that they are reprinted and shown in Appendix 5. These necessary and rigorous guidelines are also valuable when predictive testing for other serious or lethal genetic disorders are considered. For all neurodegenerative or other disorders for which no cure or meaningful treatment can be anticipated in the foreseeable future, questions inevitably arise as to the wisdom of having a no-hope test.

Howard clearly decided that he did not wish to know whether he had inherited the culprit gene. Others whom I have seen in consultation have almost invariably also chosen not to know. Couples contemplating marriage who have come for genetic counseling have reacted in a number of different ways. In some, I have witnessed dissolution of their evolving relationship, even in the absence of testing—simply in the face of risk! Some have decided not to have any children, and yet in others I have seen marriages dissolve, sometimes even without testing.

Rarely, identical twins may appear for genetic counseling and considering predictive testing. First league trouble emerges when one twin decides not to know and the other twin wishes to have a predictive test. Clearly, in such a poignant situation, even without communicating the actual test result, the actions and reactions of the tested twin would be revealing. An important ethical tenet in such a case is to do no harm. In consideration of the balance of benefit, declining to test the twin who wishes to know would be an acceptable position in my view. Certainly, that twin has the right to seek and request such a test, but the physician and/or laboratory is not compelled to accept such an analysis. This cautious approach is additionally vested in the recognition of increased suicide rates among individuals at 50% risk of having inherited the Huntington disease gene mutation. A Vancouver group study of 107 centers in 20 countries assessed data on 5,781 individuals at risk for Huntington disease. Suicide was attempted by 21, with some 5 individuals having succeeded. Moreover, this was not a long-range study.

A further concern relates to those who chose predictive testing and were happy to hear that they had not inherited the Huntington disease gene mutation. In one study of these "happy" individuals, some 40% subsequently required psychotherapy! Survivor guilt is an issue with considerable mental health consequences. Fortunately, the vast majority in this situation can be helped with appropriate psychological counseling and can attain equanimity and ultimately deal well with their numbed emotions and problems in developing a lifeplan.

Just prior to the development of a predictive DNA test for Huntington's disease, one individual at 50% risk decided that he was clearly destined to develop the full-blown disease. Maintaining that he had no future, he spent, borrowed, and embezzled money only to discover when the test became available that he was in fact negative! In another case, the wealthy parents of a young child requested testing because the husband proved positive on a predictive test. Their purpose was effectively part of estate planning, stating that they would have another child if their current only child proved positive. Since the testing of young children for a genetic disorder for which there is no meaningful treatment or to determine their carrier status for no good reason is regarded as taboo, the option of preimplantation genetic diagnosis for the couple in question seemed more sensible.

Included among the important reasons not to test asymptomatic children for the Huntington disease gene mutation is the potential impact on the emotional and nurturing interaction with their parents. Knowledge that your child is destined to die prematurely may lead to a subconscious withdrawal of those many indefinable moments and gestures made by all parents with their growing children. An unexpected hug or kiss, a loving caress or word, a special treat, an expression of concern, a word of caution, a phone call to wish good luck, and on and on. During my care of seriously ill children with fatal chronic disease, I have seen, for example, mothers and fathers withdraw and not accompany the child to their appointment. An uncle or aunt might be called on to bring the child for the scheduled appointment and, when an important question about medication has arisen, I have directly called to discover both parents at home and the mother simply stating that she couldn't bear to bring the child to the clinic. The pain that mothers and fathers endure in these situations is heartbreaking to witness, as is the feeling of rejection experienced by the child.

Once a DNA diagnosis has been established and the child made aware of the condition, the emotional environment becomes tainted and is likely to seriously impair educational achievements and eventually have major implications for college and career success. Given the profound impact of a diagnosis made in childhood, the emotional burden for the parents is such that the information is almost impossible to contain. Consequently, others both in and outside the family learn the grim news, and eventually, both within and outside the family, a certain stigmatization eventuates. After all, how many of us are strong enough to befriend and hold close someone who is destined to die young? Once again, the child at the receiving end is bound to bear yet another despairing burden, with consequences on behavior, mental health, and educational attainment. Of course, performing a predictive test on a child prior to majority removes the choice of whether or not to have a predictive test. Given how difficult this decision is at older ages, a teenager cannot be expected to muster any sage-like wisdom that would adequately inform decision making.

Indeed, any such decision to be tested, which concluded with a positive result, might immediately reverse any plan for further education and career development. Since advances in human genetics have been so profound in recent years, imagine if some form of meaningful treatment (and it does not have to be gene therapy) emerges and a child has made irrevocable decisions not to pursue an education or commits suicide?

Given the rarity of a brand new mutation, an occasional family is encountered where neither parent appears to harbor the mutant Huntington disease gene. In such cases where the adult affected son or daughter has sought parental testing to track the mutation through the family for the benefit of those who could possibly avoid having children with this disorder, a finding that neither parent has the mutation raises questions of paternity or even undisclosed adoption.

Since no effective treatment currently exists, families might well first consider avoidance of this disease using preimplantation genetic diagnosis or, if not available, routine prenatal genetic diagnosis. The awesome realization that prenatal diagnosis can accurately detect a fatal genetic disorder that might only manifest many decades later can at least provide opportunities for preventing the later pain and suffering that can be anticipated. Thankfully, Huntington disease is not common. For those of Western European descent, the prevalence is somewhere between 1 in 14,500 and 1 in 33,000. Huntington disease occurs less frequently in Japan, China, and Finland and among African Blacks. In some smaller population groups of Western European descent, the frequency might reach 1 in 6,600.

The importance of confirming a clinical diagnosis by DNA analysis aimed at demonstrating the precise number of triplet repeats in the Huntington disease gene cannot be overemphasized. Simply having a clinical diagnosis based on neurological examination and imaging studies (magnetic resonance imaging) of the brain is not good enough. I recall one such case where the diagnosis was based only on the neurological examination and brain imaging study. The unfortunate middle-aged single woman then decided to give away most of her money and worldly possessions after receiving the grim prognosis for survival. More than a year later, feeling better and certainly not deteriorating, she sought another opinion, only to discover that a DNA test was negative for Huntington disease. The legal case that ensued did provide some redress. Yet additional caution is appropriate when precise testing for the Huntington disease gene proves negative in someone who is Black or of Black ancestral origins. There is another extremely rare disorder called Huntington disease-like II, which may be clinically indistinguishable from the classical type of Huntington disease. A completely different gene is involved, albeit also with triplet repeats (of the type CTG) as the mutation. This condition is also inherited as an autosomal dominant and all of the discussion on Huntington disease applies to this disease as well.

Treatment generally is aimed at managing symptoms, including the involuntary repetitive movements, stiffness and rigidity, and the psychiatric problems that are so common. Considerable promise is vested in the well-used mouse model of Huntington disease, where efforts have been ongoing to use pharmaceutical intervention aimed at the aggregation of toxic protein in the brain cells of those affected.

The other genetic disorders with triplet repeat expansions in their genes listed in Appendix 3 are dominantly inherited, except for Friedreich's ataxia in which the inheritance is autosomal recessive. The diagnostic, counseling, preventive steps, and therapeutic options are similar to those described for Huntington disease.

THE DETERMINATION TO HAVE A
HEALTHY CHILD

It was an exciting time of discovery in human genetics. New technological developments were enabling the discovery of precise localizations of an increasing number of genes related to serious genetic disorders. It was then that I saw Victoria and heard her story. I vividly recall her sitting on the edge of her seat, nervously clasping and unclasping her fingers. She was strikingly beautiful, with long flaxen hair, and was impeccably groomed. She was accompanied by her fiancé Harold, who was smart and well-dressed.

She planned to marry, Victoria related, but was extremely anxious because of her family history. Her maternal grandmother's brother had died at age 14 years from Duchenne muscular dystrophy (DMD). Her grandmother had one son and three daughters, including Victoria's mother. One of her aunts had a son who died at age 16 years from the same type of muscular dystrophy. Another aunt had a living son with the same diagnosis. Victoria, therefore, was worried that she might be carrying a gene with a fatal flaw and needed to determine whether she was a carrier and at risk for having an affected child.

I explained that the gene for DMD was carried on the female (X) chromosome. Because of the family history, it was clear that her maternal grandmother was a carrier and must have transmitted the gene with its mutation to at least two of her daughters (Victoria's aunts) because they each had affected sons. It was, however, uncertain whether Victoria's mother was a recipient of the same lethal gene, her risks being 50%. It was possible then to track the gene through linking markers through the family as long as we would be able to obtain a blood sample from all members of the family.

Victoria was dismayed and hesitant about this recommendation, more especially since her aunt who had lost her son had become reclusive after his death, while the other aunt with the affected son was not close to Victoria at all. I strongly urged Harold to help Victoria contact her relatives and arrange for them to come down to have blood drawn. It did take some 4 months to convince all family members and to obtain blood samples from the grandmother and her living unmarried sister, Victoria's uncle and two aunts, as well as her own mother, the affected first cousin, and his sister as well as her grandfather.

We proceeded with the linkage analysis and determined that Victoria was almost certainly a carrier, as of course were her mother and her living affected first cousin's sister. The family came for a group consultation, at which time I explained the results and the implications.

Victoria, who was only 21 years old at the time, returned 2 years later, married and wanting to start a family. We discussed the fact that if she conceived a male, there would be a 50% risk of DMD. A female offspring would have a 50% likelihood of being a carrier but would be otherwise unaffected. Moreover, because the gene had been cloned by Dr. Louis Kunkel in Boston, it was possible to make a precise determination of whether or not a fetus would be affected. The catch, however, was for this direct DNA test, we would have to determine the precise mutation in the DMD gene that caused the disorder in her first cousin, whose DNA we still had. This we accomplished with no great difficulty, and Victoria and Harold indicated their intention to have prenatal diagnostic studies when they achieved a pregnancy.

About 6 months later, Victoria called to arrange her prenatal DNA studies given that she would soon be 11 weeks along in her first pregnancy. A tiny pinch of the placenta was obtained by the procedure called chorion villus sampling (see Chapter 7) and we proceeded with the DNA studies. Sadly, it revealed that the fetus was male and affected. Victoria and Harold had indicated at the time they had the prenatal studies that they would terminate the pregnancy if affected. In her mind's eye, she had the constant image of the suffering first cousin who died and the wheelchair-bound living cousin who was racked by recurrent pneumonias and was slowly dying.

Later that year, Victoria returned pregnant again and planning for the prenatal genetic studies. Once again, we performed the mutation analysis and determined that the fetus was male and affected again. Victoria and

Harold were decimated. We discussed adoption and even obtaining a donor egg. They heard the alternative opportunities, knew the future risks, and were simply drowning in anguish. I provided as much understanding, support, and encouragement as was possible.

About 6 months later, Victoria called and yet again arranged for prenatal genetic studies for her third pregnancy. Their hopes were dashed again, when we discovered that the third pregnancy was an affected male fetus. For the third time, she terminated the pregnancy, was again filled with anguish and sadness, but expressed determination to have her own family.

Thankfully, in the next 2 years, with the assurance provided by prenatal diagnosis, she accomplished just that, first with an unaffected son, James, and a subsequent healthy daughter, Sandy.

For 16 years, I have received a Christmas card with photographs of their handsome son James and their beautiful daughter Sandy and have never failed to respond in acknowledgment of their joy, happiness, and determination.

Victoria's determination to succeed exemplified the triumph of the maternal urge over anguish. She displayed remarkable courage in the face of the adversity she suffered but was rewarded with two spectacular children. Her effort to marshall her entire family to provide blood samples was yet another measure of her will to succeed. The difficulty she encountered was mild compared to some of the experiences I have seen first-hand. Sad to say, completely intact and cooperative extended families are not as common as one might hope or expect. Family disputes, estrangements, divorce, distance, and many other factors all complicate situations where cooperation, as sought by Victoria, is necessary. I have even encountered two families where the mother of a daughter refused to provide a blood sample. One's initial dismay at such an act gives way to an understanding about guilt. In this X-linked disorder, DMD, women carry and transmit the culprit gene and its mutation.

Women carriers transmit the mutated gene to 50% of their male offspring who are affected and 50% of their daughters who are carriers. Although they, too, have inherited the gene mutation, genetic counseling may be necessary to ensure their understanding and assuage their feelings of guilt. Moreover, issues of personal health need consideration.

Women who carry the DMD mutation on one of their X chromosomes are at considerable risk themselves of developing heart rhythm abnormalities or heart failure caused by involvement of their heart muscle. Hence, mothers who are known carriers should have a thorough cardiac evaluation and thereafter at least every 5 years, or sooner, if there are symptoms or signs of heart trouble. On occasion, even heart transplantation is necessary if medical treatment fails and heart failure is intractable.

The major motivation for Victoria's persistent actions was her acute memory of her deceased first cousin. She recalled how, at age 3 years, he began to stumble when he ran and could not climb stairs, after having been perfectly well and physically able before that. She noted how he had difficulty standing up from a sitting position on the floor using his hands on his thighs to "climb up on himself." She painfully remembered how he became progressively weaker, even though his calf muscles seemed larger than normal, until he required a wheelchair when he was 10 years old. Thereafter, he had intermittent episodes of chest infection, and signs of heart failure supervened, until he died prematurely from pneumonia.

MUSCULAR DYSTROPHY

Duchenne muscular dystrophy is not rare, occurring in about 1 in 5,600 live male births. Victoria's memory of her cousin vividly captured the inexorable progressive deterioration in muscle strength that her deceased first cousin experienced. Diseased muscle may leak an enzyme, creatine kinase (CK), which is then found in above normal concentration in an affected person's blood. This test provides an early clue when the diagnosis is suspected. It is not, however, a good test to determine whether someone is a carrier of a DMD mutation.

The *DMD* gene, which of course we all have, is the largest in our genome. In DMD, a tiny deletion at a critical site in the gene is the common mutation, occurring in some 65% of boys with this disorder. The other 35% are accounted for by various other types of mutations that all interfere with the production of a protein called dystrophin. This protein also expresses its action in the brain, albeit originating in muscle. In some way, this accounts for the fact that boys with DMD frequently might also have learning difficulties and speech problems with demonstrable deficits in working memory and executive function. A general shift downward in the spectrum of IQ scores has been noted among boys with DMD.

Female carriers of a DMD gene mutation experience muscle weakness in about 20% of cases, and 20% to 25% develop potentially serious heart muscle problems (called cardiomyopathy). Early detection of heart involvement in both boys and carriers is important to preserve heart muscle function. Most commonly, a drug (ACE inhibitor) to improve muscle function is used together with a beta-blocker. Standard treatment is provided if heart failure occurs. Heart transplantation is offered to carriers with serious decompensation of heart muscle (called dilated cardiomyopathy). A cortisone drug such as prednisone is now routinely offered in the treatment of boys with DMD. However, a considerable number of untoward side effects have to be considered. These include excessive weight gain, decreased growth, marked acne, increased frequency of bone fractures in the long bones and spine, and behavioral changes.

Mothers who have had two boys with DMD and have no family history may have the gene mutation in their own ovaries, which may be made up of a mixture of both cells with a normal gene complement and some that house the DMD gene mutation. In this situation (called germline mosaicism; see Appendix 2), the mother's egg possessing the gene mutation may be fertilized and result in an affected boy or carrier daughter.

A less severe and more slowly progressive disorder, Becker muscular dystrophy (BMD), is transmitted precisely the same way as DMD. Indeed, all of the signs and symptoms are similar but appear a little later and have a slower progression. Hence, being wheelchair-bound usually occurs sometime after age 16 years. In contrast to DMD, where survival rarely reaches beyond the third decade, in BMD survival into the mid-40s is not uncommon. The identical gene mutations, including deletions, account for BMD.

Victoria used prenatal diagnosis and DNA tests to achieve her dream of a healthy family. Preimplantation genetic diagnosis is also an option that enables avoidance of abortion, as long as the precise mutation in the gene is known.

For Victoria, knowledge of her family history, the finally cooperating family members, availability of DNA from the affected living first cousin, and her determination made it possible for her to successfully have her two beautiful children, despite the overwhelming anguish she experienced.

Hank ("don't call me Henry") was a high-powered hedge-fund manager who ironically disliked personal risk. On a business trip to Boston from his home base on the West Coast, he arranged for a consultation because of his concern about his family history. Further, he had just married and plans were afoot to start a family. He was smart, aggressive, and possessed of an obsessive-compulsive personality. He stated that he was in good health and with the exception of some "morning stiffness," he had no complaints. However, from his days in biology in college, he remembered the importance of family history, which was why he had made the appointment. His maternal aunt had myotonic muscular dystrophy and had died suddenly at age 51 years. His own mother was diagnosed at age 45 years with cataracts in both eyes. His maternal grandmother apparently had some type of muscle disorder diagnosed when she was 57 years old. Hank had a sister who he said was in good health but who he had not seen for 2 years. They did not speak often. Apparently, she had a prolonged labor during her first and only pregnancy. Her daughter was born not breathing and required emergency resuscitation in the labor ward. The child was now apparently about 5 years old and clearly mentally retarded.

I explained that myotonic muscular dystrophy was the most common inherited muscle disorder among adults and that, besides muscle, it involved multiple organ systems including the eye, heart, nervous system, and the glands (endocrine) that produce hormones. His mother's early appearing cataracts, his sister's prolonged labor, and her child's failure to breathe at birth were typical for this dominantly inherited disorder. Moreover, his maternal aunt's sudden death may well have resulted from a heart rhythm abnormality, which is also typical for this disorder.

His physical examination only revealed a perceptible myotonia (delay in letting go of an object or of instantly unfurling clenched fingers).

He readily accepted the recommendation for DNA studies, given my clinical conclusion that he, too, had myotonic muscular dystrophy. He also understood that in this autosomal dominant condition, he had a 50% risk of transmitting the disorder to each of his offspring. He wondered why he and probably his sister had signs of this disorder so much earlier than his mother and maternal aunt as well as his maternal grandmother. I recall his look of incredulity when I told him about the phenomenon called anticipation. This occurs in a number of disorders (see Appendix 4 and Chapter 12) where the signs of a genetic disorder appear earlier and earlier over the generations. He left shaken and worried.

DNA studies we performed confirmed the diagnosis.

A few weeks later, he returned from California with his wife, having arranged prenatal studies for a pregnancy about which he had remained silent. They came for prenatal genetic studies, which quickly revealed that the fetus was affected. They decided to terminate the pregnancy. About 6 months later, he called to schedule yet another prenatal diagnostic study on his wife's pregnancy. Once again, a positive diagnosis led them to terminate the second pregnancy. About 9 months later, he called to say that tissue from a third pregnancy was being sent for prenatal diagnostic studies. Despite the 50% risk, the fetus in the third pregnancy was also affected, and the pregnancy was again terminated. A year elapsed before I next heard from him, seeking an appointment for him and his wife, now desperate to succeed, to discuss their options. Artificial insemination by donor was rejected outright. He wanted "his own child." Preimplantation genetic diagnosis was not yet available, and they were both unwilling to consider adoption. They both seemed very determined so it was no surprise to hear from them a few months later when he called excitedly to relate that his wife was pregnant again—this time carrying twins!

The excitement was short-lived. Chorion villus sampling of the placental tissues (see Chapter 7) from both twins revealed that one of the twins was affected. This result led to a flurry of consultations and a final decision to attempt pregnancy reduction. This process is performed by introducing a needle directly into the heart of the affected fetus and injecting heart-stopping medication. This was performed, and fortunately the pregnancy with the other twin remained intact.[1] Their daughter was born without complications, and I still have a photograph of this beautiful little girl that they had sent me for "the years of encouragement and support."

Typically for dominantly inherited disorders, there is considerable variability of symptoms and signs, even within the same family and the same gene mutation. An added dimension in myotonic muscular dystrophy is the potential for increasing severity of the disorder over the generations, seen in Hank's family with his sister's child born not

1. Fortunately the body resorbs the deceased twin. This is a common process. In 20% to 40% of all twins diagnosed in the first 12 weeks of pregnancy, one twin dies and is resorbed—called the vanishing twin.

breathing. Hence, there is this tendency for the disorder to manifest at progressively earlier ages with increasing severity.

Hank and his wife had to address the deeply distressing question of whether to seek fetal reduction or to have one of the twins born affected. The reader might be surprised to know that this is a procedure that is not infrequent, with specialized centers having done well over a thousand cases. Instances in which the one twin has a profound abnormality, such as most of the brain absent (called anencephaly), the procedure may well save the life of the healthy twin. Other instances of severe chromosome abnormality associated with likely death in the womb and a strong possibility of losing the entire pregnancy, including the healthy twin, may pose less of a significant dilemma. Much greater difficulty, however, is encountered when a viable but chronic disorder affects one of the twins (or triplets or quadruplets). Conditions such as Down syndrome or, in this case, myotonic muscular dystrophy are more problematic to many couples.

Given the frequency of assisted reproduction and the common result of multifetal pregnancy, reduction of the number of normal fetuses from 4 to 2 or 1 or from 3 to 2 or 1 is not uncommon. This step is predicated upon the realization that multiple pregnancy (especially high multiples) often end with prematurity. Even with today's technologies, very premature infants are at serious risk of major complications that bring lifelong burdens. For example, in a well-known quintuplet pregnancy, one was blind, one had a brain hemorrhage, two had cerebral palsy, and one was mentally retarded.

An analysis of 1,000 consecutive cases of multifetal pregnancy reductions at the most experienced center in the United States[2] showed that the entire pregnancy was lost in 4.7% of cases. More than 95% delivered after 24 weeks of pregnancy. Lower rates of loss (2.1%) were noted when reduction was done from twins to a singleton. Higher-order pregnancies (triplets, quadruplets, etc.) clearly have higher risks than twin pregnancies for most of the important maternal and newborn complications, including fetal and neonatal death, without any procedures. As expected, survival is more likely in nonidentical twins (in two sacs) than in identical twins sharing the same enveloping sac.

---

2. Mount Sinai Medical Center, New York

MYOTONIC MUSCULAR DYSTROPHY

This type of muscular dystrophy belongs to a small group of well-known disorders (Appendix 3) that share a single mutational mechanism. The single nucleotide bases (ACGT) discussed in Chapter 5 occur in expanded runs of repeated triplets. For this disorder, CTG repeat triplets occur as if "stuttering repeatedly" to constitute a remarkable length (even several thousand) and thereby interfere with the function of the myotonic dystrophy gene. Generally, the greater the number of these triplet repeats, the more severe the signs of the disorder. The diagnosis is of course made by DNA analysis that demonstrates the precise number of CTG repeats. Normally we each have between 5 and 34 CTG repeats in this gene, but when there are more than 50, signs of this disease can be expected. Repeat numbers between 35 and 49 are not likely to be associated with symptoms or signs, but that individual's children are at risk of inheriting a larger repeat size and being affected. Hank and his family were able to benefit from the molecular diagnosis that assessed these repeat numbers and that were clearly elevated in the affected twin.

The characteristic signs of myotonic muscular dystrophy were mostly exemplified by the various members of Hank's family. The early appearance of cataracts even without myotonia (sustained muscle contraction) is noteworthy for this disorder, but of course there are many other causes of cataracts. The sustained muscle contraction interferes with an individual's inability to quickly release their hold on an object or a hand grip. Many will complain of muscle weakness, especially in the leg, hand, and neck. Frequently the facial muscles are expressionless. In an affected newborn (almost invariably from an affected mother), the infant is floppy and weak, may have a club foot, and may not breathe spontaneously. The latter situation is an emergency and, if not immediately recognized and treated, can lead to irreparable brain damage and mental retardation. In such cases, mental retardation occurs in more than 50% of infants born affected.

Myotonic muscular dystrophy usually becomes obvious between ages 20 and 40 years. Diabetes also occurs more frequently, and heart rhythm disturbance may occur in as many as 90%. Hence, an affected person experiencing palpitations or irregular heart beats should seek immediate attention as these cardiac conduction defects can be fatal if not remedied immediately. In some affected individuals, there is progression of the weakness to the point of wheelchair confinement.

During pregnancy, women with myotonic muscular dystrophy have an increased risk of pregnancy loss, prolonged labor, and even excessive bleeding after birth. Some report diminished kicking and moving by the fetus. Affected women should seek pregnancy and delivery care with maternal-fetal medicine specialists.

Thankfully, the average worldwide prevalence of this disorder is only about 1 in 20,000, although in some areas, such as Quebec, it is more common.

Although there is no specific cure or treatment, attention to the various potential complications can save lives. For example, consultations with a cardiologist and early and prompt treatment of cardiac rhythm disturbances are important. Cataracts can be removed and diabetes treated. Physical therapy and occupational therapy are important, and wheelchair and other assistive devices may ease the burden. Considerable care needs to be exercised for anyone with myotonic dystrophy requiring anesthesia, where complications occur more frequently.

Finally, it is important to contact family members once a diagnosis has been established so they may have the option of being tested, treated, and able to consider prenatal genetic diagnosis.

14

IRREVOCABILITY AND ACCEPTANCE

Among the first patients I ever saw after arriving in Boston decades ago was a warm-hearted, loving mother named Angela, who adored her children. She had brought her second son Sal (short for Salvatore) for his continuing care in the cystic fibrosis (CF) clinic that I had inherited from a predecessor. I systematically reviewed Sal's health status at the time with special reference to his productive cough and the state of his stools. I remember that Sal already had a chronic cough productive of yellow-green sputum, cultivation of which yielded the feared bacteria.[1] This lung infection was resistant to all oral antibiotics at the time and could only be successfully treated by intravenous antibiotics, which rarely banished the infection. He also took three enzyme supplements to aid his digestion of fats to counter the insufficient function of his pancreas. Angela was also administering chest percussion therapy to help rid his lungs of the tenacious and highly viscous mucous that was so difficult to expectorate. His physical examination showed him to be small for his age, underweight, and with a moist chest. Angela was well-informed about the necessary care Sal needed and was also aware of the severely limited life expectancy known at that time.

A few weeks later, Angela was back at the clinic with her fourth child, Bruno. Prior to having Sal, she had a son Alex, and between Sal and Bruno, she had a daughter Nadia. Bruno, at that time 1 year old, also had CF. Once again, I reviewed his health and current treatment and we spent considerable time revisiting the facts of CF with special reference to the high mortality for this autosomal recessive disorder and the 25% risks in each

1. Pseudomonas Aeruginosa

pregnancy for having an affected child. It was then that she impressed upon me that whatever happened to her reproductive life was simply her destiny. She and her husband Mario were staunch Catholics and "believed that the Lord had a purpose for everything." Prenatal diagnosis was not available in those years.

The following year, she became pregnant again and delivered a beautiful baby girl. It was evident on the first day of life that this child too had CF. This baby girl's first stool did not emerge,[2] because she had an intestinal obstruction that required surgical intervention. Recovery initially was uneventful, but within a week of surgery, an overwhelming staphylococcal pneumonia took hold and the baby died at age 9 days. That was the first wake I attended, and it simply broke my heart. It also seemed too much for Mario, who I learned later began to drown his sorrows in alcohol. Angela, the rock of their household, confided about her worst fears for Mario who, she said, could not bear the dawning reality that the lives of Sal and Bruno would also be truncated.

The ensuing years with endless visits to the clinic, punctuated by hospital admissions for both Sal and Bruno, saw a steady deterioration in their health. Angela had been spending virtually all her time caring for these two sick children, while her eldest son, Alex, who received comparatively scant attention, became a juvenile delinquent. Bruno, then 8 years old, became critically ill with an intractable pneumonia and died despite heroic efforts to save him. A year later, Mario was diagnosed with cirrhosis of the liver caused by alcohol, and he went into liver failure soon thereafter and also died. Angela's stoicism in the face of such overwhelming tragedy was nothing less than awe-inspiring. In those years. she cried often when she was in the consulting room without Sal. He had insisted on being seen without his mother in the room. I, too, had tears at the overwhelming sadness that enveloped the family.

At age 15 years, Sal came down with yet another bout of pneumonia, which, this time, proved resistant to all treatment, and he too died.

Angela moved out of state but would call me at least twice a year for many years thereafter, simply to say hello and keep in touch. During one such call, she confided that a diagnosis of breast cancer had just been made and that she faced a mastectomy. We spoke frequently during those awful months. Sadly, her cancer had spread and when I visited her at home

---

2. Called meconium ileus

2 weeks before she died, we talked at length about her life and her children. She never regretted having them, but had always been anguished by their suffering. A dozen years after her passing, she remains for me a model of a strong, loving, caring, and deeply religious mother.

Chronic serious illness has the potential for eroding the very fabric of a family. It is a tribute to Angela that even in the face of overwhelming sadness, she was able to keep the family together and move forward. She was ably assisted by Mario's mother, herself a model of love and kindness. The stress, however, was ever-present and touched the lives of everyone in the family. Mario had told me years before his death that he could not face the anticipated early death of his two boys with CF. No amount of talking helped. Referral to a psychotherapist was declined. The solace he found in alcohol provided no solution either and he admitted it gave but brief respite.

As Sal entered his teen years, he became progressively more isolated. Earlier friends seemed to melt away as his chronic cough produced increasing volumes of yellow-green infected mucous. Because of his diminished lung function, he was unable to participate in sports and again felt excluded. The sicker he became, the greater the isolation he experienced. Fortunately, Angela and Sal's paternal grandmother remained close and caring. The reader might find this parental and grandparental response perfectly normal and not worth mentioning. However, and not infrequently, I have witnessed in similar situations an emotional withdrawal by a parent, sibling, or grandparent. It is as though, in anticipation of loss, emotional support is withdrawn subconsciously, almost as a self-protective mechanism to lessen personal pain.

Certainly the all-pervasive effects of chronic illness not infrequently tear the family apart. The list of troubles will be readily acknowledged by families with children suffering chronic serious illness. Recurrent hospitalizations and repeated visits to the doctor prove time-consuming and tension-producing, let alone exhausting. Demands for attention, including schoolwork by the other children, add another level of concern. Very often, even in the face of adequate medical insurance, money issues can become serious. Exhaustion, tension, anger, and frustration singly or together frequently predispose to sexual dysfunction, thereby breeding even more upset and anger. When one parent fails to share the burden (not uncommon), managing becomes even harder. Exhaustion over years without respite is especially dangerous to the continuing integrity of the family. Inevitably, attention to personal health of each parent gets ignored, occasionally with grievous consequences.

Lack of attention to the healthy children in the family may lead to acting out, as was the case with Alex and juvenile delinquency. No matter how dedicated, there are only 24 hours in a day, and parents are not inexhaustible engines.

My care of this family occurred before the discovery of the CF gene (*CFTR*) in 1989. Subsequently, from DNA that we had banked from Sal and Bruno, we determined by analysis of the CF gene (*CFTR*) that both boys carried two copies of the common severe mutation in the *CFTR* gene.[3] We subsequently showed that their daughter Nadia and some of her nieces and nephews on either side of the family were carriers of this common mutation. All those found to be carriers were advised to have their partner tested in the fullness of time when they planned to have children. Alex proved not to have the mutation.

CYSTIC FIBROSIS

Cystic fibrosis is a multisystem disease involving multiple organs, but with special reference to the respiratory tract, the pancreas, intestine, liver, and gall bladder system. The main problem relates to faulty movement of ions, such as sodium and chloride, and water through channels within cell walls, especially where mucous is made. As the primary consequence of this defect created by mutations within the *CFTR* gene, mucous in the lungs becomes highly viscous and difficult to cough up. In the intestine, the sticky mucous admixes with the meconium (the first stool of a child) and causes obstruction in 15% to 20% of newborns with CF, as it did in Angela and Mario's baby who died. Defective movement of ions also occurs in the sweat glands, resulting in abnormally

---

3. The common mutation is the ΔF508, which occurs in about 7 of 10 people with CF. When one copy is inherited from each parent, the more severe form of CF occurs. There are "milder" mutations among the more than 1600 that have been discovered thus far.

high levels of salt in the sweat. Indeed, measurement of sodium and chloride in the sweat facilitates the diagnosis of CF in the vast majority of cases.

I recall an undiagnosed 21-year-old patient with CF who worked as a truck driver. He told me that in summer, he became very hot and sweaty in his truck with salt crystallizing on the steering wheel! He had ascribed his chronic cough to smoking since age 12 years.

Many of the chronic complications of CF develop as a result of the sticky mucous. First in the lung, the mucous provides a ready medium for bacteria to flourish and over time to cause irreparable damage to the airways. The sinuses almost invariably become involved as well, with chronic sinusitis. Sticky mucous causing obstruction in the pancreas destroys the architecture of that organ and not infrequently leads to diabetes. About 90% of those with CF suffer pancreatic insufficiency that impairs their digestion of fats and fat-soluble vitamins and that requires the taking of enzyme supplements with every meal. Sticky mucous in the gall bladder increases the formation of gall-stones and associated complications.

Greater than 95% of males with CF are infertile. The cause is obstruction in the tubes (the vas deferens) through which the sperm is transmitted from the testes out to the penis. Affected men simply have no sperm in the ejaculate, but they are not sterile. For men intent on having their own children, sperm can be recovered through a procedure in which a needle is introduced into the testes[4] and sperm is aspirated. Fertilization can then be accomplished in a dish after harvesting an egg from their partner (a process called in vitro fertilization or IVF).

A married male patient with CF I saw some years ago announced during one of his routine visits that he was the proud father of a newborn daughter. Keeping in mind the dictum to *do no harm*, I simply communicated hearty congratulations. Almost 1 year later, during a routine visit, he mentioned that he had been scouring the Internet and discovered that most men with CF are infertile. I did confirm that this was usually the case. I learned later that he discovered his wife's infidelity, which led to the dissolution of his marriage.

There is also a well-known condition in which the vas deferens is absent or not properly formed, again resulting in the delivery of semen without sperm. These men invariably have at least one recognizable CF mutation and in up to

---

4. A procedure called epididymal sperm aspiration and used in IVF for the procedure called intracytoplasmic sperm injection.

two-thirds may have two "mild" mutations. Curiously, they have no lung or pancreatic disease and no evidence of multisystem CF. Nevertheless, it is important if they wish to have a family that their partner have an analysis, first for mutations in the *CFTR* gene and, if negative, sequencing of the entire gene.

Cystic fibrosis is the most common lethal genetic disease in Whites. About 1 in 3,000 Whites[5] and between 1 in 4,000 and 1 in 10,000 Hispanic-Americans are born with this disorder, and there are at least 30,000 affected individuals in the United States. The frequency of carriers among Whites ranges between 1 in 22 and 1 in 28.

Six common founder CF gene mutations are shared among Ashkenazi Jews, and as a consequence, analysis of these most common mutations yields a detection rate for carriers that approximates 98%. After testing for the most common 40 to 100 mutations in Whites, the detection of carriers reaches 90% and goes up to 95%; for African-Americans, the detection rate is 69%. The detection rate for Hispanic-Americans approximates 57% and is unknown for Asian-Americans. Sequencing of the entire *CFTR* gene and analysis for any deletion or duplication in the gene enables recognition of more than 98% of all mutations.

Because CF is such a serious debilitating disorder, testing for carriers in a couple **planning** to start a family is important. If both partners are found to be carriers, there is a 25% risk of having an affected child. In such instances, options include preimplantation genetic diagnosis, prenatal diagnosis, artificial insemination from a tested donor, adoption, or not having children. Abortion should not be the option of choice when preconception testing is the standard recommendation. However, about 50% of pregnancies are unplanned, and consequently, carrier couples are discovered not infrequently already with established and even advanced pregnancies.

Care of those with CF is best provided in CF clinics, where the assembled expertise can assure appropriate care of the lungs, sinuses, malabsorption, diabetes, liver disorder, gallstones, infertility, and very careful attention during pregnancy. Avoidance of dehydration and excessive salt loss is important, especially in the summer, when salt tablets might even be necessary. Smoking in the household in which a CF patient lives should be avoided. Fortunately, life expectancy has improved dramatically over the past few decades. The U.S.

---

5. The frequency among African-Americans is 1 in 15,000 and among Asian-Americans 1 in 31,000.

Cystic Fibrosis Foundation's projected life expectancy exceeded 37 years in 2007. Today many patients are in their 40s and 50s, and some are even in their 60s. On occasion, however, in the face of severe lung disease, heart or heart/lung transplantation becomes a consideration. This should be considered as a desperate step and not a primary option. Hopefully continuing research will provide opportunities for the development of gene therapy in the not-too-distant future. Meanwhile, every effort should be made to maintain the lungs in as best a condition as possible for as long as possible. Avoidance of CF can be achieved by preconception carrier testing of a couple, informing relatives of the need to be tested if a carrier is found in the family and considering the options discussed above, including preimplantation diagnosis.

He was tall and handsome, with blonde hair, blue eyes, and rippling muscles. As his wife Jean told me, Bill was the life of every party and since his army days had indulged in drinking more than he should. "Just like his father," said Jean, on repeated visits when she shepherded each of her three adult sons separately in to see me for a consultation. Bill's father died at age 52 years with a diagnosis of cirrhosis of the liver complicated by liver cancer and diabetes. An autopsy was never done. Given his fondness for the bottle, it was always assumed that he had developed an alcoholic cirrhosis.

At Bill's 45th birthday party, Jean told me that she had watched him cavorting around the dance floor with what seemed to her to be some difficulty. She also noticed that his skin color seemed darker than it used to be, although he had no significant sun exposure through the cold Northeast winter. She had also realized that his sexual ardor seemed dampened and quite out of character, compared to his previous "appetite." She also thought that he was intermittently impotent. Jean finally convinced Bill to see their family doctor.

Bill was referred to me for a genetics consultation by his family doctor who, after a few liver function tests, began to suspect a genetic disorder. On direct questioning, Bill admitted to being more fatigued than usual in the past year or two and that his joints ached but were never swollen. He occasionally had abdominal pain and he admitted to a diminished libido. He ascribed his symptoms to "drinking too much," which he said probably explained the increased levels of liver enzymes that his doctor had noted when the blood test results returned from the lab.

Physical examination was not especially remarkable. Having never seen him before, I could not know with any certainty that his skin color had changed to a darker shade. His joints were fine and his liver was not enlarged. Systematic examination was effectively unrevealing.

Bill mentioned his three brothers who lived in-state and who were apparently well. Bill and Jean also had three sons, all in their teens.

I explained to Bill that his family doctor had noted an increased level of iron in his blood, raising the question of an alcohol-damaged liver or the autosomal recessive condition called hemochromatosis. I remember him feeling certain that the latter genetic suggestion was absurd but well recall a deep frown when he remembered the cirrhosis and liver cancer that took his father. He was not particularly keen to provide another blood sample for DNA analysis, until I reminded him that while it was in his best interest, it was definitely important for his boys' sake.

Analysis of the hemochromatosis gene (HFE) soon revealed that Bill had inherited the common HFE mutation from each of his parents. During a subsequent visit to discuss these results, Bill pointed out that his mother was and continues to be healthy. Slowly he began to understand how recessive genetic disorders are transmitted and that his mother must be a carrier with one copy of the HFE mutation, while his late father may have had hemochromatosis and two copies of the common mutation. Bill therefore understood that his father, if he had hemochromatosis, would have passed one copy of the common mutation to Bill and his three brothers. The fact that his mother was a carrier and his father probably affected meant that Bill and each of his three brothers had a 50% likelihood of developing hemochromatosis. Further, Bill would automatically pass one copy of the common mutation to each of his boys. For a brief moment, he expressed relief that they would only be carriers and not affected. That brief moment dissipated in a minute, when I drew attention to the fact that his wife, Jean, had about a 1 in 10 to 1 in 12 likelihood of being a carrier of a mutation for hemochromatosis.

In due course, Jean brought the boys in for testing, one by one. Two were indeed revealed only as carriers, but the third turned out also to have hemochromatosis, having received the mutation from both Jean and Bill. Discovery of the common gene mutation in Jean provided the expected confirmation. Over the next few months, DNA mutation analysis of the HFE gene in Bill's three brothers revealed that all actually had hemochromatosis and did not know it. Between them, the brothers had 10 children, all of whom would automatically be carriers at the very least and would require confirmatory testing. Jean's siblings were also tested and two of the four were found to be carriers. Their children were also to be tested. Jean's parents had died—her father from non-Hodgkin's lymphoma and her mother from kidney failure.

When Bill's father died, it was assumed that his cirrhosis was caused by alcohol and that the liver cancer was a consequence. No one recognized the possibility that the cirrhosis, liver cancer, and diabetes were typical features of hemochromatosis. Moreover, the lack of an autopsy delayed the recognition of hemochromatosis in Bill's father's four sons. This was unfortunate, particularly for one of Bill's brothers, who, upon testing, was found to not only have hemochromatosis but also established cirrhosis and was therefore at risk for developing liver cancer. This was especially unfortunate given the availability of very effective treatment for hemochromatosis (*see* below).

Over the past few decades, there has been an increasing failure by physicians to recommend autopsies when there is a lack of clarity or precision about a diagnosis. Families, too, have often not been keen to subject their loved one to an autopsy. The fact is that it is not uncommon for diagnostic surprises to emerge at the time of autopsy and, not infrequently, have implications for the health of other family members.

HEMOCHROMATOSIS

Hemochromatosis is the most common genetic disease, with somewhere between 1 in 200 and 1 in 400 Whites being affected. Between 1 in 10 and 1 in 12 Whites carry an HFE mutation. This disorder is much less common among African-Americans and is extremely rare among Asians. About 1 in 35 Hispanics are carriers.

The symptoms and signs evidenced by Bill were typical. The test his doctor did initially not only indicated liver dysfunction but also an elevated level of serum iron and iron-transporting proteins (ferritin and transferrin). These tests are not specific, hence, a precise diagnosis by DNA analysis of the *HFE* gene is usually necessary. This would be important because initiating treatment should be based on an exact diagnosis.

Additional problems that emerge are caused by the primary defect in this disorder. Normally, the intestine has a barrier that prevents most of the iron in our diet from being absorbed into the body. In hemochromatosis, it is as if the body's barrier has become a leaking sieve, enabling much larger quantities of iron to enter the bloodstream and be deposited, especially in the liver, pancreas, heart, testes, joints, and skin. Excessive deposits of iron interfere with organ function, and consequently, in addition to the features already described, heart failure and rhythm disturbances resulting in death may occur, as well as testicular dysfunction with resulting impotence and/or loss of libido.

When routine blood tests reveal elevated iron, ferritin, and transferrin levels in the absence of any definitive symptoms or signs, continuing monitoring twice a year is usually adequate. However, when symptoms and signs are present, the usual treatment is to remove excess iron by weekly phlebotomy, taking a pint of blood each time until the concentration of ferritin has reached an acceptable level. The initial period of bloodletting may continue for 2 or 3 months and, thereafter, every 3 to 4 months for men and perhaps once or twice a year for women.

Liver transplantation is the only available treatment for cirrhosis of the liver if liver failure has supervened. Affected individuals should be advised to avoid eating raw shellfish.[6] Avoidance of iron-containing medicines or mineral supplements is also advised, as well as high doses of vitamin C (which enhances iron absorption). Minimal alcohol (if at all) and reduced red meat consumption (iron content) is advisable. Early and appropriate monitoring and treatment would allow a normal life expectancy. While prenatal diagnosis is possible for this highly treatable disorder, it is hardly ever utilized. Bill's symptoms and signs were subtle, and but for an observant and caring wife, a timely diagnosis would have been missed. His brother was not as fortunate. Bill's father almost never consulted a physician until his final fatal illness. His sons copied that risky behavior, avoided annual visits, and one son is destined to prematurely lose his life, too.

Although we may be born with a genetic disorder, it may take decades to manifest. That is a common reality for a remarkable number of inherited diseases, thereby making for a cogent imperative to always ask, "Is it genetic?"

---

6. Shellfish can contain a bacterium called vibrio vulnificus, which could cause death in a person with high iron levels.

15

ANCESTRAL GENETIC BURDENS

They were an interesting, if not improbable, couple. Jim was the son of a Presbyterian minister of Scottish descent whose wife had been a nurse with uncertain ancestral origins. He had become a child psychiatrist. He had a somewhat disheveled appearance, a droopy right eyelid (called ptosis), a small goatee, and prematurely graying hair. Jim's wife, Anna, on the other hand, was a go-go realtor—loud, ostentatious, with an infectious laugh and an Oscar de la Renta pant suit. She had been advised by a physician client to whom she had recently sold a house that preconception testing for Tay-Sachs disease for those of Ashkenazi Jewish ancestry was a must, after she confided that it would be her last sale since she had just discovered her first pregnancy. Jim came along with Anna under considerable protest, stating vociferously, even in the office, that his Presbyterian roots made testing unnecessary to determine whether he was a carrier of a gene mutation for Tay-Sachs disease. Anna was having none of it and simply insisted that he yield and provide a blood sample, which he duly did.

Given the frequency of Tay-Sachs disease carriers among those of Ashkenazi Jewish ancestry (1 in 25 to 1 in 30), it was no surprise that Anna was found to be a carrier of a common mutation in the Tay-Sachs disease gene. I well recall a sense of dismay when Jim's result also revealed that he, too, carried a different mutation in the same Tay-Sachs disease gene. Did someone in the laboratory mislabel a sample or confuse Jim's sample with another individual since many samples were run simultaneously? Double-checking the laboratory worksheets and repeating the analysis still left me with a sense of unease. I communicated the results but strongly recommended that Jim return for a second sample. This time, Jim arrived with considerable indignation and absolute certainty that some mistake had been made in our laboratories.

The repeat analysis showed the identical Tay-Sachs disease gene muta-tion noted in the original sample from Jim. The tense counseling session that followed 2 weeks later focused particularly on their 25% risk of having a child with Tay-Sachs disease. They opted for prenatal studies that were performed at 16 weeks of pregnancy via amniocentesis-derived amniotic fluid cells, which yielded a result indicating that the fetus was a carrier of Jim's mutation but not affected by the disease. At 9 months, almost to the day, Anna delivered a beautiful daughter, whom she named Audrey "in everlasting appreciation."

Following my recommendations, Anna saw to it that her three siblings and both her parents were tested. One of the three siblings proved to be a carrier of the Tay-Sachs disease gene mutation that Anna carried, as did her mother. Her mother was an only child whose parents had perished in the Auschwitz concentration camp. Jim's siblings declined testing, as did both his parents.

Jim proffered the opinion that he probably represented a brand new mutation in the Tay-Sachs disease gene but quickly reconsidered when the uncertainty of his mother's ancestral origins came into focus. It is indeed highly likely that his mother too had inherited the same gene mutation, which in all likelihood had been transmitted over a number of generations and originated in someone of Ashkenazi Jewish origin[1] in the past. For all the ethnic-related genetic disorders, it is important to recognize that they also occur in many other racial or ethnic groups, albeit uncommonly or rarely. At the time of Anna's pregnancy, the standard was to offer testing for the carrier state for Tay-Sachs disease only. Today, the requirement is to also test for another neurodegenera-tive disorder called Canavan disease, which also occurs with increased frequency among those of Ashkenazi Jewish origins. We and other genetic diagnostic centers routinely test (preferably at preconception) primarily couples of Ashkenazi (Eastern European) ancestry for at least 11 different disorders,[2] in addition to cystic fibrosis. The guideline we use

---

1. Although there is still some argument, recent multicenter population genetic studies led by geneticist H. Ostrer recognized distinctive Jewish population clusters, each with shared Middle Eastern ancestry and variable degrees of European and North African admixture.

is to test for the carrier state when the frequency approximates 1 in 100 (*see* Table 15.1).

Founder effects, as was probably the case for Jim's mother's origins, are not uncommon, especially for the rarer genetic conditions. Not too long ago, for example, a frequency approximating 1 in 25 for Tay-Sachs disease carriers was noted among non-Jewish French Canadians. Initial speculations included a story that once upon a time, a Jewish salesman came sailing down the Saint Lawrence waterway and dropped his genes a number of times (!). Years later, following the cloning of the Tay-Sachs disease gene and recognition of three common mutations among Ashkenazi Jews, it was realized that the common mutation among French Canadians was completely different.

Jim and Anna, who initially had no idea about Tay-Sachs disease, became especially anxious when I explained the signs and consequences of this lethal disease. Sadly, I have seen a number of children with Tay-Sachs disease, and memories of them have never faded. These affected babies are often beautiful, with porcelain- doll-like features (probably resulting from the deposition of complex fats called gangliosides in their tissues). For the first 3 to 6 months, normal development of skills are seen, and babies may get to a sitting position. Thereafter, however, they become increasingly floppy, topple over, cannot seem to focus, and startle easily to a sudden noise or movement. Despite their floppiness, their reflexes may be brisk. Steadily, they deteriorate with increasing spasticity, difficulties in swallowing, seizures, blindness and eventual unresponsiveness, lapsing into a vegetative state, never having spoken. Death invariably supervenes from pneumonia between ages 2 and 4 years.

Fortunately, prenatal diagnosis was available for Jim and Anna, and they were spared the need to address the question of whether to terminate a pregnancy with an affected fetus. Today, early diagnosis by preimplantation genetic diagnosis is available at 11 weeks of pregnancy, or by prenatal diagnosis at 15 to 16 weeks when amniocentesis would otherwise be performed.

---

2. Tay-Sachs disease, Canavan disease, Niemann-Pick disease Type A, Gaucher disease, Bloom syndrome, Fanconi syndrome, familial dysautonomia, maple syrup urine disease, mucolipidosis IV, glycogen storage disease I, and Factor XI.

Anna realized the importance of tracking the mutation through her family, thereby discovering that one of her siblings was also a carrier. That sister had not yet had children and had the advantage of being put on the alert to be certain that her partner would also be tested. In the fullness of time, Jim and Anna's offspring would be informed about her carrier status so that they, too, would be in a position to avoid an unnecessary tragedy.

TAY-SACHS DISEASE

Despite the increased frequency of Tay-Sachs disease among Ashkenazi Jews, this disorder has occurred in children of virtually all ethnic, racial, and religious groups. While the carrier rate among Ashkenazim approximates 1 in 30, for non-Jews and Sephardic Jews, the carrier frequency is between 1 in 250 and 1 in 300. Some originally genetically isolated population groups such as French Canadians in the eastern Saint Lawrence River Valley area of Quebec, the Cajuns of Louisiana, and the Old Order Amish in Pennsylvania have all been found to have carrier frequencies for Tay-Sachs disease similar to those observed among Ashkenazim.

While more than 100 different mutations have been reported in the Tay-Sachs disease gene (called *HEX-A*), analysis of the three most common mutations enables determination of 94% of carriers among Ashkenazi Jews. Among French Canadians, there is a characteristic mutation represented as a deletion within the gene. Of course, that is not the only mutation that might occur. Fortunately today, the frequency of infants born with Tay-Sachs disease has been cut by 90% because of the systematic offer of screening or testing prior to or early in pregnancy. It is now likely that more infants with Tay-Sachs disease are born to non-Jews in the United States as a consequence of systemized, focused testing. The *HEX-A* gene produces an enzyme (called hexosaminidase), and when mutated, production fails and hexosaminidase A deficiency occurs, resulting in the accumulation of excess complex fats (gangliosides) in the brain and nervous system causing Tay-Sachs disease.[3] Analysis of

---

3. Warren Tay was a British ophthalmologist who in 1881 noted the typical cherry-red spot in the retina at the back of the eye. Bernard Sachs was a New York neurologist who reported the cellular changes and increased frequency of the disease among the Ashkenazim.

Table 15.1 Examples of Genetic Disorders that Compromise Health and That Are Found More Commonly in Various Ethnic Groups

Ethnic Group	Genetic Disorder	Typical Features
Africans (Blacks)	Sickle cell disease and other disorders of hemoglobin	Anemia, pain, crises, strokes
	Alpha- and beta-thalassemia	Anemia, heart failure
	Glucose-6-phosphate dehydrogenase deficiency	Anemia, jaundice in newborn
	African-type adult lactase deficiency	Milk intolerance
	Benign familial leucopenia	Infection
	Hypertension (in females)	High blood pressure
Afrikaners (White South Africans)	Variegate porphyria	Neurological problems, abdominal pain, and sun sensitivity
	Fanconi anemia	Anemia; leukemia
American Indians (of British Columbia)	Cleft lip or palate (or both)	Facial defect (hare-lip)
Amish/Mennonites	Ellis-Van Creveld syndrome	Dwarfism, extra digits, heart abnormalities
	Pyruvate kinase deficiency	Anemia
	Hemophilia B	Bleeding
Armenians	Familial Mediterranean fever	Fever, abdominal pain, joint pain, rash

(Continued)

Ethnic Group	Genetic Disorder	Typical Features
Ashkenazi Jews	A-beta-lipoproteinemia	Nervous system degeneration and fat malabsorption
	Bloom syndrome	Lymphomas, growth problems, sun sensitivity
	Breast cancer	Breast or ovarian cancer
	Canavan disease	Degenerative brain disease, mental retardation
	Congenital adrenal hyperplasia	Genital abnormalities; adrenal tumors
	Dihydrolipoamide dehydrogenase deficiency	Developmental delay, seizures, large liver, blindness
	Dysferlinopathy (limb-girdle muscular dystrophy 2B)	Progressive weakness of limbs and pelvic muscles
	Dystonia musculorum deformans	Progressive disabling muscle twisting spasms and movements that impair speech and swallowing
	Factor XI (PTA) deficiency	Blood clotting
	Familial dysautonomia	Development problems, medical crises, feeding/swallowing problems, pain insensitivity, seizures
	Familial hyperinsulinism	Low blood sugar, seizures, poor muscle tone, sleep disorders
	Fanconi anemia (type C)	Birth defects, anemia, high risk of leukemia and other tumors
	Galactosemia	Developmental delay, ovarian failure, cataracts, newborn illness and death (untreated).
	Gaucher disease (adult form)	Blood and bone problems
	Iminoglycinuria	Amino acids in urine, no clinical problems
	Joubert syndrome	Developmental delay, jerky eye movements, unsteady gait, rapid breathing
	Maple syrup urine disease	Feeding problems, vomiting, lethargy, coma in first week of life, seizures, low blood sugar

	Meckel syndrome	Multicystic kidneys, brain anomaly, extra digits
	Niemann–Pick disease	Progressive brain degeneration; enlarged liver and spleen
	Tay-Sachs disease	Progressive degenerative brain disease, seizures, blindness
Chinese	Thalassemia (alpha)	Anemia
	Glucose-6-phosphate dehydrogenase deficiency	Anemia
	Adult lactase deficiency	Milk intolerance
	Deafness (Connexin 26 gene)	Hearing impairment to deafness
Eskimos	Congenital adrenal hyperplasia	Genital abnormalities; adrenal tumors
Filipinos	Cleft lip and palate	Birth defects (harelip) of lips, mouth, and other anomalies
Finns	Congenital nephrosis	Kidney failure
	Aspartylglucosaminuria	Neurodegeneration and mental retardation
	Progressive myoclonus epilepsy	Epilepsy
	Diastrophic dysplasia	Dwarfism
	Dystrophic retinae dysacusis syndrome	Blindness
French-Canadian	Familial hypercholesterolemia	Coronary heart disease
	Spastic ataxia	Muscle and balance disorder
	Tay-Sachs disease	Degenerative brain disease
	Neural tube defects	Brain or spinal defects (e.g., spina bifida)
Irish	Neural tube defects	Brain or spinal defects (e.g., spina bifida)
	Phenylketonuria	Mental retardation
	Schizophrenia	Psychosis
Italians	Fucosidosis	Mental retardation

(Continued)

Table 15.1 Examples of Genetic Disorders that Compromise Health and That Are Found More Commonly in Various Ethnic Groups (*Continued*)

Ethnic Group	Genetic Disorder	Typical Features
Japanese	Fukuyama congenital muscular dystrophy	Muscle disease
Japanese and Korean	Congenital Plasminogen deficiency	Blood clotting
	Fundus albipunctatus	Blindness
	Acatalasia	Severe oral ulcers
	Oguchi disease	Night blindness
	Dyschromatosis universalis hereditaria	Skin disorder
Maori (Polynesians)	Clubfoot	Foot deformity
Mediterranean peoples	Thalassemia (mainly beta)	Anemia
(Italians, Greeks,	Glucose-6-phosphate dehydrogenase deficiency	Anemia
Sephardic Jews,	(Mediterranean-type)	Fever, abdominal pain, joint pains, rash
Armenians, Turks,	Familial Mediterranean fever	Fever, abdominal pain, joint pains, rash
Spaniards, Cypriots)	Glycogen-storage disease (type III)	Liver disease
Norwegians	Cholestasis-lymphedema	Liver problems
	Phenylketonuria	Mental retardation
Yugoslavs (of the Istrian peninsula)	Schizophrenia	Psychosis

Note: This table simply provides some perspective on the extent of hereditary ethnic disorders. Any specific concern is best discussed with your doctor.

hexosaminidase in serum can be used to detect most carriers as long as there is not an ongoing pregnancy or use of oral contraceptives.

In such cases, analysis of hexosaminidase A is performed only with white blood cells—and not serum.

Less well-known is the juvenile later-onset form of Tay-Sachs disease, which results in survival into adolescence. An adult form is rare but well-known, with the diagnosis not infrequently missed. The adult form is characterized by progressive stiffness and balance loss with weakness and a bipolar form of psychosis.

Avoidance of this lethal disorder is best achieved by preconception testing for carriers in the population groups just noted. Couples who are both carriers have a 25% risk of having an affected child and can choose to have either pre-implantation genetic diagnosis or prenatal diagnosis. When ancestral origins are uncertain, it might simply be wiser to have the hexosaminidasc A enzyme carrier test.

Other recessively inherited biochemical genetic disorders are discussed in Chapter 25.

It was a spectacular and typical Mediterranean summer day. Rome was extremely hot and very crowded as hordes of tourists clamored and climbed over the many ancient sites and ruins of this remarkable city. Marco remembered that day well, since it marked a turning point in his life. He had been trying to obtain a green card to immigrate to the United States, and on that day, he made his way to the U.S. consulate and was finally rewarded with what he described as "a card to his passage to freedom and joy." The "joy" had everything to do with Fiona, whom he had met and fallen madly in love with in their last year in high school. When her family emigrated to Boston, taking Fiona away from him, he thought his heart would break. They had remained in touch by phone and internet, but neither had the travel funds to visit.

Through Fiona's family, Marco soon found employment as a salesman, and a year later, the anticipated marriage was celebrated. Pregnancy followed almost immediately, and the young couple looked forward to starting their own family.

Their son, Leonardo, was born without complication and looked the spitting image of his father. Although development was normal, by age 9 months, Leonardo appeared small, not thriving, and particularly pale. After repeated visits to their family doctor, who opined that Leonardo was pale because of the long Boston winter and that "he would be fine," they sought an opinion from a pediatrician. Paying attention to their ancestral origins, the pediatrician quickly obtained the necessary blood studies that enabled a diagnosis of a disorder called beta-thalassemia.

Marco and Fiona were devastated to hear about the long-term care that was going to be necessary and the possibility of Leonardo's shorter lifespan.

Neither Marco nor Fiona, and certainly not their families, had ever heard of thalassemia. Even though they were of Mediterranean ancestry, no one in the family knew of a person with this disorder. However, their parents came from Sardinia, an island in southern Italy, where the population had a high frequency of thalassemia. Marco and Fiona were stunned to hear from me that the likelihood of each of them being a carrier of a gene mutation for this disorder was at least 1 in 30.

I explained that the word thalassemia derived from the Greek "thalassa," meaning "sea," and haema, meaning "blood." As carriers, they unwittingly had a 25% risk of having a child with this serious chronic anemia. The basic problem in this disorder revolves around hemoglobin, which is an iron-containing protein almost exclusively found in red blood cells and whose function is to ferry oxygen from the lungs around the body and release it to all tissues. I elaborated further that when red blood cells are lost (because of bleeding), broken up too early (by disease), or not made in sufficient quantity by the bone marrow, anemia results. The worse the anemia, the less oxygen available to the tissues and the more breathless and tired we become. Appetite is lost, growth halts, weight loss occurs, and eventually heart failure and even death may ensue if treatment is not provided or successful. Hemoglobin is made up of two protein (globin) chains, and disease results when there is a reduced rate of manufacture of one of the globin chains or when a defect occurs in a chain. The hemoglobin then becomes abnormal, resulting in the early destruction of red blood cells, the loss of hemoglobin, and resultant anemia. The future treatment that they could anticipate being necessary provided no comfort whatsoever.

Once significant anemia has developed, regular blood transfusions given every 2 to 3 weeks are started. Extensive blood group testing of donors precedes that regimen and includes testing for viruses including hepatitis and HIV/AIDS. Over years, this regimen of blood transfusions deposits excessive amounts of iron in many vital tissues, including the liver and the heart. Efforts at bone marrow transplantation succeed if a very good match is achieved from an identical twin or a very well-matched sibling. Survival in about 90% of cases is achieved as long as there is no serious liver involvement and not excessive deposition of iron. Where those factors are not present, survival might not reach 60%. Moreover, if a good bone marrow match is not achieved, rejection may occur with potentially fatal results. Cord blood taken at birth from the parents' next child (or stored from a previous child) may provide a stroke of luck and a successful cure. There are reports of couples who went ahead to have another child with the express purpose of hoping to conceive a child who would be blood group- and tissue-compatible with the affected child and thereby save their thalassemic child.

The excessive iron deposition is dealt with by chelation therapy involving the use of drugs that help the body get rid of iron. Unfortunately, the drug needs to be administered 5 to 7 days a week by 12-hour continuous infusions under the skin via a portable pump. Needless to say, there are a series of unwanted side effects that may complicate chelation therapy. After years of treatment and excess iron deposition into the heart muscle, cardiac disease also becomes a threat to survival. Osteoporosis is also a common complication in adults with thalassemia.

THALASSEMIA

Thalassemia is among the most common serious genetic disorders that occur worldwide. The beta-thalassemia that Leonardo inherited is especially common in populations along the Mediterranean and especially in southern Italy, Sardinia, and Cyprus, where between 1 in 7 and 1 in 8 of the population are carriers of a mutation in the beta-thalassemia gene. In the Maldives Islands, 1 in 6 are carriers. In India, with a population exceeding 1 billion, there are approximately 45 million carriers of the various thalassemia types and disorders affecting hemoglobin. The high gene frequency of beta-thalassemia in these regions is thought to most likely be related to their increased resistance to malaria, which is endemic in those very same areas. You can imagine the difficulty and cost of managing such a heavy genetic load in a developing country, given the need for frequent blood transfusions and sophisticated, costly medical management.

Affected infants fail to thrive, have feeding problems, and experience diarrhea and recurrent bouts of fever while their abdomens become more prominent because of enlarging liver and spleen. After age 10 years, affected children are at serious risk of developing severe complications resulting from iron overload from the many transfusions and the complications of chelation therapy. Iron deposition in the heart muscle is the most important life-threatening complication, accounting for some 71% of deaths.

Given Mediterranean ancestry, it is now expected that couples be tested to determine their carrier status for beta-thalassemia. Discovery that a couple both carry a gene mutation for beta-thalassemia provides various options. They may opt not to have a child, choose artificial insemination by donor from a male shown not to be a carrier, elect adoption, or (as is most often the case) choose early prenatal diagnosis around 11 weeks in any future pregnancy (or prenatal studies by amniocentesis around 16 weeks), and terminate the pregnancy if the fetus is affected. Where available, preimplantation genetic diagnosis is an important but expensive option, in which the status of the fertilized egg can be determined and, if affected, not implanted in the womb, thereby avoiding abortion. Those who oppose abortion would probably find the latter procedure equally unacceptable. However, much suffering of many for a lifetime can easily be avoided by preconception genetic screening. Such has been the experience, for example, in Sardinia, led by Professor Antonio Cao, with a remarkably successful program. Of course, prenatal diagnostics can proceed only once definitive mutations have been found in both prospective parents. Professor Cao was initially faced with 1 affected child in 250 births. Once the program was established, that rate fell to 1 in 4,000. As is the rule, Marco and Fiona were urged to contact and inform their siblings, uncles, aunts, and cousins on both sides of the family about the importance of having carrier tests for beta-thalassemia.

Without treatment, affected children have a shortened lifespan, and with treatment, life expectancy is likely to extend into the third to fifth decade. It is important to note that there are milder forms of beta-thalassemia (called intermedia and minor), where signs may begin later and the course of illness is not as severe. Diagnosis is usually accomplished by relatively simple blood tests, DNA mutation analysis being necessary only in the context of future childbearing and for carrier testing in at-risk relatives.

There are a large number of variant forms of hemoglobin, many of which are benign. Some, however, are critically important and may be carried by one partner while the other partner is a carrier of the beta-thalassemia gene. If, as is not infrequent, the abnormal hemoglobin in one partner is the sickle hemoglobin (*see* discussion below), then the offspring could be born with sickle-beta-thalassemia, which would require the same treatment as noted earlier and would also lead to a truncated lifespan.

Another disorder resulting from an abnormal hemoglobin structure is the common alpha-thalassemia. There are two very significant forms of this disorder, the first being severe enough to cause fetal death or death in the newborn. Profound anemia may occur in the fetus, resulting in awesome and lethal swelling of the entire body. Massive enlargement of liver and spleen, a large head and heart, and other defects are common. The second form is milder and similar in its manifestations to beta-thalassemia. Carriers are detected by relatively simple blood tests, while DNA analysis is required for more sophisticated prenatal diagnosis or preimplantation genetic diagnosis.

Alpha-thalassemia is found in a huge swath of the world, including Africa (with very high gene frequencies in Nigeria, Ivory Coast, and Kenya), the Mediterranean countries, the Arabian peninsula, India, and Southeast Asia. In one province in China (Guangxi), 11.19% of the population are carriers of alpha-thalassemia and 6.8% carry the beta-thalassemia gene. In Egypt, 9% are carriers of the alpha-thalassemia gene. You don't have to be reminded that your risks relate to your ancestral origins and not to where you currently live.

All of the exhortations relating to preconception testing, carrier detection, prenatal diagnosis or preimplantation genetic diagnosis discussed above apply equally to the avoidance and management that is necessary for alpha-thalassemia.

ANCESTRAL GENES

We all have advantageous and potentially harmful genes that are mostly inherited. The advantageous genes may, for example, protect us from developing various disorders such as heart disease, asthma, allergies, and even malaria. Disadvantageous or potentially harmful genes may make us susceptible to a wide range of human diseases that include certain cancers, heart disease, diabetes, and many other common illnesses. The vast majority of the advantageous and harmful genes act in concert to benefit or impair our health. In this chapter, we are focused on ancestral genes that are particularly passed down through the generations and that cause genetic disorders due to involvement of a **single** gene. Someone inheriting a mutation in a single gene that causes recognizable genetic disease is regarded as a carrier when that disorder essentially manifests only when a mutated copy of the gene is inherited from *both* parents.

These mutated ancestral genes are passed down through endless generations, usually having begun as a spontaneous mutation long ago. Once a mutation has occurred in a small isolated population—especially if in-bred—more and more of that population group come to be carriers. The founder mutations spread in that population group, as has been the case for many originally isolated groups (*see* Tables 15.1, 15.2, & 15.3). The Eastern European ghettos for Ashkenazi Jews fostered the spread of a series of different mutations now tested for routinely in pregnant women in that group (*see* Footnote 3). Dr. Oliver Sachs, in his book *The Island of the Colorblind*, describes that one in three inhabitants of the Pacific Atoll, Pingelap, carry the gene mutation for achromatopsia. In 1775, a typhoon decimated the island and most of the population died. Those that survived and their subsequent generations intermarried, resulting in an amazing 6% to 10% of the people having achromatopsia. In this recessively inherited disorder, there is total absent color vision, as well as poor eyesight and difficulty with bright light. Legend has it that once upon a time, a marooned Irish sailor added his genes (!) containing the mutation in the achromatopsia gene, thereby acting as the founder. The French Canadians noted earlier, as well as the Acadians in Louisiana, inherited and harbored the gene mutation for Tay-Sachs disease at a rate similar to that found among Ashkenazi Jews but mostly due to a different and characteristic mutation.[4]

Ellis-van Creveld syndrome is another, albeit rare, condition occurring in an isolated population, the Old Order Amish, who live around Lancaster, Pennsylvania, in the United States. Characteristic features include short-limbed dwarfism, extra fingers, heart defects, and dental and/or oral defects.

---

4. An example of a **dominantly** inherited disorder from a founder is exemplified by the genetic condition called Variegate Porphyria in South Africa. A Dutch settler in the Cape is believed to have been affected and transmitted the specific gene mutation to 50% of his offspring. Affected adults are very sensitive to the sun, hairy, and subject to severe attacks of abdominal pain, hypertension, paralysis, disturbances of sensation, confusion, and even psychosis. Today, as many as 1 in 400 White Afrikaans-speaking South Africans—especially in the Eastern Cape—may be affected.

Table 15.2 Likelihood of Being a Carrier for Various Ethnic Groups[1]

If You Are	The Chance is About	That you Carry a Gene Mutation For
Afrikaner (White South African)	1 in 400	Porphyria[2]
Armenian, Jewish (Sephardic) Turks, Arabs	1 in 3 or 1 in 8	Familial Mediterranean fever[2]
Black	1 in 8 to 1 in 10	Sickle cell anemia[2]
	7 in 10	Milk intolerance as an adult
Black and male or	1 in 10	Hereditary predisposition to develop
Black and female	1 in 50	hemolytic anemia after taking sulfa or
	1 in 4	other drugs[3]
		High blood pressure[3]
Finns	1 in 36	Aspartylglucosaminuria[2]
French-Canadian	1 in 49-90	Aspartylglucosaminuria[2]
Italian-American or Greek-American	1 in 10	Beta-thalassemia[2]
Jewish (Ashkenazi)	1 in 111	Bloom syndrome
	1 in 40 (women)	Breast/ovary cancer gene mutation
	1 in 40	Canavan disease
	1 in 26	Deafness (non-syndromic)
	1 in 96	Dihydrolipoamide dehydrogenase deficiency
	1 in 127	Galactosemia
	1 in 18	Gaucher's disease
	1 in 32	Dysautonomia
	1 in 8	Factor XI deficiency
	1 in 5 to 1 in 7	Familial Mediterranean fever
	1 in 66	Familial hyperinsulinism
	1 in 92	Fanconi anemia
	1 in 71	Glycogen Storage disease type 1A (Von Gierke disease)
	1 in 92	Joubert syndrome
	1 in 122	Maple syrup urine disease type 1B (MSUD)
	1 in 81	Mucolipidosis type IV
	1 in 90	Niemann-Pick disease Type A
	1 in 25–30	Tay-Sachs disease
Asian	1 in 1	Milk intolerance as an adult[3]
White	1 in 25 to 1 in 29	Cystic fibrosis[2]
	1 in 31	Deafness[2] (non-syndromic)
	1 in 10	Hemochromatosis[2]
	1 in 40 to 1 in 60	Spinal muscular atrophy[2]

[1] These disorders can occur in any ethnic group but are more rare.

[2] DNA carrier and prenatal diagnostic test available.

[3] No DNA test available.

Table 15.3 Chances of Genetic Disorders in a Child for Various Ethnic Groups

If You Are	The Chance that You Could Have Been Born with a Defect Leading To	Is About
Black	Sickle cell anemia	1 in 300 to 500
	Beta-thalassemia	1 in 125
White	Hemochromatosis	1 in 200 to 1 in 250
	Cystic fibrosis	1 in 2,500 in 3,000
	Phenylketonuria	1 in 14,000
Jewish (Ashkenazi)	Tay-Sachs disease	1 in 3,600
	Familial dysautonomia	1 in 3,600
	Canavan disease	1 in 6,400
	Niemann-Pick type A disease	1 in 32,000 to 1 in 40,000
Italian-American or Greek-American	Beta-thalassemia	1 in 400
Armenian, Jewish (Sephardic), Turks, Arabs	Familial Mediterranean fever	1 in 250

Since we know that genes are shared in closely knit populations through marriage, it is no surprise that the closer the relationship of the couple, the greater the likelihood that they each carry a mutation in the same gene, resulting in a one in four risk of having a child with a specific disorder. Hence, marriages between first cousins are noted to have about double the risk of having a child with a birth defect, mental retardation, or genetic disorder, approximating 6% to 8%. Increased risks are also recognized for uncle–niece unions, but marriages between second cousins are not clearly recognized as having significant increased risks.

Consanguinity is especially common in a number of countries, including the United Arab Emirates, the Middle East, Pakistan, and India. Rates of consanguinity range between 25% and 70%! One study from the United Arab Emirates of 2,200 women concluded that there was a significant increase in the occurrence of cancer, birth defects, mental retardation, and physical handicaps in the offspring of consanguineous couples.

The rate of genetic defects alone was 5.8%. A Jordanian study came to similar conclusions and also pointed out increased rates for infant mortality, stillbirths, and birth defects. The birth of a child with a rare genetic disorder in the absence of a family history of such a defect always raises the question of consanguinity somewhere in the ancestral background. Genetic counseling is advised for all related couples, not only for risk assessment and carrier detection tests but because of increasing possibilities for prenatal genetic diagnosis.

Charles Darwin raised the question concerning the advisability of first-cousin marriage. Ironically, he married a first cousin, and together they had 10 children. He questioned the wisdom of his close marital union after 3 of his children died.

Carriers of autosomal recessive disorders rarely show any symptoms or signs of these conditions. Sickle cell disease carriers participating in military basic training have been reported to have an increased incidence of sudden, unexplained death, possibly because of exertional heat illness. About 5% of carriers may occasionally have some blood in the urine, and most cannot concentrate their urine. In one rare recessive disorder known as Bardet-Biedl syndrome (the main features of which include obesity, extra digits, mental retardation, eventual blindness, and small or poorly functioning gonads), carriers may show a tendency toward obesity, high blood pressure, diabetes, and various kidney defects.

Following the discovery of male infertility, couples may choose artificial insemination by donor. Care should be taken to check the ethnic origins of the donor so that ethnic-specific carrier tests can be performed prior to insemination. Sperm banks differ markedly in their genetic testing of donors. Potential recipients are advised to confer with a genetic counselor prior to any planned insemination. Once again, adopted individuals are at a disadvantage, and caution should attend any consideration of having a donor without known ethnic origins.

Parents who have a child (or a prenatally detected fetus) with a recessively inherited disorder will be informed that there is a two-thirds risk that their other children are carriers of the same gene mutation. Since these carrier children will invariably be healthy, carrier testing is appropriately postponed until their late teens, when genetic counseling should be offered.

SICKLE CELL DISEASE

Another disorder due to an abnormal hemoglobin is sickle cell disease. Just as for the thalassemias, this disorder is also inherited as an autosomal recessive. Where both parents are carriers, there is a 25% risk of having an affected child. There is a single mutation in one hemoglobin chain, which the parents might share, or one parent may have another hemoglobin abnormality that, in combination with their partner results in a condition such as sickle/thalassemia disease. All manner of permutations of these abnormal hemoglobins are well-known.

Sickle cell disease occurs most commonly among persons of African, Mediterranean, Middle Eastern, and Indian ancestry, as well as among those from the Caribbean and Central and South America. Between 1 in 8 and 1 in 10 African-Americans are carriers of the sickle cell trait, and about 1,100 infants with sickle cell anemia are born annually in the United States. Between 1 in 300 and 1 in 500 African-Americans born in the United States have sickle cell disease, resulting in more than 70,000 affected individuals. In many countries in Africa, between 25% to 35% of the population are carriers, with more than 15 million Africans actually affected by this serious disorder. In some parts, more than 1 in 100 children are born with sickle cell disease.

Once again, the red blood cells are fragile, sickle-shaped, and break up easily, causing a veritable plethora of complications in potentially every organ system. Not only may anemia develop, but episodes of sudden unheralded break up of red blood cells may literally clog blood vessels. In the blood vessels to the brain, a stroke occurs; to a kidney, there is function failure; to the bowel, there is tissue death (infarction); to the penis, there is painful constant erection (called priapism), which requires immediate specialist attention; and on and on. Affected individuals are also at increased risk of infections, as over years their spleens may be compromised by repeated episodes of being clogged with red blood cell debris, which steadily disables the protective function of the spleen. Extremely painful crises are experienced when clogging occurs in blood vessels in the chest or the abdomen, in particular, and much care is necessary to try to avoid these severely disabling episodes. Maintenance of hydration, avoidance of extreme heat or cold or very high altitude without oxygen supplementation, and quick medical attention if a complication arises all constitute judicious steps. One pharmacologic agent, called hydroxyurea, has been approved since it was shown to reduce the frequency of painful crises resulting from blocked blood vessels and the need for frequent blood transfusions. Moreover, recent data point to a decreased mortality in those using hydroxyurea and a safety record thus far of 17.5 years.

The management of the endless possible complications requires involvement of well-informed physicians and centers. Fortunately, screening of all newborns in the United States enables very early diagnosis and prospective care and treatment, which includes penicillin prophylaxis and immunizations against certain bacteria. Nevertheless, it is obviously much wiser to avoid the condition entirely if parents so wish. Carrier detection is simple and requires a tiny blood sample. At the very least, all African-Americans should have a carrier test. Where both partners in a couple are carriers, the usual options apply, including prenatal diagnosis and preimplantation genetic diagnosis, as discussed earlier.

Life expectancy may be seriously curtailed in this disease, but careful attention and early constant medical treatment has effected major improvements in longevity. Once again, as soon as a diagnosis has been made, all relatives should be contacted, informed, and have the recommendation to seek a carrier test. Currently, the **average** life expectancy approximates 53 years for men and 58.5 years for women.

Across the enormous swath of continents and countries in which the abnormal hemoglobin disorders are highly prevalent and in which malaria is endemic, there exists yet another common hereditary defect that leads to red blood cell break up. This disorder, called G6PD deficiency,[5] is inherited as an X-linked trait, mainly affecting males.[6] At least 400 million people worldwide carry a gene mutation for G6PD deficiency! Fortunately, G6PD deficiency is thought to protect against malaria. The highest frequencies are found on the African continent, Asia, the Mediterranean countries, and the Middle East. Owing to population migrations, G6PD deficiency is also found in North and South America and in northern European countries. Ingestion of fava beans may also precipitate acute red blood cell disintegration and severe anemia, while ironically, anti-malarial drugs may do the same. A number of other drugs may precipitate the red blood cell breakdown, the most common of which belong in the sulfa-category (such as sulfonamides).

Babies born in any of these countries or as the offspring of immigrants elsewhere need to be observed for the development of jaundice, especially within the first 24 hours of life. Their yellow color develops rapidly as a consequence of red blood cell breakdown and critical attention is necessary to avoid the

---

5. Glucose-6-phosphate dehydrogenase deficiency.
6. The X-linked mode of inheritance is as discussed for hemophilia (Chapter 6) and Duchene muscular dystrophy (Chapter 6), with all the relevant caveats about transmission and symptoms and signs in gene mutation carriers. Affected individuals are usually asymptomatic and without testing have no idea that they harbor a G6PD gene mutation. This defect makes their red blood cells vulnerable to stressors such as certain drugs or infection, which can result in a rapid break up of red blood cells and acute, even life-threatening, anemia. Diagnosis may be prompted in the newborn if jaundice associated with acute anemia develops as a result of rapid breakdown of red blood cells.

pigments that emerge from the red blood cells and which deposit in the basal ganglia of the brain, causing brain damage.[7] In some cases, the baby's blood is exchanged by transfusion with normal red blood cells. In countries where G6PD deficiency is very uncommon, immigrant parents, if well-informed, may need to prod their physicians about their ethnic origins and the risk of this disorder. Distant to the newborn period, complications are confined only to exposure to certain drugs, fava beans, and infections, with no curtailment of life expectancy.

---

7. Called kernicterus, in which the features resemble cerebral palsy, together with deafness.

16

PUZZLING FEVERS

It was a tough, rough-and-tumble game. The two elite boys high school rugby teams had been competing for years, and there was much prestige being a member of the winning team. Andre was one of the star players and, as a consequence of his position at center, was a marked man. Less than halfway through the game, he was felled by two burly opposing players. His mates later said they could hear his thigh bone fracture at the time of impact. He screamed out in pain and could hardly move. The medics rushed out with a stretcher and carried him off the field and into an ambulance. He was rapidly admitted to the hospital and, because of the associated bleeding, was rushed into surgery.

He was speedily anesthetized, and the superb trauma surgeons got to work on his shattered thigh. Just over an hour into the surgery, the anesthesiologist became extremely concerned because he noticed a rapid rise in Andre's body temperature. At the same time, Andre developed a fast, irregular heartbeat and his blood pressure dropped precipitously. To his complete dismay, the anesthesiologist recorded a temperature that exceeded 107°F. Shortly thereafter, Andre's heart simply stopped, and he died without regaining consciousness. The mandated autopsy did not reveal a definitive diagnosis.

Later, the only clues that became apparent in the family history were that his mother had surprisingly large calf muscles, which nevertheless did not stop her from complaining about how weak she was. And one of her brothers had died suddenly during surgery on his gallbladder. A specific cause for that death was never established, but she did recall the surgeons discussing infection as the cause in view of a sudden high fever.

Blood samples taken from Andre immediately before surgery started and during his collapse under anesthesia revealed extraordinary high levels

*of an enzyme called creatine phosphokinase (CPK). The sudden develop-
ment of incredibly high fever during surgery, the extraordinarily high
level of CPK, and the family history led to a clinical conclusion that
Andre had died as a consequence of a genetic disorder called malignant
hyperthermia.*

I was a highly impressionable medical student then and have never for-
gotten the desperate sadness that enveloped the family and the entire
surgical and nursing teams. Little was known then about this disorder
and nothing was known about the effective and preventive treatment
that emerged later. The relatively low penetrance[1] of the genes involved
in malignant hyperthermia make it difficult to recognize subtle, or at
least not obvious, signs in family members. Hence, the prominent calf
muscles of Andre's mother would have passed without notice, as did the
sudden death of his uncle—the only such death in the family.

The reason for the extraordinary response of the body to overheating
was not understood for years. Now we know much about the complex
mechanism that results in the release of calcium within the channels of
skeletal muscle cells—a mechanism controlled by no less than seven
genes. The released calcium activates the internal energy-producing
mechanism within the cell, initiating chemical reactions that cause heat.
This in turn steps up the entire cell machinery to chew up glucose stores,
making more heat. All of these events cause muscular contractions that
eventually result in actual rigidity of the muscles, leading to production
of even higher temperatures. The factor that initiates this cascade of
responses is the body's reaction to anesthesia, such as halothane,[2] and
certain muscle relaxants, such as succinylcholine, either of which individuals may receive when undergoing surgery. Only rarely is the initiating factor vigorous exercise and excessive heat.

MALIGNANT HYPERTHERMIA

Estimates of the incidence of malignant hyperthermia range between 1 in 5,000
and 1 in 50,000 anesthesias. However, some estimate the prevalence of actual

1. The observable expression, or lack of it, of a mutant gene.
2. Also sevoflurane and desflurane.

gene mutations to be as frequent as 1 in 3,000. The difficulty lies in the absence of a simple, inexpensive, and effective screening test. Currently, detailed sequencing of about seven genes enable detection of mutations in only about 50% of cases. The actual clinical diagnostic test depends on obtaining a muscle biopsy and then exposing the muscle to halothane, caffeine, or other drugs and assessing in the laboratory how that muscle contracts.

One particular gene (*RYRI*) is linked to about 50% of cases of malignant hyperthermia, and more than 100 mutations have been identified in this gene. However, given the fact that a number of different genes may cause malignant hyperthermia, international societies[3] have recommended that both the muscle contraction test and DNA analysis be used to achieve the most reliable diagnosis. Even using both tests, successful recognition might only reach about 80% at present. In families clearly recognized as having malignant hyperthermia, DNA tests may reveal a mutation, and muscle contraction tests would not be necessary. In those cases, of course, all family members at risk would be advised to have the DNA test, thereby saving their lives should they have to undergo an unexpected surgical operation. Another salutary realization is that the muscle contraction test may occasionally provide a false-positive result, and this may in fact be due to an unrelated muscle disorder.

Malignant hyperthermia is inherited as an autosomal dominant condition with an affected person having a 50% risk of transmitting the mutant gene to each of his or her offspring. There is also a recessively inherited malignant hyperthermia type that occurs mostly, but not only, in boys and is associated with a number of birth defects, including spine curvature (scoliosis), unusual facial features, a webbed neck, a prominent breast bone, low muscle tone, slightly delayed motor development, hyperextensible joints, muscle weakness, and undescended testes, to constitute a condition called King syndrome. Curiously, malignant hyperthermia also occurs in pigs, dogs, horses, and probably other animals. In pigs, the disorder is recessively inherited.

Malignant hyperthermia may also occur in several inherited muscle diseases.[4] Hence, families in which any of these disorders occur should be wary of the possibilities of malignant hyperthermia, more especially if there has been

---

3. European Malignant Hyperthermia Group and the North American Malignant Hyperthermia Group.
4. Including Duchenne or Becker Muscular Dystrophy, central core disease, paramyotonia, myotonia congenita, and periodic paralysis.

any unexplained death or someone with elevated levels of CPK. The wrong time to first start thinking about the possibilities of malignant hyperthermia is on the gurney, being wheeled into the operating room for urgent or emergency surgery. The signs triggered by the anesthetics include rapidly developing rigid muscles, and development of high acid levels in the body together with high levels of potassium, with muscles falling apart. Fortunately today, every operating room is supplied with the remarkable drug Dantrolene. This drug decreases the release of calcium from muscle, thereby relieving muscle contractions and rigidity. Crisis treatment will also include sophisticated care focused on the body chemistry and anticipating the danger of clotting, kidney failure, and brain damage.

Although a malignant hyperthermia crisis may occur at the very first anesthetic, on average, three anesthesias may be given before triggering the hyperthermia reaction. Malignant hyperthermia has been described in newborns and has been diagnosed as late as age 78 years. About 40 years ago, the mortality rate exceeded 80%, whereas today it is probably less than 5%.

Clearly, the potential for fatality due to malignant hyperthermia requires families to be alert to their histories. Attention should be paid to family members with increased muscle bulk (not caused by weight lifting), those with chronic muscle weakness or muscle cramps, and definitely those with an elevated level of CPK. Affected individuals may appear entirely normal, showing no signs whatsoever. In susceptible individuals where surgery is necessary, spinal or epidural anesthesia would be best if possible. Otherwise, there are other, probably safer, combinations of anesthetics available.

Hagop was a psychologist who had done well in college, graduated magna cum laude, and received his Ph.D. following superb work on his thesis. Soon after receiving his doctorate, he met and married Seta, whose career was in business management. On their honeymoon, Hagop developed a fever associated with severe abdominal pain. The emergency department physician who examined his belly remarked on his abdominal scar. Hagop explained that when he was 9 years old, he had an episode of severe abdominal pain, which resulted in surgery. Later he was told that the tentative diagnosis of appendicitis was not confirmed at the time of surgery but that they did take out his appendix all the same. Since that time, in response to questions by that physician, he had had occasional episodes of fever, sometimes associated with a red rash. At other times, he had experienced episodes of joint pains, with or without fever. His own primary care doctor had given him analgesics and told him to rest, and sure enough, all symptoms disappeared, usually within days.

With this history and no clear indication of an acute abdominal emergency, Hagop was simply observed, and within days his symptoms and signs had subsided and they were able to return home, albeit with a truncated honeymoon.

Despite his protestations, Seta insisted on a visit to a specialist. The academic physician they consulted quickly recognized Hagop's history of intermittent, but recurrent, short episodes of fever, abdominal pain, joint pains, and the rash, suggesting a diagnosis of Familial Mediterranean Fever (FMF). His clinical conclusion was virtually clinched when he recognized the Armenian ancestry of both Hagop's parents.

Subsequent testing of the FMF gene (MEFV) revealed two different mutations that he had inherited, one from each parent, confirming the diagnosis of this autosomal recessive disorder. Because Seta was also of Armenian ancestry, she was subsequently tested and found to be a carrier of a single MEFV mutation.

Treatment with an anti-inflammatory drug called colchicine soon did away with all his symptoms and signs, and he has remained well years later on this medication, with only an occasional symptom.

The cause of any illness characterized by intermittent symptoms and signs may not be easily determined. A major clue was Hagop's Armenian ancestry, the importance of which was only recognized after years of significant intermittent illness. None of the signs he had, taken alone, was specific for any particular disorder. The combination of recurrent fevers with and without abdominal or joint pain (or chest pain) and a red rash should have alerted his pediatricians.

Recognition of his ethnic origin should immediately have alerted them to the fact that between 1 in 3 and 1 in 8 Armenians carry a mutation in the *MEFV* gene. Incidentally, the same frequency of carriers can be expected among Turks, North African Jews, and Iraqi Jews. A rate as high as 1 in 5 among Ashkenazi Jews is also recognized, except that the predominant mutation in the *MEFV* gene codes for a milder form of FMF and in many might simply be a polymorphism (*see* Chapter 5).

The carrier frequency among North African Arabs approximates 1 in 100. About 1 in 1,000 people of Mediterranean descent have FMF.

Since Hagop had FMF and Seta was a carrier of an FMF mutation, their risks of having an affected child in any pregnancy was 50%.[5] They had the option of using preimplantation genetic diagnosis or prenatal diagnosis to avoid having affected children. Artificial insemination by donor was also an option they could have considered. A child born affected and eventually symptomatic would be placed on a medication (colchicine) for life.

Acute attacks may be triggered by infection or stress, but often no precipitating factor is recognized. In about 50% of cases, symptoms begin in childhood, the majority being diagnosed by the age of 20 years. Fortunately, the frequency and severity of attacks decrease with age. At least 85% of those with FMF achieve complete remission or major improvement on colchicine. Sometimes higher doses are necessary, and occasionally even weekly intravenous administration is required. For non-responders to colchicine, a few other drugs can be tried.

A critically important concern in long-standing FMF is the deposition of a complex protein called amyloid, mainly in the kidneys. In undiagnosed or untreated FMF, amyloidosis will result in kidney failure and death without dialysis or kidney transplantation. Once again, simply paying attention to the family history, this time with care to determine ancestral origins, can save a life. I never cease to be amazed when a patient tells me that although their parents are living, they have no idea about their ethnic origins.

Today, routine testing for mutations in the *MEFV* gene or actually sequencing the gene provides a precise diagnosis in at least 95% of cases. In rare instances where only one mutation has been discovered and the symptoms and signs are consistent with FMF, a trial of therapy with colchicine is warranted. Only rarely does amyloidosis develop in the kidneys in a person without any other signs.

A certain lack of clarity still exists for some patients known to have signs of FMF but in whom only one mutation in the *MEFV* gene has been found.

---

5. Much more often, a couple is found with each carrying an FMF mutation. Their risk of having a child with FMF is 25%.

In one of the extremely puzzling and challenging families I saw recently, both of their boys had symptoms typical of FMF with intermittent fevers, abdominal pains, and lethargy. Mutation analysis by sequencing the *MEFV* gene revealed that the 12-year-old son had a mild mutation (often described as a variation), and the younger son had a more significant mutation. Analysis of both parents' DNA revealed no mutation whatsoever in the mother, but **both** mutations seen in the boys were present in the father, who was perfectly well! Emerging data suggest that there might well be a substantial number of individuals in whom only a single mutation has been recognized but who still show clinical symptoms of FMF. A trial of colchicine is recommended now in these situations. One likely implication is that there is a second gene with a mutation elsewhere in the genome acting in concert with the mutation in the *MEFV* gene, causing actual FMF. This phenomenon of a mutation in two different genes resulting in a particular disorder is called digenic inheritance and is recognized for some other disorders, such as the common form of inherited non-syndromic deafness.[6]

PERIODIC FEVERS

Besides FMF, there are a number of other rare hereditary recurrent periodic fever syndromes.[7] These disorders are also characterized by intermittent periods of fever, invariably unexplained red, sometimes itchy rashes; and joint, muscle, abdominal, or chest pains. Some of these conditions make their appearance in the first year of life and may be extremely worrisome to both patient and family. Fortunately, none of these periodic syndromes are common. Like FMF, the hyperimmunoglobulin IgD syndrome is inherited as an autosomal recessive disorder. Dominant inheritance is characteristic for TRAPS and CAPS, as well as cyclic neutropenia. One clue to the diagnosis of these initially worrisome syndromes is the possibility of consanguinity or an affected parent. In busy pediatric practice, it is not uncommon for repeated bouts of fever to be treated with antibiotics, despite negative bacterial cultures. The possibility of a periodic fever syndrome should always be kept in mind.

---

6. Resulting, for example, from mutations in the common connexin 26 and 30 genes.
7. Including tumor necrosis factor (TNF)-receptor-associated periodic syndrome (TRAPS), cryopyrin-associated periodic syndrome (CAPS), hyperimmunoglobulin IgD syndrome, and cyclic neutropenia.

BLEEDING AND CLOTTING

Pregnancy had been a breeze. Bernice had gained 27 pounds and felt well and more energetic than she could ever remember. All of her visits to her obstetrician were unremarkable and he, being conscientious, took a family history, inquiring particularly about any birth defects, mental retardation, or genetic disorders in any family member. Bernice answered in the negative but did say that she had been living on the East Coast for the past 15 years and had not seen much of her family in the Midwest. Her husband's family history was also devoid of any recognizable genetic conditions.

For this long, lanky, loose-jointed woman, labor and delivery were easy. However, within hours of giving birth to her beautiful daughter, she suddenly complained of feeling dizzy, nauseous, and faint, even though she was in bed. The alert nurses noted that her pulse rate had risen to 110 per minute, and her blood pressure had dropped to 90/40. She had broken out into a sweat, and the obstetric resident on call quickly discovered that Bernice was in the process of having a large postpartum hemorrhage, originating from the placental site. Despite immediate attention by the medical staff, Bernice collapsed in shock, even before the first bottle of plasma was started intravenously. Bernice slowly recovered consciousness to find that she had already received 1 pint of blood, which was followed by 2 more. Her bleeding was controlled, and she was able to return home a few days later with her newborn daughter.

Prior to her discharge from hospital, her attending physicians had closely questioned her about any history of bleeding. She described how she bruises sometimes without even knowing that she might have bumped herself. As a child, she remembered having quite a number of nosebleeds that seemed to go on interminably. She admitted that sometimes her gums bleed on brushing or after flossing her teeth. She thought her menstrual periods were not unusual, but her description indicated that they were heavier than normal.

Phone calls from her siblings and parents in the Midwest provided additional information. Her one sister and her brother both had suffered prolonged nosebleeds in childhood and both bruised very easily. That sister was currently pregnant and expressed fear once she heard the details about Bernice's postpartum hemorrhage. None of Bernice's three siblings had children thus far. Bernice's mother also reported that she bruised very easily and had experienced heavy menstrual periods. She also related that Bernice's brother had continuous and persistent bleeding after his circumcision several days after his birth.

At her 6-week check-up, Bernice underwent additional blood tests, which concluded with a diagnosis of an autosomal dominant genetic condition called Von Willebrand disease[1](VWD). Subsequently, diagnostic tests revealed that her brother, one sister, and her mother all had this bleeding susceptibility disorder.

So often now in the world in which we live, families reside far from one another. Even though the clues of a bleeding disorder (*see* Table 17.1) were evident in Bernice's family, no one could fault the lack of exchange of information about prolonged nosebleeds and their potential implications. The heavy menstrual bleeding Bernice experienced is typical for VWD. Between 5% and 20% of women with excessive menstrual bleeds have undiagnosed VWD. The first choice of treatment for adolescents or those women not planning pregnancy is hormonal contraceptives. The excessive bleeding following circumcision is also typical for this disorder but did not trigger any diagnostic evaluation (although it should have). The fact that multiple family members bruised easily without even noticing any trauma was recognized by them all as an inherited tendency. None of them would have predicted a near-death experience for Bernice from this very same bleeding disorder. Certainly her sister (and her attending physician), being put on notice about VWD, was able to seek care in a tertiary care center where expert management was available. The typical bruising, bleeding, and heavy menstrual periods are characteristic of VWD.

---

1. This genetic disorder is named after Erik Adolf von Willebrand, a Finnish pediatrician who described this condition in 1926.

222 YOUR GENES, YOUR HEALTH

Table 17.1 Clues to an Underlying Bleeding Disorder that Warrant Evaluation if Any of These Indicators Are Present

- Heavy menstrual periods from the time menses began (menarche)
- A family history of a bleeding disorder
- A personal history of one or more of the following:
  1. Nosebleeds that last more than 10 minutes that require packing or cauterization
  2. Easy bruising
  3. Bleeding for more than 5 minutes from minor wounds
  4. Bleeding from the mouth or the anus without an obvious cause
  5. Prolonged bleeding after tooth extraction
  6. Unexpected bleeding after surgery
  7. Bleeding from an ovarian cyst even during ovulation
  8. Bleeding that requires a blood transfusion
  9. Bleeding after delivery of a child that occurs even 24 hours later, or more

VON WILLEBRAND DISEASE

Many patients are surprised to learn that VWD occurs in between 1 in 100 and 1 in 1,000 of the population. Von Willebrand disease is the most common inherited bleeding disorder. VWD is caused by a gene defect resulting in a deficiency or dysfunction of a blood clotting factor called the Von Willebrand factor, which is a plasma protein that acts in concert with blood platelets (the small cells that accompany our white and red blood cells in the circulation) and another clotting factor called Factor VIII. For the most part, the bleeding tendency is mild. However, one study from Duke University Medical Center reported the death of 5 women, reflecting a mortality rate some 10 times higher than that for unaffected women. They noted that bleeding during pregnancy occurred some 10 times more often than in other women.

Autosomal dominant inheritance accounts for most cases, and various types are recognized. An affected individual has a 50% likelihood of transmitting the VWD gene to each of his or her offspring. In some rarer cases, the inheritance is autosomal recessive and neither of the affected individual's parents, who are carriers, show any signs of the disorder whatsoever. Even though an affected person is born with VWD, symptoms and signs may only become apparent in adulthood and may only be diagnosed in midlife or later!

Not infrequently, because of excessive menstrual bleeding and development of anemia, women with VWD may elect to have a hysterectomy. They need to be aware that there is at least a three times greater risk of bleeding during and after surgery and of needing a blood transfusion.

The Von Willebrand factor levels increase during pregnancy, peaking during the last 3 months and then dropping off precipitously after delivery. This drop is potentially hazardous and levels need to be monitored for 2 to 3 weeks post-delivery. This was the potential danger and the origin of Bernice's sister's fear. Fortunately, armed with the established diagnosis because of Bernice's experience, her sister, albeit already pregnant, was able to seek specialist care in the 11th hour. Analysis of her levels of the Von Willebrand factor and Factor VIII were carefully monitored, and immediately upon delivery, she received the medication Desmopressin. This drug releases stored Von Willebrand factor and is a mainstay of treatment for this disorder. It can even be given by inhalation through the nose.

Ideally, once the diagnosis of VWD is made (preferably prior to conception), specialist attention by a hematologist would be recommended. This is important given the on-going clinical trials of new and better clotting factors. Because there is a potentially serious bleeding tendency, most would advise against the use of forceps during delivery or vacuum extraction. Spinal anesthesia (epidural) should only be used after checking that the Von Willebrand factor and Factor VIII levels are close to normal. Concentrates of these factors are given to women to raise these factors to normal levels.

Women with VWD who plan to become pregnant should link up with a hematologist, a high-risk obstetrician, and a knowledgeable anesthetist in a center that has a blood bank on site and has experience in coping with sudden, serious bleeding. At delivery, two large-bore intravenous needles should be in place,[2] and levels of the Von Willebrand factor and Factor VIII should be known ahead of labor and delivery. Necessary medications such as Desmopressin should also be on hand. Bernice was lucky, but women have died from postpartum hemorrhage caused by VWD.

Given the multiple types and subtypes of VWD, both specialist attention as well as highly dependable laboratories are required for evaluation, diagnosis, and monitoring. Von Willebrand factor levels are affected by various genetic factors and also by hormones as a result of stress, exercise, pregnancy, and estrogen levels. DNA analysis is not straightforward either and, again, is best accomplished by a specialist hematologist or a clinical geneticist.

Since effective treatment is available, prenatal diagnosis is only rarely a consideration for the most severe form (autosomal recessive) of VWD.

---

2. In shock, veins collapse, making intravenous access difficult.

It should be obvious that someone with VWD should avoid contact sports, with special attention to preventing head injury. Medications such as aspirin or non-steroidal anti-inflammatory drugs can aggravate any bleeding tendency. Circumcision should only be arranged after consultation with a specialist.

Von Willebrand disease represents yet another important genetic disorder where a family member may not recognize symptoms or signs among their close relatives. For all families, a high degree of vigilance is necessary to avoid unnecessary consequences of an undetected genetic disorder. A lifelong awareness that all of us harbor a considerable number of harmful genes and that the vast majority of our serious/chronic illnesses have their origins not only in single mutated genes but in the actions of multiple genes acting in concert is important. Once again, know your family history, seek consultations in the face of uncertainty, and thereby secure your health and that of your loved ones and even save a life.

It was a Sunday afternoon, and 40-year-old Luis, his wife Cathy, and three of their five children were enjoying time together at a bowling alley. Luis was on the top of his form and had just scored a spare. The moment that his next ball left his hand, he suddenly clutched his chest and coughed up what seemed to be about a pint of blood. He fell to the floor and into the pool of blood, coughing and spluttering blood in all directions. It did not take long for an ambulance to arrive, and he was quickly managed by the EMT team, an intravenous line was placed, and he was transferred to hospital.

Luis had never had any such episode nor, in fact, any bleeding problem that he could recall. In hospital, immediate imaging studies of his lungs revealed at least three arteriovenous malformations[3] (AVMs) in his lungs. A careful examination revealed only tiny, spider-like capillaries appearing like red spots around his lips and nose. Only on direct questioning did he recall having brisk and prolonged nosebleeds in his teens.

Following a blood transfusion, a catheter was introduced into his arteries and maneuvered into the clearly seen feeding blood vessel of the still bleeding AVM. That vessel was blocked by insertion of a platinum coil through the catheter in the process called embolization.[4] This procedure promptly

---

3. An arteriovenous malformation is a mesh and tangle of tiny arteries and veins without intervening capillaries, which connect directly and are subject to rupture.
4. Sometimes a tiny inflatable balloon is used.

stopped his bleeding, and recovery thereafter was swift. Further discussions and additional evaluation resulted eventually in embolization of the other AVMs in his lungs. Meanwhile, Luis and Cathy were referred to us for a genetic evaluation and counseling. Only then did they realize the importance of Luis's family history.

His brother Alfred, then 46 years old, had a son with a brain hemorrhage in his late teens who had died suddenly. His brother Alfred had no other children and no evaluation followed. Moreover, no geneticist was consulted. Luis's sister Carmen, then 44 years old, had complained of intermittent periods of fatigue, dizziness, and palpitations. She had repeatedly been found to be anemic and was treated with iron tablets, but again she was never fully evaluated. She had one daughter who, on one occasion after coughing vigorously, produced some sputum with about a teaspoon of blood. That had happened about 10 years ago, and there had been no further episodes. Luis's late father had died in his 60s from "a stroke," and because no autopsy was done, the family did not know if a hemorrhage or thrombosis had occurred. Luis was not aware of any history of bleeding. Luis's mother had a heart attack and died in her 70s. Luis and Cathy's two oldest boys had both had a history of significant nosebleeds. Subsequent evaluation by imaging of the lungs of all five children and vascular imaging of their brains, including Luis's, revealed that one of the boys had a cerebral AVM that was promptly embolized. Their second son had a single AVM in his right lung and that, too, was embolized. Initially, when Luis and Cathy and their two eldest sons came for their appointment, I explained the autosomal dominant mode of inheritance of this condition called Hereditary Hemorrhagic Telangiectasia (HHT).[5] Each affected family member would have a 50% risk of transmitting this disorder to each of his or her offspring.

I have had the privilege of caring for thousands of families in my career. Endless families among them reflect a common theme. Different health problems appear in various family members and seem to bear no relation one to another. In the family of Luis, for example, was a nephew

5. Also termed Osler-Weber-Rendu disease.

who had a brain hemorrhage, a niece who had a lung hemorrhage, a sister with iron deficiency anemia,[6] a father who had a stroke, and two of Luis's boys, who experienced significant and recurrent nosebleeds. Neither Luis nor the family members could be expected to come up with a diagnosis of HHT. However, it is the mindset of needing to think "genetic" that I am trying to communicate as important. The critical question to be asked by a family member noticing significant adverse health events, as in Luis's family, is whether there may be a genetic basis for the family's problems. A clinical geneticist would have immediately suspected the diagnosis of HHT, and there may have been a chance to have saved the life of the nephew.

HEREDITARY HEMORRHAGIC TELANGIECTASIA

Hereditary hemorrhagic telangiectasia is not rare and affects at least 1 in 5,000 individuals. Multiple AVMs may occur in the lungs, intestine, brain, or liver from which catastrophic bleeding can occur.

Tiny AVMs or spider-like capillaries seen in the skin that blanch on pressure with a finger may also rupture and bleed after mild injury. Hereditary hemorrhagic telangiectasia rarely affects an infant and mostly becomes apparent in adolescence or later in adulthood. Recurrent nosebleeds represent one of the most common occurring clinical signs. About 80% of affected individuals have serious nosebleeds by the age of 20 years and 90% before the age of 30 years. Note that before blood transfusions became available, deaths from blood loss caused by nosebleeds were not uncommon. About 30% of affected individuals suffer lung AVMs, while about 10% have brain AVMs. A bleed into the spinal canal may cause paralysis. Women with HHT should have imaging of their lungs and brain prior to having children, especially since AVMs tend to increase in size and number during pregnancy. Otherwise, they could risk hemorrhage and other complications in the lungs and brain. Women with HHT have a higher incidence of lung and liver AVMs.

One well-recognized additional hazard, fortunately uncommon, is that blood may shunt directly from arteries to veins, thereby increasing the work of the heart, which could even result in heart failure. These direct open channels, if

---

6. Caused by cryptic intestinal bleeding

occurring in the lung, establish an avenue for clots or bacteria to pass directly into the arterial circulation and then even into the brain, causing an abscess or stroke.

Mutations in three well-known genes[7] cause HHT. In 1%-3% of people with HHT, a mutation is found in the SMAD4 gene. Mutations in this gene are also associated with juvenile polyps in the intestine with the risk of cancer. In accordance with International Guidelines, colonoscopy should begin between 15-18 years of age. Those with HHT should undergo testing of their entire intestinal tract from the age of 25 years.

At least two other genes, yet to be identified precisely, are also thought to be causal. Prenatal diagnosis is possible once a mutation has been recognized.

Special anticipatory care is necessary for a person with HHT to pre-emptively treat a potentially dangerous complication. Annual visits to a specialist familiar with HHT are important. Annual testing for blood in the stool and for checking the blood count would be a standard requirement. For those with lung AVMs, chest X-rays or CT scans and even echocardiograms may be necessary. This attention is also important, even for those who have had a lung AVM embolization. A CT scan at least every 3 to 5 years is recommended to assess whether or not AVMs in the lung have grown or new ones have appeared. A brain MRI should be done at least once. Needless to say, all family members, including asymptomatic children, should have a DNA mutation analysis and, if positive, seek the kind of management just described. This way, families can secure their health and often save lives.

Wilhelm and Petra were in my office to discuss the results of DNA tests we had done. It was then that she related their story, which could have been taken directly from a medical textbook. Wilhelm and Petra had the entire family come for Thanksgiving dinner. This was the first time that her four siblings and her parents, their own two children, and six nieces and nephews had come together since they left the Netherlands some years earlier. Wilhelm described how Petra had put together a table heavily laden with typical Thanksgiving fare. Everyone had comments to make about the tasty turkey, the spectacular pumpkin pie, the blueberry tart, and the other special dishes Petra had prepared. She had a feeling of peaceful contentment as she watched and listened to the happy talk around the table. Suddenly, without warning, her brother Pieter, who was a physician and the eldest of

---

7. ENG, ALK I, and SMAD4.

the five siblings, asked if anyone around the table had noticed a health problem in the family. An uncomfortable silence descended on the festive table, Petra recalled. His four sisters, almost in unison, tried to shush him. They all knew that Pieter was the brightest among them, but he also was awkward, insensitive, difficult, and single-minded. Undaunted, he launched forth with a breathless recounting of the family's ills.

He began by pointing out that their mother had a deep vein thrombosis (DVT) in her early 50s and that their mother's sister had a stroke and died at age 59 years. His one sister Dottie, who had been on hormone replacement therapy, also had a stroke at age 51 years. She had remained with a mild paralysis on one side of her body. His other sister Denise, within days of giving birth to her second daughter, had suffered a pulmonary embolus[8] and had almost died. Petra had suffered three miscarriages in the second or third month of her pregnancies before giving birth to her son and daughter. Pieter himself had no children and was not married.

Pieter went on to explain that he thought there was some type of clotting susceptibility gene in the family and that everyone should be tested.

Petra's contentment gave way to agitation and felt that her effort to have the whole family over for a celebratory Thanksgiving dinner had been ruined by Pieter. Despite his good intentions, his sisters apparently let him know in no uncertain terms what they thought of his poorly timed outburst. It took the quiet but commanding voice of their mother to call for quiet and to listen to Pieter's recommendations.

Pieter related that he had listened to a superb lecture just before leaving the Netherlands, specifically on the subject of clotting susceptibility genes. That's where he learned of the high likelihood that his family harbored a gene mutation in a key clotting gene that would explain the strokes, deep vein thrombosis, the pulmonary embolism, and the miscarriages. He said he would arrange for those of his siblings who would be willing to be tested to have a DNA analysis of what he called the Factor V Leiden and Prothrombin genes. Not all agreed to follow his recommendations, but Dottie, who had suffered a stroke and was concerned for her two children, was the first to have the necessary tests. She discovered that she carried a mutation in the Factor V Leiden gene, and thereafter her three sisters went

---

8. A blood clot from a vein, most often from a leg, that breaks loose, and is carried in the bloodstream to the heart and out into the lung. If large enough, sudden death could occur; otherwise, pain in the chest and some breathlessness may be experienced.

for testing. Petra and Denise were found to have the same mutation, as did the youngest sister Anna. Pieter, never short on tact or hyperbole, said that Anna was sitting "on a keg of dynamite" and that "tomorrow is too late." The reason he gave was the fact that she was taking "the pill," which was "dangerous" because it could cause a stroke in someone with the Factor V Leiden mutation, and he suggested that she stop taking "the pill" immediately. Pieter himself was the last to be tested and, needless to say, proved negative.

Pieter's sudden exposition about the family's likely genetic burden may well be regarded by most as inappropriately timed. He may, however, have realized that once dinner was over, it would have been difficult to keep them all together and get their attention. Either way, his intercession was critically important to Denise and Anna and may have been life-saving. Most of us would think that a family history of deep vein thrombosis, strokes, and pulmonary embolism would be noted by the different physicians taking care of Petra and her sisters. The facts are that even today, in the golden era of genetics, physicians have little time to take a detailed and extensive family history. Throughout this book, it will have become obvious that genetic disorders with considerably different manifestations may not be recognized as linked and, hence, the information not shared with a health care provider.

Anna was unwittingly taking an oral contraceptive and unaware of her significant risk of having a stroke. When a woman has a mutation in a clotting susceptibility gene, she should not take oral contraceptives. Women having hormone replacement therapy who carry this mutation also face a two- to fourfold increased risk of thrombosis.

FACTOR V LEIDEN

When we have a nosebleed or sustain a cut, we are unlikely to ponder the fact that dozens of factors are involved in making our blood clot and the bleeding end. There is indeed a clotting cascade involving these many factors that is controlled, of course, by many different genes. Inheritance of a mutation in one of these genes, such as the Factor V Leiden gene, conveys a genetic susceptibility to clot more easily. Many of these clotting factors operate syner-gistically and are frequently influenced by extraneous factors. Dehydration or taking long trips by air or by car without moving from a sitting position for many hours leads to slowing of the circulation in the legs. Someone with a genetic predisposition to clot may well develop a thrombosis in a leg vein. Later they may have the significant risk that a piece of the clot may break away and shoot into the lung, causing a pulmonary embolus, which could result in sudden death. In fact, some have called this sequence of events the "Economy Class Syndrome," which is precipitated after having sat for hours without moving and squished up in a tightly packed airplane.[9] There is a threefold increased risk of pulmonary embolism after long-distance (more than 8 hours) air travel. However, if the individual has a Factor V Leiden mutation, then the risk increases 14- to 16-fold and is further compounded by use of oral contra-ceptives.

Occurrence of the Factor V Leiden mutation is not uncommon, being pres-ent in about 1 in 20 (5.2%) Whites in the United States. Frequencies are less in other ethnic groups, including 2.2% in Hispanics, 1.2% among African-Americans, about 0.5% among Asian-Americans, and 1.25% among Native Americans. In some regions of the world, such as in southern Sweden and Greece, the prevalence may exceed 10% of the population.

All of these figures apply to situations where only one Factor V Leiden muta-tion is inherited. However, if a Factor V Leiden mutation is inherited from each parent, an even greater risk of clotting would exist. In someone such as Pieter's mother, who had a deep vein thrombosis, the likelihood is 15% to 20% that a Factor V Leiden mutation is present.

DNA analysis of the Factor V Leiden gene should be performed to discover the common mutation in a number of different circumstances. These would include pulmonary embolism at any age, deep vein thrombosis, clotting at unusual sites (brain, gut, liver), family history of an affected first-degree rela-tive (sibling, parents, or children), and unexplained early recurrent miscar-riages. Many of us would also recommend testing after a diagnosis of unexplained severe preeclampsia[10] in pregnancy, placental abruption (tearing of the placenta away from the uterine wall), or growth restriction of a fetus. Testing women under age 50 years who have had a heart attack or stroke is also

9. No difference in the frequency of pulmonary embolism was noted for travelers in business class versus economy class in one study.
10. Hypertension and protein in the urine.

judicious. Women who sustain a deep vein thrombosis or a pulmonary embolus while using Tamoxifen to prevent breast cancer (*see* Chapter 8) should also be tested. Women in families with a known Factor V Leiden mutation should be tested if they plan to use oral contraceptives. In those rare cases where children have suffered clotting within an artery, Factor V Leiden and other clotting susceptibility genes should be tested. Needless to say, individuals can live an entire lifetime with the Factor V Leiden mutation and never have any clotting issues whatsoever.

In pregnancy, there is an increased propensity to clot because levels of clotting factors rise,[11] other factors that normally prevent clotting decrease; and blood flow in the legs decreases. If another disorder such as obesity, diabetes, sickle cell disease, lupus, or heart disease is present, or if the maternal age is older than 35 years, then Cesarian section is often recommended.

Thus it is no surprise that pregnancy poses even more significant risks of clotting for women who carry a Factor V Leiden mutation. There may be as high as a 30% increased rate among women with unexplained recurrent pregnancy loss, as well as a two- to threefold increased risk for a range of pregnancy complications. In addition, significant risk occurs after delivery where special attention and anti-clotting medications may be necessary, especially if there is a history of deep vein thrombosis or pulmonary embolism. Mutations in any one or more other genes involved in the clotting cascade may act in concert with the Factor V Leiden mutation. The effects are additive, and risks are considerably higher as a consequence. For example, the clotting susceptibility Prothrombin gene mutation (which occurs in about 1 in 50 Whites) should also be tested in the circumstances described above. This gene mutation, when present together with the Factor V Leiden mutation, is associated with a 20-fold increased risk and a 150-fold recurrence risk of thrombosis. Individuals with high levels of clotting Factor VIII, when present together with the Factor V Leiden mutation, experience a two- to threefold higher incidence of pulmonary embolism. When thrombosis does occur in Factor V Leiden mutation carriers, the likelihood of an extraneous risk factor approximates 81% in women and 29% in men. These risk factors include three or more previous pregnancies, maternal age older than 35 years, smoking, multiple pregnancy, preeclampsia, Cesarian section, obesity, and varicose veins.

Factor V Leiden carriers who also have an elevated level of the normally circulating amino acid called homocysteine have about a 22-fold increased

---

11. Including factors II, VII, VIII, and X.

risk of thrombosis. Hence, a fasting level of homocysteine should be checked in anyone found to have either thrombosis or a Factor V Leiden or Prothrombin gene mutation. Any thrombosis that occurs in childhood should result in testing multiple clotting genes.

Because clotting factor susceptibility genes act in concert, once someone is found to harbor a Factor V Leiden or a Prothrombin gene mutation, additional tests for mutations in other genes should be pursued.[12] The usual treatment for an acute episode of thrombosis is anticoagulation, usually starting with the drug heparin given intravenously and followed by anticoagulant tablets (such as Warfarin) as the level of anticoagulation is monitored. Since about 30% of individuals with deep vein thrombosis/pulmonary embolism suffer a recurrence within 10 years, the tendency to clot is regarded as a chronic disorder. Generally, anticoagulation medication will be given for between 6 and 12 months if no clearly determinable precipitating factor (such as oral contraceptives or surgery) is identified. Where a clearly identified factor is recognized, the course of anticoagulants may be considerably shorter. For those who have had a deep vein thrombosis, compression stockings are usually recommended for about 2 years thereafter.

Anticoagulants are inherently dangerous and, if not carefully monitored, may result in a serious—if not fatal—hemorrhage, especially into the brain. Therefore, a person at risk of thrombosis and on anticoagulants should be paying close attention to factors that can precipitate thrombosis on the one hand and dosage and level of anticoagulation on the other hand. Clearly, there is a need to seek a balance between the obvious benefits and the real risks. Both the Chinese and Japanese show increased sensitivity to Warfarin and may require lower dosage. Home monitoring with personal dose control provides much relief. Women who plan to become pregnant should not be on Warfarin as that drug has the potential for interfering with cartilage development in the fetus. When planning pregnancy, a switch to heparin is necessary if anticoagulation has to continue. The hormone pregnancy test after each cycle could help time the needed switch.[13] Women should be reminded that pregnancy itself and especially immediately after delivery are periods that promote clotting. Given other options, pregnant women requiring anticoagulation therapy

12. These would include mutation analysis in the Prothrombin gene if not yet done, antithrombin III activity, protein C activity, lupus inhibitor, anticardiolipin antibodies, protein S activity, and Factor VIII level.

13. Pregnant women with certain high-risk mechanical heart valves who are at risk of clots forming on valves should not switch.

should be in the care of maternal–fetal medicine high-risk specialists. This point requires emphasis because 11% of maternal deaths in the United States result from pulmonary embolism.

A review of Petra's family will remind all of those at risk to have all first-degree relatives tested once a mutation has been detected in either the Factor V Leiden or Prothrombin gene. Children at risk (a parent with a mutation in the Factor V Leiden gene) are not usually tested because thrombosis rarely occurs before age 18 years. Testing would proceed only if, in those rare instances, thrombosis has occurred. In this context, it is important to note that strokes might even occur in the fetus or the newborn, thereby emphasizing the need for specialty care when a prospective mother knows about her carrier status. Prenatal diagnosis is possible whenever a gene mutation is known but for Factor V Leiden and Prothrombin would rarely be requested.

There need be no fear for a well-informed family receiving appropriate monitoring and care. Paying attention to the warning signs and facts as the family did to Pieter's forthright exposition can secure people's health, reassure those not at risk, and indeed, save lives.

Charles had met Adrienne in their advanced placement biology class in the final year of high school. While they went to different colleges, they saw each other as often as possible and the whole family predicted that they would marry. They decided that a marriage certificate would simply represent a piece of paper and not capture the deep feelings they had for one another. After college, they lived together for 2 years before deciding to start a family. Charles had a mild form of hemophilia A. This sex-linked bleeding disorder had been in his family for generations on his mother's side. Charles experienced some type of bleeding about twice a year and was actually diagnosed only in his teens when he was hit by a soccer ball and sustained a surprisingly large hemorrhage in his thigh muscle. Over the years, he had some significant bleeding following a tooth extraction and one episode of bleeding in his right knee joint after a fall.

They both had a complete understanding of the mode of sex-linked inheritance and recognized that Charles' mother was almost certainly a carrier of a gene mutation in the hemophilia Factor VIII gene (F8). Further, Charles' maternal uncle, who was born prematurely, had a hemorrhage in his brain and died a few days after his birth. It had always been unclear whether he actually had hemophilia A or that the hemorrhage was a complication of his prematurity. Charles had a brother who also had mild hemophilia A and who had only occasional episodes of bleeding, including two episodes in his knee joints. Charles and his brother were also color-blind.[14] Charles' sister, after testing, was shown to be a carrier of a mutation in the F8 gene, as was the case in her daughter. Upon hearing that she was a carrier, she had decided to only have girls and actually stopped trying to get pregnant after having one daughter. Charles' brother and his wife had one son. Because the F8 gene mutation cannot be passed from father to son, he and his wife were overjoyed when they discovered that they would have a son who, of course, could not inherit his father's hemophilia A.

Charles and Adrienne pursued their dreams of having a family and, in due course, were blessed with the birth of a boy they named Jimmy. He, too, was not affected. They gave much thought to planning their second pregnancy and simply hoped that they would have another son. Obstetrical ultrasound studies at 18 weeks in her second pregnancy revealed that Adrienne's fetus was female. They were both pleased with this result, albeit recognizing that their future daughter would be an obligatory carrier of the F8 gene mutation but would not otherwise be affected.

At term, Adrienne delivered their daughter, Margaret. There were no bleeding problems, and they were delighted. However, they did note that although they were tall, Margaret was a surprisingly short 18¾ inches in length. Compared to their son Jimmy, they also thought that the backs of her hands and the tops of her feet seemed puffy. At Margaret's 6-week check-up, their pediatrician noted a short, broad neck, rather low-set ears, and a broad chest with widely spaced nipples. Upon recalling the puffy hands and feet, he recommended a chromosome analysis to determine whether Margaret had a disorder called Turner syndrome.[15]

Fifteen days later, they learned that Margaret did indeed have Turner syndrome, characterized mostly by the presence of only one X chromosome

---

14. Color-blindness is a genetic trait in which the gene is carried on the X chromosome. Therefore, mothers who are carriers, as must have been the case with Charles' mother, will transmit one X chromosome to each child. For male offspring, there is a 50% likelihood of inheriting the gene for color-blindness when the mother is a carrier. This form of color-blindness, which prevents the affected individual recognizing red and green colors, is the result of a mutation in the color-blindness gene, which travels closely linked to the hemophilia A gene near the very tip of the long arm of the X chromosome. It is therefore no surprise to find that Charles and his brother were also color-blind. Generally, about 8% of all males have this form of color-blindness.

15. Discussed fully in Chapter 3. Features include short stature, tiny uterus, non-functioning ovaries, and frequent heart and kidney abnormalities.

rather than two. It was not clear then whether Margaret had retained the X chromosome transmitted from her father or from her mother. They both immediately realized the need for testing the F8 gene, as the mutation was known in the family. This they accomplished in the next few months and discovered that Margaret actually had mild hemophilia A, despite being female. She had inherited and retained her father's X chromosome (curiously, in Turner syndrome, it is usually the father's X chromosome that "gets lost").

In sex-linked inheritance (*see* Chapter 6), the gene mutation on the X chromosome is usually transmitted by a female carrier to 50% of her daughters, who would also be carriers, and to 50% of her sons, who would be affected. In about 90% of carriers of the *F8* gene, no bleeding issues arise, but in about 10%, prolonged bleeding may occur. This might include heavy menstrual periods, bleeding after surgery, or bleeding after delivery of a child.

Affected boys may be severely, moderately, or mildly affected. Clearly, Charles and his brother were mildly affected, as is the case with Charles' daughter Margaret. The severity of hemophilia A[16] remains fairly constant in transmission over the generations and, if severe, will result in severely affected males generation after generation.

Although Turner syndrome is not rare, occurring in about 1 in 2,500 female births, the concurrence of hemophilia A and Turner syndrome is well-described but rare. Hemophilia A in a female may also occur in rare circumstances where a husband has hemophilia A and his partner is unwittingly a carrier of a gene mutation in the F8 gene. The consequence could be a 50% likelihood of having a daughter with two X chromosomes but also hemophilia A.

---

16. There is another form called hemophilia B caused by deficiency of the Factor IX clotting factor. This disorder is rarer (about 1 in 20,000) than hemophilia A. The various symptoms and signs, however, are much the same. The Factor IX gene (*F9*) is also transmitted on the X chromosome, and hence the mode of inheritance is exactly the same as hemophilia A. Treatment of course is intravenous infusion of Factor IX concentrate. Hemophilia B was originally called Christmas disease and named after a 5-year-old boy with the first diagnosis of Factor IX deficiency.

HEMOPHILIA

Severe hemophilia A is usually detected during the first year of life, and sometimes an affected infant may have a major bleed in the head following birth. As the child becomes mobile, bleeding into joints occurs with increasing frequency unless preventive treatment is initiated. At a time when effective treatment was not available, boys would have between two and five bleeding episodes each month, with the joints most commonly affected. Bleeding would also occur through the kidneys, the gut, and the brain. Serious pain and swelling is experienced when there is bleeding into joints and muscles. About 1 in 4,000 to 1 in 5,000 males born have hemophilia A in all countries and in all races.

With moderately severe hemophilia A, diagnosis is usually made by age 5 or 6 years. Bleeding episodes might occur less frequently than in the severe form. Mild hemophilia A is reflected in Charles' family history. Although this educated couple understood sex-linked inheritance, they did not recognize the fact that about 10% of carrier females manifest mild hemophilia. Of course, they could not have anticipated the relatively rare event of coincident Turner syndrome with hemophilia A.

The medical history of the British royal family provides a typical "pedigree" for this sex-linked disorder (*see* Chapter 6). Affected sons of a female carrier undergoing circumcision may have serious bleeding if no preventive measures have been instituted. Hemophilia, in fact, is one of the oldest recognized genetic disorders, mention being made in the Talmud (*see* Chapter 6).

Bleeding inside the head, mostly due to injury, is a leading cause of death in hemophilia A. The main cause of serious disability results from recurrent bleeding into joints. Even today, in some developing countries where proper treatment is not provided, life expectancy may only reach age 11 years. In France, and some other European and African countries, catastrophes occurred when hemophiliacs were transfused with blood infected with the HIV virus, causing AIDS. Similar experiences occurred in the United States and also included the hepatitis C virus. Many hemophiliacs died from either or both infections, mostly between 1975 and 1985.

The diagnosis of hemophilia A is made by assessing the product of the F8 gene, which is the Factor VIII clotting factor. The varying severity of hemophilia is due to the abnormality in the gene product. Hence, there may be virtual absence of detectable Factor VIII, leading to severe hemophilia A. Or the level of the protein product may be normal but seriously dysfunctional.

Alternatively, the levels of Factor VIII clotting activity may be diminished and a milder form of the disorder would emerge.

A precise diagnosis, however, is made by DNA mutation analysis of the *F8* gene. Once a precise mutation is determined, prenatal diagnosis or preimplantation genetic diagnosis becomes available in a future pregnancy.

Enormous strides have been made in the successful treatment of severe hemophilia A. Affected children are usually treated with prophylactic infusions of Factor VIII concentrate three times a week or even every other day to maintain an effective Factor VIII clotting activity level. In this way, and with appropriate care, almost all joint bleeding can be avoided. These children should not be given intramuscular immunizations, which should be administered simply under the skin.

For older children and adults, much disability has now been avoided with the availability of intravenous infusions of Factor VIII concentrate at home. Since 1990, plasma-derived concentrates have been used in which viruses have been eliminated. It is clear that treatment should be initiated as quickly as possible after any bleed and certainly within 1 hour. Desmopressin (as discussed earlier with Von Willebrand's disease) can be used in mild hemophilia because this medication often doubles or triples Factor VIII clotting activity.

Fortunately, in pregnancy, the level of Factor VIII clotting activity normally rises and is partly protective. However, immediately after birth, Factor VIII clotting activity can drop precipitously within 48 hours, and bleeding might ensue. Women are advised to determine their carrier status for hemophilia prior to starting a pregnancy. With careful care and specialist attention, vaginal delivery should not be problematic.

After receiving Factor VIII concentrates, some hemophiliacs develop an immune response (called inhibitors) to the administered protein. This obviously can complicate care and make the control of bleeding more difficult. Hemophiliacs certainly don't need to be reminded to avoid medications that may cause bleeding, such as aspirin or aspirin-containing products.

At least in the United States, all patients with hemophilia A should attend a federally funded hemophilia treatment center at least once, where assessment, education, genetic counseling, and instruction about treatment can be provided.

Hemophilia is a prime example of a genetic disorder in which awareness of a detailed family history and knowledge about the disorder can assure the health of an affected person and certainly save their life. Indeed, medical and genetic advances have made a world of difference to the lives and life expectancy of hemophiliacs.

––––––––––––––––––––––

The aforegoing family histories provide some insight into the complex arena of genetic disorders characterized by bleeding or clotting. These disorders can be considered to arise as a consequence of:

1. Deficiencies in one (or more) of more than two dozen coagulation factors in what is called our clotting cascade.
2. Abnormalities in the structural integrity and function as well as actual number of circulating platelets in our bloodstream; a whole range of disorders exist in this category, often with serious risks of hemorrhage as a constant hazard.
3. Weakness or abnormality in the walls of arteries and veins, resulting in bruising, bleeding or rupture (*see* Chapter 18).

18

BLOOD VESSELS THAT BURST

An Arctic-like wind whistled through the canyons of the city, which appeared encased in ice following a blizzard-like snow storm. Boston's Logan airport was closed, and the only brave souls who ventured out were emergency crews and crazy people. That was how Eric vividly remembered the telephone call in the dead of night from his sister-in-law, Jill. Through constant sobbing, Eric learned that his brother Paul, a few hours earlier, had suffered a brain hemorrhage and was semi-comatose. Jill said that Paul had been working in their garage and failed to come in for supper when called. Jill discovered Paul lying on the floor, difficult to rouse, and unable to speak. Jill quickly summoned the ambulance, and Paul was rushed to the hospital. An MRI of his brain immediately revealed a large hemorrhage involving the left hemisphere of his brain. Eric and his wife Dawn flew out to Colorado 3 days later, at which time there had only been slight improvement in Paul's level of consciousness. A very guarded prognosis had been provided by Paul's physicians.

Jill related that Paul had known about his hypertension for at least 10 years but had not told any of his three siblings. He had only intermittently seen his primary care physician and not faithfully taken his antihypertensive medication. Jill said that Paul often cursed his hypertension that he said he inherited from his late father, who had been killed in an automobile accident at 51 years old. Paul had also had some kidney stones that had caused him considerable abdominal pain. He had ascribed the stones to the hot, dry climate and his failure to remain well-hydrated.

Soon after their return from Denver, Dawn insisted that Eric see his primary care doctor. "Tomorrow is too late," she would say, to no avail. It took 4 months of nagging for Eric to actually appear for a routine physical. To his dismay, he discovered that he too had hypertension. The trigger that led to Eric making an appointment with his doctor was the news that Paul's brain hemorrhage resulted from a ruptured aneurysm—a small localized bubble or ballooning of an artery in his brain. Upon hearing this history, his physician ordered a magnetic resonance arteriography (MRA), which enabled clear visualization of the arteries in Eric's brain.

To his further dismay, a small, unruptured aneurysm the size of a berry was also discovered along the course of his middle cerebral artery, a key vascular channel. Consultation with a neurosurgeon followed, and not long after, Eric underwent surgery to place a clip on the neck of the aneurysm to prevent it from rupture. At the same time, as part of further evaluation to determine the cause of his hypertension, imaging of his kidneys followed. This showed multiple cysts in both kidneys, leading to the conclusion that he had polycystic kidney disease, also confirmed later in his brother Paul. Imaging studies of both the brains and kidneys of their two siblings yielded entirely normal results.

Paul regained consciousness but never spoke again and was left with paralysis on the right side of his body following the left brain hemorrhage.

Eric and Dawn were referred to a clinical geneticist for genetic counseling. They learned that polycystic kidney disease was dominantly inherited and that there was a 50% risk for each of their four children to inherit the mutated gene (PKD1) from Eric. The age range of their children was from 8 to 16 years.

Paul's approach to his own health proved almost fatal and left him severely disabled and incapacitated. His phlegmatic attitude toward his hypertension and the required medication left him seriously vulnerable. Moreover, had he been more vigilant, a fuller evaluation for the cause of his hypertension might have been accomplished and his polycystic kidney disease revealed. His disinclination to inform his siblings about his own hypertension also placed them at potentially serious risk. Perhaps, because he was the eldest son, he might have felt that admitting to a chronic disorder might make him appear weak to his younger siblings. Whatever the reason, it is extremely common for families not to share information about each other's illnesses. While it might be easy to understand for any of a myriad number of possible reasons, from time to time failure to share and inform close relatives can lead to preventable catastrophes.

Fortunately, Eric (lucky to have Dawn as his wife) eventually sought care and discovered that he too had polycystic kidney disease and a cerebral aneurysm. Ironically, Paul's misfortune saved Eric's life. How much better it would have been for the family to have been well-informed and for all of the siblings to have taken appropriate steps for evaluation. At the very least, it is highly likely that Paul would not have ended up totally disabled.

Eric's father, who died in an automobile accident at age 51 years, was known to have had hypertension. Given the subsequent family history, it is a virtual certainty that he too had polycystic kidney disease. An affected person has a 50% risk of transmitting this dominantly inherited disorder to each of his or her children. Consequently, all of Paul and Eric's offspring, following genetic counseling, had the necessary tests for polycystic kidney disease (*see* discussion below).

The concurrence of a cerebral aneurysm and polycystic kidney disease is well-known. Those with a positive family history of an aneurysm in association with polycystic kidney disease (with or without a hemorrhage into the brain) have about a 22% risk of having an aneurysm themselves. Those without such a history have about a 6% risk. Since the average age of rupture of a cerebral aneurysm approximates 39 years, delaying brain imaging is really unwise.

POLYCYSTIC KIDNEY DISEASE

It may come as a surprise to many that autosomal dominant polycystic kidney disease (ADPKD) is the most common potentially lethal genetic disorder caused by mutations in a single gene. ADPKD occurs in 1 in 400 to 1 in 1,000 persons, with approximately 600,000 affected in the United States alone. Knowing the family history is really important, because symptoms and signs may not be obvious or sufficiently notable to alert the individual or the physician to this diagnosis. Hypertension might only develop later in the disease course. Pain emanating from the kidneys may result in back or abdominal pain and is not uncommon. Kidney stones occur in about 20% of those affected, as it did in Paul. Invariably, the occurrence of severe pain as a kidney stone passes will result in imaging studies of the kidney, leading in most cases, when present, to a diagnosis of ADPKD.

Progressive kidney failure, unfortunately, is the major problem in ADPKD. At least 50% of those affected have serious kidney failure by age 60 years. At that stage, only kidney dialysis and transplantation remain as options. Earlier diagnosis and appropriate treatment may avert and delay kidney failure and leave time to arrange for kidney transplantation.

Other manifestations may occur in ADPKD. Multiple cysts in the liver occur in at least 94% of persons affected and are mostly symptom-free. Estrogen hormone replacement therapy may aggravate and increase the size of liver cysts in affected women. The usually silent cysts may occur in other organs such as the pancreas. Widening (dilatation) of the upper parts of the aorta (the largest artery exiting the heart) should always be checked by imaging given occasional situations of rupture. A heart murmur may signal the presence of a floppy mitral valve (the valve between the upper and lower left chambers of the heart) and be associated with potential rhythm disturbances or panic attacks. Caffeine is best avoided because it may promote growth of kidney cysts. Smoking is not recommended since it may diminish blood flow to the kidneys.

Collagen, the universal connective tissue of the body, is found in all tissues and organs. The walls of our arteries and veins can stretch, thanks to the structural characteristics of collagen. Not surprisingly, then, that collagen is found throughout the kidneys, including the filtering apparatus (the basement membranes). However, weakness in collagen fibers will allow a blood vessel to balloon (called an aneurysm) and rupture, and cysts may occur in the kidneys, liver, and elsewhere. The ADPKD genes have an important role in the development of the kidney tubules as well as involvement in maintaining the integrity of blood vessel walls.

Two genes are associated with ADPKD: *PKD1* accounts for more than 80% of cases, and *PKD2* is responsible for more than 10% of cases. There may well be a third gene, but proof is lacking. One reason for suspecting a third gene is that full sequencing of both the *PKD1* and *PKD2* gene in seeking mutations achieves a detection rate approximating 92%. A precise DNA diagnosis is desirable, and once a mutation is recognized, the analysis of all family members can be concentrated simply on that one mutation and not require sequencing of the entire gene. The initial diagnosis may be achieved by ultrasound studies of the kidneys that may, however, miss 10% to 15% of cases. The much more expensive CT or MRI scans will be invariably diagnostic, but DNA testing will provide precise diagnosis by mutation analysis before the presence of any obvious cysts. Mutation detection is extremely important if future preimplantation genetic diagnosis or prenatal diagnosis is desired. Moreover, in families where kidney transplantation becomes necessary for an affected individual, a sibling offering to be a donor of a kidney may become a match. It is critically important then for the molecular diagnosis to have been made. I am aware of two different instances where the DNA test was not done. A sibling donor provided a kidney and only later was discovered to be affected, with the donated kidney also being defective.

When a tiny portion of the *PKD1* gene is deleted, along with a subjacent gene (called *TSC2*) that otherwise results in a condition called tuberous sclerosis (*see* Chapter 20), both conditions co-exist and are detectable in the fetus in early pregnancy. A rarer disorder already evident at birth and called infantile polycystic kidney disease is transmitted as an autosomal recessive condition with risks of recurrence of 25%.

Once again, knowledge of the family history; sharing medical information with siblings, parents, and children; seeking genetic counseling and testing where appropriate; evaluating the cause of hypertension; and excluding the presence of cerebral aneurysms will enable the affected person to secure their health as much as possible and certainly save their life.

A brisk, unremitting wind blew across the island, the palm trees lining the shore bowing in unison as if in deference to the power of the wind and the sea. Despite the balmy early evening temperature of Hawaii, the Yamaha family, cozy in their family room, watched a movie. Besides the parents, two of their sons and their daughter were present. One of the sons, age 15 years, had severe mental retardation and epilepsy. He had no intelligible speech and his communications were mostly by gesture. Suddenly, and without warning, he stood up and began banging on his chest and screaming uncontrollably. The family had never seen such behavior from him and being unable to control or quiet him down, they hustled him struggling into their car and rushed to the hospital. Still screaming and tearing at his chest, he was impossible to examine until four emergency department staff grabbed hold of his limbs, placed him on a gurney, and tied him down with a strait jacket, upon which he instantly died.

A mandated autopsy revealed that his aorta had ruptured, with blood filling his chest cavity. Examination of his brain showed a congenital blood vessel malformation in one location and the probable cause of his seizures.

A precise cause for his mental retardation remained unclear. The family was devastated and at a loss to understand how this could have happened to a 15-year-old child. Their family doctor opined that some type of rare syndrome accounted for his mental retardation, vascular malformation in his brain, and his ruptured aorta.

About 2 years later, the second son, Ted (age 14 years at the time), was sitting in the same living room watching television when he began to complain of pain in his chest and back. Without a moment's hesitation, this time, the parents quickly rushed him to the hospital, told their story of their previous child, and waited anxiously while the immediately ordered CT scan for Ted was performed. A leaking aortic aneurysm was detected, and Ted was rushed to the operating room, where he died before surgical repair could be accomplished.

Ted's grieving family was overwhelmed, and it took many weeks for them to begin to address questions raised by the emergency room physicians. Aortic rupture in two siblings must be genetic, they said, and they advised a genetics consultation, with special reference to the surviving daughter. In due course, they consulted with a clinical geneticist and reviewed the tragedies that had taken their boys' lives.

Discussions ranged over genetic disorders such as Marfan syndrome and other disorders (see discussion) in which dilatation of the aorta may result in rupture. At that time, no molecular diagnosis was available, and no definitive absolute diagnosis could be made. Their key question about why they had not been referred to a clinical geneticist after the loss of their first child was not satisfactorily answered and resulted in a medical malpractice lawsuit.

A safe rule is that unusual, remarkable, or unexpected adverse health events—especially in the young, but in all under age 50 years—should be considered genetic in origin until proved otherwise. This rule would have led to the recommendation of a CT scan of the aortas of Ted and his sister and would have enabled recognition of early dilatation of Ted's aorta. That, in turn, would have led to careful surveillance and measurement of the dilatation, leading to elective surgery to replace the defective part of his aorta without waiting for spontaneous rupture. That would have saved his life and resulted almost certainly in a close to normal life expectancy.

There had been no family history taken, with the paternal grandparents still alive but the maternal grandparents having died young. Both of Ted's parents were otherwise healthy, but neither had a scan of the aorta. Neither of the sons had hyperextensible joints with lax ligaments, long arms, long fingers, short-sightedness, scoliosis, or heart murmurs. These are some of the typical features of the dominantly inherited connective tissue disorder called Marfan syndrome, discussed below.

ANEURYSMS OF THE AORTA

There are a number of genetic disorders in which dilatation of the aorta may occur (*see* Appendix 6). Rupture or tearing of the aorta, which is almost invariably fatal, may occur in all but is a greater risk in disorders such as Marfan syndrome, familial aortic aneurysms, or the Loeys-Dietz syndrome. In all of these disorders, it would be wise to check the dimensions of the aorta from adolescence to adulthood and beyond and, for some, to maintain a schedule to monitor any progression of dilatation. At a certain size, recommendations are made for elective surgery.

Ted and his brother both suffered rupture of an aortic aneurysm, typical for a condition called Thoracic Aortic Aneurysm and Dissection (TAAD). The frequency of this disorder is not known, but only about 20% of those with TAAD have an affected parent or sibling. Ted's parents had not yet agreed to the recommendation of having their aortas imaged. This, at first glance, might sound surprising, but it is the kind of response I have seen quite often. In some, simple fear of discovering a serious or life-threatening defect may paradoxically be followed by the illogical response, "I'd rather not know." Even when the potential life-saving benefit is emphasized, some choose not to know. The negative response to testing by others may be motivated by a feeling of guilt when, for example, one or more of their children are affected. I have even encountered situations where issues of paternity are suspected.

Not well-recognized is the fact that aortic aneurysms rank as the 13th major cause of death in the United States, resulting in about 15,000 deaths annually. About 20% of the thoracic aortic aneurysms are due to a clear genetic flaw. The cause of the ballooning in a portion of the aorta is a weakening or tearing in one or other location in the wall of this great artery. Weakly constructed collagen forming the scaffold of this great artery is the likely fault. At least 10 genes thus far are known to be associated with aneurysm formation of the aorta and all can be tested in highly specialized molecular genetics laboratories. Once an affected person has been diagnosed, siblings and parents should be tested by cardiac ultrasound (echocardiography) or, when necessary, by magnetic resonance imaging (MRI). The size of the aneurysm needs to be monitored as the best indication for when to offer surgical repair and replacement of the section of the defective aorta. Once monitored and operated on in a timely fashion (and not when a tear or rupture has begun), a close to normal life expectancy can be achieved. Again, the family history is key.

Ted and his brother showed no signs of connective tissue abnormalities caused by abnormally constructed collagen, as seen in other disorders in which dilatation of the aorta may occur (*see* Appendix 6). Typical features, as seen in the more common Marfan syndrome (*see* below), were not present.

Incidentally, the jury found the primary care physician negligent for not having referred the family to a clinical geneticist after Ted's brother died.

Cecil C. (or CC, for calm and cool, as the girls called him) was certainly not a doctor. He was the first to profess his limited knowledge of medical matters, although he had been an emergency medical service technician before becoming the high school girls basketball coach.

All of his charges were tall, lanky girls. To his trained eye, one girl stood out. Shanika was 16 years old and in her stockings measured 6 feet, 2 inches in height. He also noted that she had flat feet and felt certain that she had a spinal curvature (scoliosis). Her long arms seemed like windmills to him, and when she sprained a ligament in her hand, he thought she had the longest fingers he had ever seen. Haunted by an image he would never forget while working as an EMT, he insisted she have a check-up with her doctor and bring him a note affirming that she was in good health. As an EMT, he was part of the ambulance crew that rushed to the home of a young mother who had collapsed on the kitchen floor. He recalled the chaotic scene around her and the attempts to resuscitate her, which culminated in her death in the ambulance. The autopsy later revealed a ruptured aortic aneurysm.

Shanika duly returned with a note stating that she was in good health and fit to play basketball. He expressed his delight to Shanika, who off-handedly mentioned that the doctor had stated she had a slight murmur but that it was "innocent" and of no importance.

That evening Coach CC called Shanika's mother, with whom she lived, and urged her to have Shanika consult a cardiologist. When she expressed doubt about the need to have a specialist consultation given her doctor's report, Coach CC related the catastrophic loss of the young mother he had witnessed who had Marfan syndrome.

Shanika's mother eventually agreed and Shanika subsequently saw a cardiologist. His evaluation included an echocardiogram, which to the family's amazement and dismay revealed dilatation of the ascending aorta. He made the diagnosis of Marfan syndrome[1] on the basis of her armspan being longer than her height, her very long fingers (called arachnodactyly), scoliosis, and of course the dilated ascending aorta. She also had joints with lax ligaments, a high arched palate, and dental malocclusion (upper front teeth extending over her lower front teeth). No dislocation of the lenses in her eyes was present.

The cardiologist immediately recommended that both of Shanika's parents come in for an evaluation including an echocardiogram. It took some time to find Shanika's father, who eventually materialized for his evaluation. He indicated that he worked as a security guard at night and slept most days. He had long parted from Shanika's mother, whom he had never married. The echocardiogram revealed a well-advanced aneurysmal dilatation of his ascending aorta at a size that demanded immediate surgical attention to avert what could have been an imminent rupture. Elective surgery was accomplished in a teaching hospital and his recovery was uneventful. Coach CC had vicariously saved his life.

Subsequently, both of Shanika's siblings were evaluated, and the youngest, then 12 years of age, was suspected to have Marfan syndrome and placed on a schedule of echocardiograms to monitor her aorta on an annual basis. Subsequently, analysis of the Marfan syndrome gene (FBN1) revealed a mutation that Shanika, her sister, and her father all harbored. Shanika's paternal grandfather had died suddenly in the South, and his death had been ascribed to a heart attack, without an autopsy having been done. Shanika's father said that he thought he had siblings but did not know any of them or where they were.

---

1. This syndrome was named after a French pediatrician, Bernard-Jean Antonin Marfan, who described the typical physical features in 1896.

But for an observant, caring coach, Shanika could well have eventually dropped dead on the basketball court—the type of incident that has happened elsewhere in other sports venues.

Marfan syndrome is not rare, affecting an estimated 1 in 5,000 to 1 in 10,000 people and without ethnic predilection. The major characteristic signs were discussed above and a number of major and minor signs are necessary for a geneticist to reach a diagnosis. One important major sign, revealed only by a CT scan or MRI, is widening of the sheath (called the dura) that contains the spinal cord in the lower back (called dural ectasia). Since there are many tall people, even with long fingers, clear and definitive signs involving the aorta, the heart, the eyes, the connective tissues, the lungs, and the musculoskeletal system have to be assessed to make a clinical diagnosis.

MARFAN SYNDROME

An absolute diagnosis depends on precise sequencing of the specific Fibrillin 1 gene. Once a mutation has been detected, other family members at risk (siblings, parents, and children of the affected) should be offered testing, even if they are asymptomatic. About 75% of those diagnosed with Marfan syndrome have an affected parent, the remaining 25% representing the consequence of a brand-new mutation in the *FBN1* gene. If a parent is affected for this autosomal dominant genetic disorder, then there is a 50% risk of transmission to each child. Rarely, the mutation in the *FBN1* gene may exist in some of the cells either in the ovary or testes of a parent (called germline mosaicism; *see* Chapter 2 and Appendix 2).

For a woman with Marfan syndrome, pregnancy can prove hazardous. Pregnancy may be associated with a more rapid dilatation of the aorta, including rupture either during the pregnancy or in the weeks after delivery. Hence, women with Marfan syndrome are advised to consult with a geneticist before undertaking a pregnancy. The single key issue is whether there is dilatation of the aorta, leading to the potential risk of rupture during pregnancy or delivery and even in the post partum period. Hence, precise monitoring by echocardiography of the aorta is critical. Rarely severe manifestations are present in a newborn or infant. Once it has been established that there is a specific mutation in the *FBN1* gene, prenatal diagnosis or preimplantation genetic diagnosis becomes possible. The requests for such tests in Marfan syndrome are positively rare.

For persons with Marfan syndrome, paying special attention to the aorta and the heart are critical, and long-term care should be vested in the hands of a cardiologist familiar with this disorder. Monitoring of the aortic size may eventually lead to a recommendation for surgery to avert a future rupture. Sometimes repair of a heart valve is necessary if leakage that could lead to heart failure is detected. Medications, such as beta-blockers, reduce stress on the aorta from blood flow.[2] Matters that are not life-threatening are dealt with in a routine way, including eye care, attention to bones and joints, repair of hernias, orthopedic attention to flat feet, and dental problems requiring orthodontic attention. Contact or competitive sports, including isometric exercise, are to be avoided, as are all activities that cause joint injury or pain. Laser correction of eye problems should be avoided, given the weaker connective tissue in Marfan syndrome. Playing a wind instrument, such as a trumpet (which requires breathing against resistance), is also not recommended, as it could burst the lung at a vulnerable spot. Positive pressure ventilation, as used in scuba diving, should be avoided.

Cleary, early diagnosis of Marfan syndrome is important if lives are to be saved and appropriate care rendered to secure a family's health.

---

2. Another drug, Losartan, which in a mouse model of Marfan syndrome was shown to inhibit aortic growth. There has not been a way to prevent aortic complications. This drug has been tried in a few patients in which the rate of progressive aortic root dilation was slowed. Clinical trials are now ongoing.

19

BRAIN CONNECTIONS AND DISCONNECTIONS

Jerry and Matilda ("Please call me Mattie") met in college and were inseparable. They married soon after graduation and carefully planned for their future. Jerry focused on information technology and over the years became a networking specialist. Mattie was more interested in medicine and trained as a nurse practitioner. Both were "compulsively neat" and, as Mattie related during one consultation, their house was so neat that a guest recently asked if anyone actually lived in it. They acknowledged that they were "obsessively neat" but loved this characteristic that they shared.

About 5 years after graduation, they planned to start a family. Mattie immediately began taking the folic acid vitamin supplement (to avoid spina bifida) and, 3 months later, happily reported that her pregnancy test was positive. The pregnancy was uneventful and free of any complication. She took no medications and was especially careful with her diet and avoided alcohol. Labor, however, turned out to be rather prolonged and unexpectedly very painful. Later, her obstetrician explained that their son Peter had a rather unexpectedly large head size, which made passage through the birth canal slow and difficult. Nevertheless, at birth, Peter was pink, vigorous, and signaled his entry into the world with a loud cry.

As a nurse practitioner, Mattie understood the importance of breast feeding, and as soon as her "milk came in" she settled down to enjoy this closeness with Peter. Only 2 years later and after direct questioning did Mattie realize that Peter never really looked her in the eye during breast feeding.

Within weeks of birth, it became obvious that Peter was frequently "cranky" and difficult to console when crying, which he did frequently.

He also slept poorly and awoke frequently through the night for months on end. The inevitable fatigue steadily wore on the nerves of Jerry and Mattie, who found themselves in arguments that they had never had before.

Peter's motor development was on track, with him sitting up unsupported at age 7 months and walking at 13 months. In retrospect, Mattie acknowledged that Peter did not seem to like being held or cuddled and did not reach out to be picked up. Between ages 15 and 18 months, he had acquired a significant number of words and appeared to be doing well. However, within weeks of receiving a routine vaccination for measles, mumps, and rubella, he seemed to lose much of his acquired language. He also stopped responding to his name.

The neurologist to whom Peter had been referred raised the possibility of autism. He was, however, concerned about the sudden change in development and the associated "big head" that Peter had. This latter observation resulted in a brain MRI, which revealed no abnormality. Peter's parents seriously questioned the role of the vaccination in precipitating Peter's loss of abilities.

The ensuing 18 months provided little comfort. Repetitive hand-flapping and walking in circles became an unrelenting behavior with an accompanying high-pitched hum. Peter seemed unable to play or interact with other children of his own age. In fact, as Mattie reported, he could literally trample on a child's hand or foot without noticing or recognizing the resultant cry of pain. It seemed, Mattie reported, that other children seemed to be like "inanimate objects." Peter also had a frantic reaction to loud noises, such as those made by the vacuum cleaner, and would rapidly exit the room holding his ears and even running into a wall. He also seemed to have a high pain threshold. He continued to dislike being touched or held, and finding foods he would eat became a major challenge. Just prior to his fifth birthday, Peter had a major seizure in the absence of any obvious precipitating fever or infection. By then it was clear to Jerry and Mattie that Peter's IQ was in the retarded range and that the diagnosis of autism was certain.

I saw them both in consultation after they had decided to consider another pregnancy. Careful review of their family history revealed that Jerry, his sister, and his father all had large heads (called macrocephaly). One nephew, then age 6 years, had experienced some speech and language delay but, following speech therapy, was doing well. Mattie herself was well and in passing mentioned that she had perfect pitch.[1] She, too, had a nephew, the son of her sister, who had been diagnosed with dyslexia after his teachers had pointed out his persistent letter reversals and difficulties in reading.

I discussed the fact that no definitive associated recognizable disorder explained Peter's autism, given that the neurologist had obtained numerous genetic tests that yielded only normal results. The risk of recurrence approximated 6% with a potential additional 4% risk for somewhat milder disorders that involve language and social development, as well as psychiatric disorders. No prenatal diagnosis would be possible, given the absence of a definitive DNA or biochemical diagnostic test. Mattie was insistent that the preservative Thimerosal (which contained mercury) in the vaccine that Peter received was the cause of his autism. She remained unconvinced about published studies that did not support any role of Thimerosal in causing autism.

There was no basis to relate Jerry's nephew's speech and language delay or Mattie's nephew's dyslexia to Peter's autism.

Jerry and Mattie decided on a second pregnancy and just over a year later delivered their son Matthew. This time, Mattie noticed the lack of eye contact that Matthew exhibited when breast feeding and many of the same features that Peter manifested over the ensuing months and years, confirming yet again a diagnosis of autism.

Thorough studies have thus far exonerated the role of Thimerosal as a causal factor for autism.[2] However, an environmental factor thus far unrecognized remains a possibility. Two avenues of research point to brain involvement, either prior to vaccination or very much earlier in

1. Perfect pitch or absolute pitch is the rare ability to identify tones with their corresponding musical note names without the help of a reference tone. Just as most of us can recognize the individual colors of a rainbow without thinking, individuals who possess the trait of perfect pitch can identify the precise pitch of a tone. Studies of identical and non-identical twins as well as families whose members have perfect pitch indicate the important role of genes in transmitting this fascinating trait. Undoubtedly, environmental factors such as early musical training have some influence on the development of this rare ability.
2. Moreover, in 2010 the British journal *The Lancet* retracted the original published paper implicating Thimerosal, citing the study as unethical. The first author, Dr Andrew Wakefield, was found to have manipulated the data.

fetal or infantile development. Studies of home videotapes of autistic compared to non-autistic children at their first year birthday parties enabled recognition of greater than 90% of autistic children by observation of their behaviors. Particularly noteworthy were the lack of pointing, showing objects, actually looking at others, and responding to their name when called. Studies of brain tissue have revealed nonspecific and variable changes that likely date back to early developmental stages.

I explained that macrocephaly is frequently inherited as a dominant characteristic, with a 50% likelihood of transmission of this trait. Given the highly successful careers of Jerry, his sister, and their father, it was safe to conclude that Peter's head size almost certainly had nothing to do with his autism. It is important to note, however, that where a child with autism has a large head in the absence of a parent or family history with macrocephaly, analysis of one particular gene (PTEN) would be recommended. Typically in autism spectrum disorders (ASDs), there is an acceleration of head circumference growth in infancy, followed by an earlier deceleration.

Peter's seizure reflected the observations in various reports that epilepsy occurs in 5% to 49% of ASD cases. Moreover, seizure patterns as seen on electroencephalography (EEG), even in the absence of actual seizures, have been reported in up to 60% of cases. The MRI Peter had apparently revealed no abnormality. Recent reports, however, indicate an unexpectedly high rate (48%) of MRI abnormalities in those with typical autism.[3] Multiple reports document about a twofold increase in the rate of various birth defects, especially when intellectual disability was present. Male preponderance (up to 8:1) persisted in these studies. Autism spectrum disorders may involve different systems, not infrequently causing (or being associated with) gastrointestinal symptoms (loose stools, constipation, abdominal aches, food reflux, food hypersensitivity or selectivity). Reports about abnormalities in the immune system have been inconsistent but may wll predispose to ear infections resulting in hearing impairment in some. Hearing deficits in autism are

---

3. Brain abnormalities included hyperintensity of white matter, temporal lobe changes, and increased spaces surrounding penetrating arteries.

common, ranging from mild to profound in at least 3.5% to 13.3% and not necessarily caused by ear infections. Hearing sensitivity or bizarre reactions to sounds are not uncommon.

Jerry and Mattie's perfectionist behaviors may be irrelevant as far as causality is concerned. Nevertheless, reports record that parents and siblings of an autistic child often show some similar manifestations, including a history of delayed language acquisition, delayed social development, absence of close friendships, being a perfectionist, or having a rigid personality type. This remains a tenuous explanation for a complex disorder.

Much has been made about the claimed increased frequency of autism in the last few years. Careful studies in different countries have reflected a prevalence ranging from 1 in 250 for typical autism to 1 in 150 that would include children with a spectrum of behavior variably called autistic-like or with pervasive developmental delay. Differences in actual prevalence rates are due to a number of factors, including variations in study methods and design, variable adherence to precise diagnosis, as well as massive media attention following the vaccine scare. Moreover, changes in classification between mental retardation, ASDs, and pervasive developmental disorders (PDD) and the use of broader diagnostic criteria have also contributed to the apparent increased incidence of autism. Most studies conclude that this increase is indeed apparent and not real. However, a large California study from the MIND institute concluded that the increase in the frequency of autism was real and that there may well be an environmental contributing factor. The difficulty of actually making a precise diagnosis is due to the absence of a definitive biochemical or molecular test. Rather, diagnostic criteria depend on imprecise and subjective signs and observations, sometimes open to variable interpretation. Diagnostic criteria focus on impaired social interactions and communication, as well as aberrant behaviors.

For impaired social interaction, criteria focus on eye-to-eye contact, facial expression, and interaction with others, including the inability to share enjoyment, interests, or achievements; impairments in communication include the lack of language, inability to initiate or sustain a conversation, repetitive use of words and language peculiarities, as well as a lack of spontaneous make-believe play or imitative play. Repetitive patterns of behavior, such as Peter's hand-flapping and walking in circles, are typical but not always evident. Persistent preoccupation with one object, and later with one subject, is common. A series of diagnostic checklists are usually used to assist in the diagnostic effort.

Asperger syndrome,[4] sometimes called high-functioning autism, is characterized by normal language development but with a range of behaviors described above. These affected children or adults are usually loners, don't do well in groups or at parties, don't usually appreciate jokes, follow a strict routine of their own, and are frequently preoccupied by a single interest, such as computers. Individuals with Asperger syndrome are often noted to be clumsy. A much rarer condition is called childhood disintegrative disorder, in which normal development is typical for at least 2 years, after which there might be loss of language as well as social and play skills. I recall one patient who, at age 7 years, following normal development (including bicycle riding), deteriorated rapidly and for a time would only bark like a dog.

Great care is exercised in trying to determine the cause of autism, which, if discovered, could influence care, risk of recurrence, prognosis, options for future prenatal diagnosis, and long-term management. At present, however, in about 85% of cases with ASDs, no definitive cause can yet be determined. Constituting the remaining 15% are individuals with autistic behavior due to a secondary cause such as a chromosome abnormality, a gene mutation, or an environmental agent.

Autistic behaviors may be seen in a wide range of very different genetic disorders but most commonly in association with mental retardation or serious cognitive disabilities. Examples include the Prader-Willi and Angelman syndromes (*see* Chapter 21), the Fragile X syndrome (*see* Chapter 10), Down syndrome (*see* Chapter 2), Rett syndrome,[5] tuberous sclerosis complex (*see* Chapter 20), and some mitochondrial disorders (*see* Chapter 22). A clinical geneticist will be able to determine the need for additional tests if any of

---

4. Named for Dr. Hans Asperger, an Austrian physician who described features of this syndrome.

5. This disorder, manifesting primarily (but not only) in females, may closely mimic typical autism while presenting with the behavioral characteristics of pervasive developmental disorder. A period of normal development is common and followed by a loss of language and typically repetitive hand-wringing movements. Analysis of the gene (MECP2) for this disorder enables a precise diagnosis. Affected males rarely make it out of the womb and, if born alive, are frequently profoundly retarded. A few, however, survive but are mentally retarded.

these disorders are to be considered in the evaluation of a child with autistic features.

Most recently and as a consequence of remarkable advances in the analysis of the human genome, it has become apparent that in typical autism, without a recognizable cause, tiny deletions or duplications occur with increased frequency in the genomes of those affected. These gaps and duplications shown by the test called a chromosomal microarray (see Chapter 5) occur about 10 times more frequently than in unaffected individuals.[6] Of particular importance is the observation that certain genes involved in the duplication or missing in the deleted areas function at the nerve interconnections (synapses) in the brain. Failures of connectivity, therefore, might occur and explain the disconnect so evident in the behavior of even autistic children without mental retardation. For at least some cases, the involvement and dysfunction of different genes may explain the wide range of signs and behaviors that are commonly witnessed. Why these gaps and duplications occur with increased frequency in autism is the subject of intense research, more especially since they may not be present in either parent. The matter is of further interest because deletions and duplications occur in all of our genomes and probably account for so many of the physical and mental differences and susceptibilities that we manifest.

Genome-wide scans of thousands of children with autism in many studies have identified particular regions in the genome that show common associations in at least 10 different chromosomes. The theory is that there might be a genetic susceptibility to develop autism in response to a thus far unknown environmental factor(s). The genetic contribution clearly remains important and is evidenced by the fact that if one pair of identical twins is affected, then there is a very high likelihood (70%–90%) that the other twin will also be affected (called concordance), compared with an approximately 10% likelihood in non-identical twins. There is up to an 8-to-1 male-to-female sex ratio for typical autism and, as mentioned earlier, the increased risk of recurrence.

The care of a child with autism and later as an adult may prove to be a lifetime challenge. The earlier the diagnosis and the earlier the intensive behavioral therapy is initiated, the better the chance for an optimal outcome. The *National Research Council* has a publication available online entitled *Educating Children with Autism*, which is highly recommended. The mainstay

6. Limited gene marker studies thus far make it likely that this may be a low estimate.

of management is behavioral and educational therapy, with actual medications still to be proven to be of value.

Mattie felt certain that Thimerosal caused Peter's autism. Despite being made aware that the risk of recurrence approximated 6% or 7%, she chose to downplay the odds, believing that the cause was an environmental agent. She failed to realize, however, that ignoring facts don't change the facts. The devastating truth of this axiom dawned on the parents with the awesome reality that Matthew was also affected—even though there was no exposure to Thimerosal. I have seen and known families with three children affected with autism and have come away with the realization that many parents in managing these challenges must be saints. It is also clear that people view risks very differently. To some, a 50% risk suggests a good chance that all will be well half the time and they are content to take a chance. For others, 25% or even a 10% risk of an adverse outcome is too great. I well remember a father pounding on my desk, exclaiming that if he had known that there was a 1 in 10,000 risk of having a child with a birth defect, he would never have had children. When I drew his attention to the fact that, on average, we all have a 3% to 4% risk of having a child with a major birth defect, mental retardation, or genetic disorder, he was stunned and wondered why no one had told him this before. The risks we take in having children are personal, but it certainly would seem wiser to be fully aware of their measure.

The scene was chaotic, as related by the police who arrived at the crash site following the emergency call by a neighbor. Apparently Phillip had been driving at high speed, rounded a curve in the road, and lost control of his car, which slammed into the side of a house. When the police arrived, they found the occupants of the house screaming at Phillip, who had extracted himself from his demolished car. Instead of responding or reacting to the vitriolic stream of abusive language that flowed from the occupants, Phillip was mumbling about people who were out to get him and were chasing him. He was not apologetic and seemed unaware of the implications of the damage he had caused. The house occupants thought he was "on drugs," and but for the timely arrival of the police, Phillip may well have been the recipient of a smashed skull, courtesy of the baseball bat carried by the male occupant of the house.

Phillip was hastily ensconced in the police car and taken to the station. His parents were called and a blood sample obtained to determine the presence of alcohol or illicit drugs. Bill and Daphne found their son sitting in a cell, rambling on unintelligibly and seemingly unaware of the situation. Phillip's distraught parents sought the help of a lawyer, who secured his release with fixed plans for immediate psychiatric evaluation.

Before this incident occurred, after 6 weeks of his first year at college, Phillip's resident dormitory assistant had telephoned his parents, advising them of the situation with their son. Phillip had only been attending classes intermittently, had leftover food all over his room and under his bed, had not made his bed in 6 weeks, and seemed to talk to himself. His parents were seriously concerned after a few phone calls in which Phillip sounded intermittently incoherent and non-communicative, abruptly cutting off their conversations with, "I have to go now." In consultation with university officials, they decided to bring him home and seek psychiatric care. After a few days at home, he seemed much improved and convinced his mother that he could safely take and drive her car. That was the prelude to the accident.

The psychiatrist elicited a history from Bill and Daphne about Phillip's tendency from his childhood to be a loner. He had few friends and had never had a girlfriend. He had occasionally voiced fears that people were against him but could never substantiate any reasons nor name any people. When he was about 14 years old, he had a number of physical fights at school. Given his above-average intelligence, Phillip managed his school-work and exams well, but school reports reflected erratic behavior and difficulties with interpersonal relations.

Phillip's family history was striking and informative. His younger sister had been diagnosed with bipolar disease (manic depression), a diagnosis that also applied to Daphne and one of her four sisters. One other sister had schizophrenia, and the son of that sister had been tentatively diagnosed as likely schizophrenic. Both of Daphne's brothers had been diagnosed with attention deficit hyperactivity disorder (ADHD), and one of them had a daughter with depression. Daphne's mother was suspected as having had schizophrenia. She was thought to have had hallucinations and had died when she jumped off a sailing boat into the sea, even though she could not swim. Phillip's father suffered from depression, as did Phillip's maternal aunt and maternal grandmother.

Phillip's psychiatrist diagnosed him as having schizophrenia in view of his paranoid delusions, social withdrawal, loss of interest, aimlessness, and idleness, together with his striking apathy and blunted emotional responses.

Phillip was referred to a psychopharmacologist who, after trying a number of antipsychotic medications, came up with a combination that provided some stability of mood, thought, and action. Phillip did not return to his distant college but to a local community college, living at home and managing to progress satisfactorily.

It may be surprising but it is not uncommon to find affected individuals on both sides of the family, either with schizophrenia or overlapping disorders such as manic depression (bipolar disease), depression (unipolar disease), or ADHD. When both sides of a family have affected individuals, the vulnerabilities transmitted will be variable and the individual risks increased but hard to assess precisely. The most important known risk factor is a positive family history of schizophrenia or related disorders.[7] The Swedish National Hospital Discharge registry was used to identify all patients with bipolar disorder (40,187 individuals) or schizophrenia (35,985 individuals) over three decades. In this, the largest study ever, first-degree relatives of those with either bipolar disorder or schizophrenia had a 3% to 4 % risk of developing either condition, whereas half-siblings had a 1.5% to 2% risk. A clear illustration of the overlap between these two diagnoses in that study was reflected by the fact that 2,543 individuals had received the diagnosis of both disorders on at least two occasions.

Schizophrenia most often becomes overt between ages 16 and 30 years, with an excess of males in the younger age range and an excess of females in the older age range. Certainly, the peak age at the onset is in the early 20s for men and late 20s for women.

Between established and new antipsychotic medications, many with schizophrenia have been able to avoid hospitalization and have been able to resume a normal to a relatively normal life. Unfortunately, many end up with repeated hospitalizations and long-term care.

Interestingly, the occurrence of bipolar disorder and schizophrenia in the same extended family is not uncommon. Bipolar disorder is

---

7. Such as schizoaffective disorder, schizoid personality disorder, and paranoid personality disorder, bipolar and unipolar disease.

characterized by alternating behavior with two emotional extremes: sadness and depression on the one side and manic behavior on the other. Also called manic depression or manic depressive disorder, the frequency approximates 1% to 2% of the population. In the manic phase, an individual may be reckless and behave inappropriately—for example, spending wildly (writing checks for money that he or she does not have) or having promiscuous sex. Such patients may lose touch with reality and be diagnosed as schizophrenic. I recall years ago, when still a medical student, seeing a patient who walked into the room in a state of absolute mania. He immediately pulled out a check book and wrote each of us in the room a check for a million pounds!

Individuals with bipolar disorder may experience vast swings in mood from the depths of depression to peaks of mania, while others have primarily depressive symptoms or mainly manic or hypomanic episodes. Those who are depressed have a despondent mood, no energy, feelings of worthlessness, and difficulties in concentration. Thoughts of suicide are not unusual, and between 10% and 15% who suffer from bipolar disorder attempt or commit suicide.

The manic person presents with a great, happy mood, speaking quickly with flights of endless ideas but with difficulty concentrating. They may also exhibit poor judgment; behave recklessly; show anger, irritability, or fear; have delusions and hallucinations; be abusive; or even engage in violent acts.

Genome-wide association studies now clearly show that the predisposition to bipolar disorder results from the action of a number of genes, while twin studies have clearly established the strong heritability of bipolar disorder. Those who have close relatives with bipolar disorder have a higher risk of developing bipolar disorder or major depressive illness themselves. Table 19.1 shows individual risks of developing unipolar or bipolar disorders. As noted, if one parent is affected with bipolar disorder, then the risk for all offspring developing bipolar or unipolar disorder approximates 28%. Adolescents who experience recurring episodes of major depression have about a 10% to 15% likelihood of developing bipolar disorder. The life-time prevalence rate of bipolar disorder was 4.5% in a United States study. This disorder ranks as one of the main causes of disability in the Western world for people 15-44 years of age.

Table 19.1 Familial Risks of a Unipolar or Bipolar Disorder

If Affected	Unipolar or Bipolar	Risk (Percent)	For Relative
One parent	Bipolar	28.0	All offspring (uni- or bipolar)
One parent	Bipolar	4.1–14.6	Parent's sibling or offspring (bipolar)
One parent	Bipolar	5.4–14.0	Parent's sibling or offspring (unipolar)
Both parents	Either	56.0–84.0	All offspring (unipolar or bipolar)
One parent	Unipolar	5.5–28.4	Parent's sibling or offspring (unipolar)
One parent	Unipolar	0.7–8.1	Parent's sibling or offspring (bipolar)
One identical twin	Bipolar	67.0–100.0	Other twin
One non-identical twin	Bipolar	20.0	Other twin
One identical twin	unipolar	50.0	Other twin
One non-identical twin	unipolar	50.0	Other twin

Many famous people lived with bipolar disorder, including the brilliant composer Ludwig van Beethoven, the famous opera star Gaetano Donizetti, the remarkable and celebrated artist Vincent van Gogh, and a long list of artists, actors, and authors. Clinical depression dogged Charles Dickens, one of the greatest authors in the English language, the Pulitzer prize-winning novelist Ernest Hemingway, the playwright Tennessee Williams, President Abraham Lincoln, and Winston Churchill (who described it as his "Black Dog"), to name but a few of the creative and successful people who were not cowed by their mood disorder.

Few realize that about 1 in 100 people are schizophrenic. Of interest is the fact that among the Amish in the United States, the rate of schizophrenia is low (about 1 in 2,000), whereas in a northern Swedish isolated group, the frequency is about 1 in 42! Schizophrenia occurs in all ethnicities, and a number of environmental factors are believed to influence the development of this disorder. Lower socioeconomic status is associated with higher incidence rates, as shown by a cross-national study by the World Health Organization of populations in Europe, Asia, and the United States. For example, in the United States, schizophrenia occurred almost eight times more frequently in the lowest compared to the highest socioeconomic groups. Even the sex hormones appear to have a role. Women are more likely to become symptomatic when their estrogen levels are low, such as immediately after giving birth or after menopause, than when such levels are high, such as during pregnancy. Estrogen also affects the function of connectivity chemicals (neurotransmitters) that have been implicated in schizophrenia. However, the heritability of schizophrenia is well-established and may account for an estimated 60% to 85% of the cause(s), susceptibility, or predisposition.

The vast majority of genetic disorders, although present biologically at birth, only manifest later. Symptoms and signs may first appear days, months, years, and decades after birth. Explanations abound for this phenomenon, including gender, mode of inheritance, the strength of the gene effects (called penetrance and expressivity), the action of modifying genes, the presence of different mutations or combinations of mutations, and of course environmental factors. For some with later-manifesting conditions such as schizophrenia, early subtle, but nonspecific signs may be retrospectively recognized to have occurred in childhood. Boys, for example, may be especially aggressive, whereas girls might be oversensitive and conforming. On average, those who do develop schizophrenia are more likely to have had developmental issues involving language, learning, physical disabilities, social skills, and emotional control.

Environmental factors may have a causal or predisposing role in schizophrenia. For example, significantly more obstetric complications involving fetal hypoxia (implying brain damage) occur in the newborn history of schizophrenics than others, including their own siblings. A Swedish study of 524 individuals with schizophrenia and 1,043 matched controls showed greater than a fourfold risk if there were signs of hypoxia at birth. Even in identical twins with only one affected, obstetric complications occur more often in the affected twin. However, as noted above, genetic factors play a key role in the genesis of schizophrenia. Various population studies antedated the more recent DNA studies. The risk of schizophrenia was noted to increase according to degrees of relatedness within a family. Studies of identical twins revealed that in 40% to 50%, both were affected, compared to non-identical twins in whom 10% to 17% were both affected. Studies of identical twins separated soon after birth and reared apart showed that in at least 62.5% of cases, both were affected. Some might argue that the identical twins were exposed to the same prenatal or perinatal (the period just before and soon after birth) environments to explain such results.

Adoption studies have been particularly valuable in providing compelling evidence of heritability in schizophrenia. The rates of occurrence of schizophrenia in adoptees, their adopting families, and their biological parents have clearly implicated a key role for genes in causation. A greater risk for schizophrenia was noted among adoptees who were offspring of schizophrenic mothers and who had been separated from their mothers at birth compared to those adopted from unaffected mothers. Similarly, lesser rates of psychosis were found among adoptees who were the offspring of healthy biological parents, whether or not these children were reared by adoptive parents with or without schizophrenia. The rates of schizophrenia in both adoptee groups were clearly lower than those found in adoptees from biological parents with schizophrenia.

Schizophrenia and related disorders have also been reported four times more frequently among biological relatives of schizophrenic adoptees. This observed increased frequency among biological relatives of schizophrenic adoptees includes schizoid and paranoid personality disorders, again suggesting gradations of schizophrenia or a variable spectrum of schizophrenic manifestations. This risk for schizophrenia and this variable spectrum of manifestations occurs some 10 times more frequently among the biological relatives of schizophrenic adoptees than among the biological relatives of unaffected individuals.

In the race to complete the mapping of the human genome, there was an intense search for a gene, or genes, in which a mutation(s) might explain the biological basis of schizophrenia. Given the acceptance that there was an environmental component to causation, the studies in multiple countries focused on a search for a genetic signature—that is, a set of susceptibility or predisposing genes that might be found in common among schizophrenics. These linkage and association studies have indeed revealed a number of genes or gene locations in common that imply risks for schizophrenia.

More critical, however, have been the advances that more recently revealed the presence of deletions and duplications at least 10 times more often than normal in those with schizophrenia. Some genes at these locations are known to normally function at connections (synapses) between neurons in the brain. Mutations in these genes would disrupt nerve interconnections and effect connectivity.[8] The same, or worse, might occur if the gene in question is missing (because of the deletion) or simply duplicated. Mutations in genes at these locations increase the risk not only of schizophrenia but also of a range of other psychiatric disorders, including autism and mental retardation, and have been revealed by the chromosomal microarray technique (*see* Chapter 5). Of interest was the realization that the same psychotic disorder could occur whether there was a deletion or a duplication. When these mutations occurred

---

8. In fact, one such gene is named *Disrupted in Schizophrenia 1*, and another is called *Neuregulin 1*.

for the first time in an individual (and not inherited from either parent), there was about an eight times greater frequency of schizophrenia compared to unaffected individuals. It appears that these brand new mutations in different genes and in different patients account for the variable manifestations and the different psychoses. Unfortunately, these various deletions/duplications are thought to account for only a small proportion of affected individuals.

Other genetic disorders—common, uncommon, and rare—may also be associated with schizophrenia or schizoid features. Women with the triple X syndrome (*see* Chapter 3) have an increased risk of having a schizoid disorder. Individuals with a deletion mutation on chromosome 22 (the Velocardiofacial syndrome discussed in Chapter 11) have the highest known risk for developing schizophrenia or schizoaffective disorder (up to 60%). There is a rare biochemical genetic disorder[9] in which the female carrier of the specific gene mutation may have psychotic manifestations after a heavy protein meal! This occurs because of the accumulation of ammonia resulting from the enzyme deficiency limiting the liver's ability to break down protein.

Table 19.2 summarizes the risk of developing schizophrenia among the relatives of schizophrenics. From the table, it can be seen that the brother or sister of a schizophrenic has a 7.4% to 10% risk of being affected. The risk to a child with two affected parents is between 45% and 50%.

Given the chronic nature of this disabling disorder, serious problems that involve education, occupation, and social functioning are common. Increased mortality rates are due to a range of factors that include a poorer quality of hygiene, safety, and medical treatment, complications of medications, violent deaths, and suicide. The reported suicide rate for those with schizophrenia is some 10 times greater than that for the general population. More than 50% of schizophrenics reportedly attempt suicide during their lifetimes, and about 10% actually succeed.

Important advances have been made in the development of new antipsychotic medications, some of which have unfortunate complicating side effects such as causing movement disorders. Nevertheless, awareness of the family history and early diagnosis and initiation of appropriate medication may help enormously and alter the long-term course of this disabling disorder. Medications used in schizophrenia have also been effective in the treatment of bipolar disorder. Among many talented people, John Nash (mathematician and Nobel Prize winner) and President Abraham Lincoln's wife, Mary,

---

9. Ornithine transcarbamylase deficiency.

Table 19.2 The Risk of Schizophrenia Among the Relatives of
Schizophrenics

Relationship to Schizophrenic	Estimated Risk of Having Schizophrenia (Percent)
Parent	6
Brother or sister	7.4–10
Brother or sister (one sibling and one parent affected)	15–17
Identical twin	40–50
Non-identical twin	10–17
Child (one parent affected)	7.4–16.2
Child (both parents affected)	45–50
Uncle or aunt	2–5
Nephew or niece	3–5
First cousin	1–2.4
Grandchild	3–5
Half-sibling	3–6
Adopted child of an affected mother	17.0
Unrelated (general population)	0.9

had schizophrenia. These observations may simply reflect notations in the lives of celebrities and have little or no other relevance. It is interesting that Albert Einstein and the Nobel Lauriat James Watson, as well as James Joyce, each had a child with schizophrenia. However, there are reports that among the non-schizophrenic relatives of patients with schizophrenia are those who are particularly creative. In fact, impressive creativity has been noted in some of the offspring of schizophrenics.

Major depressive disorder that occurs usually without mania has a lifetime incidence of more than 12% in men and 20% in women. Twin studies indicate a much lower degree of heritability than seen in schizophrenia and bipolar disorder. Once again, multiple genes and environmental components are thought to be causal.

Established and newer medications and early intervention have made significant inroads in the treatment of schizophrenia, bipolar disorder, and major depressive disorder. In addition, new anti-psychotic medications have reduced the mortality rate in schizophrenia, and together with a multidisciplinary team of health professionals, a remission rate of 80% can be achieved.

SKIN

A MIRROR TO THE BRAIN

Olga was a patient woman, subservient to her husband and, for all intents and purposes, a slave to her children. But there came a day when she felt she had had enough. Her husband's frequent demand for unprotected sex left her vulnerable for a third pregnancy that she desperately wished to avoid. Her husband Peter ("named after Peter the Great," he would frequently and repeatedly claim) had no such misgivings. He did janitorial work and was satisfied with his steady employment, albeit with a modest income. He had dropped out of high school, which he hated and where he had considerable difficulty learning. He had a few marble-sized lumps on his arms and torso and at least a dozen variably sized spots that resembled coffee stains (café au lait spots) on his abdomen, back, and thighs. He took pride in being able to avoid seeing doctors for most of his 40 years.

Peter and Olga had two boys, both of whom clearly had learning difficulties, with the eldest also suffering from attention deficit hyperactivity disorder (ADHD). As Olga would frequently say, "The village policeman could easily conclude that both boys inherited their problems from their father." Moreover, she had observed that both boys, as well as Peter, had rather large heads. Neither of the boys had any lumps at ages 6 and 8 years, respectively. Peter's sister had been diagnosed with breast cancer in her late 40s. She, too, had those tell-tale lumps and multiple coffee-stain spots. When her breast cancer was diagnosed, one of those lumps was also biopsied, and a diagnosis was made of neurofibromatosis type I (NF1). Peter's father had had a brain tumor, which they later learned was an astrocytoma.

Following his sister's diagnosis, Olga convinced Peter to see their family doctor. The diagnosis of NF1 was made without difficulty on physical examination. In addition to the lumps, the café au lait spots, and his learning disorder, Peter also had a curved spine (scoliosis), a large head, and freckles in his armpits and groins.

Upon hearing the news of Peter's diagnosis, Olga issued an ultimatum. No more sex until he had a vasectomy. After weeks of grumbling and arguing, Peter assented and made an appointment to have a vasectomy. Barely a year later, and to her horror, Olga discovered that she had become pregnant. She quickly sought an appointment with their family doctor who seemed unfazed by the vasectomy failure, simply saying, "It happens." Despite her Catholic beliefs, she requested that the pregnancy be terminated, and her physician duly complied. The first trimester termination was uneventful, and she returned home the same day with a feeling of great relief. About 3 months later, and dismayed by her weight gain, she returned to see the family doctor, who this time seemed flustered when announcing that Olga was indeed pregnant. The D and C[1] had failed, and all her doctor could say was that he was amazed. Olga duly delivered a very premature infant at 32 weeks gestation. Her newly born daughter suffered multiple complications of prematurity and was later diagnosed with cerebral palsy and mental retardation with seizures. Even later, a diagnosis of NF1 was also made.

It is inconceivable for one family to experience a failed vasectomy, a failed first trimester abortion, and have a pathologist fail to recognize the absence of fetal tissue following abortion. The frequency of vasectomy failures depend on the experience of the surgeon and the various techniques used. Published failure rates range from 0.2% all the way to 13%. Standard practice requires that a sperm count be performed twice between 2 and 4 months after the procedure to confirm the absence of any sperm. The appearance or reappearance of sperm may occur if the tubes recanalize. The requirement is for the physician to inform the patient of the potential failure rate and to check the sperm count as just

---

1. Dilatation and curettage.

noted. Peter's physician did neither. Failure to abort after a D and C is known but rare. Certainly the pathologist would have been expected to recognize the absence of fetal tissue. Needless to say, a lawsuit claiming medical negligence ensued.

It is very common for pediatricians and family doctors to see the children in a family without ever even meeting the father. The diagnosis of NF1 would have been made much earlier in their boys as well as in Peter if he had materialized even once together with his children in the doctor's office. The cerebral palsy and mental retardation in their daughter had nothing to do with NF1 but was a consequence of marked prematurity and associated complications. Much the same can be said for women receiving antenatal care, when the husband meets the delivering physician for the first time in the labor ward after delivery of a child with a genetic condition not previously diagnosed in the husband but clearly evident by his physical appearance. Peter's family history was also instructive. His sister, who had NF1, developed breast cancer, which occurs five times more frequently in women with this disorder. Also, Peter's late father had a brain tumor, which is typically found in NF1.

NEUROFIBROMATOSIS

Peter's family was typical for NFl, but about 50% of the time there may be no history whatsoever, and the affected person is the first in the family to be born with a mutation in the *NFl* gene. Thereafter, however, there is a 50% likelihood that he or she will transmit this dominant genetic flaw to each of their offspring. For those born with an NFl mutation, signs may not be clearly apparent during childhood but may become obvious in the teens and later years. Few realize how common NFl really is, occurring in about 1 in 3,000 persons.

The signs manifested in Peter and his children were typical and included the lumps that were visible (they may also occur within the body), the large head, the learning disorder, scoliosis, the multiple café au lait spots, and the freckles in the armpits and groin. Tiny little nodules[2] are common, as are other features

2. Called Lisch nodules, seen usually in the iris (colored part of the eye) by slit-lamp examination by an eye specialist.

within the eyes. Bones and joints may also be involved. In about 50% of adults with NFl, a tangled mess of nerves and tissues[3] occur mostly internally (not visible under the skin), grow slowly over many years, and have the potential for causing disfigurement or interfering with, for example, limb function. Surgical removal can be nightmarish for the surgeon and the patient and is ill-advised if it can be avoided. A wide range of other manifestations of NFl do occur primarily in adulthood and fortunately are not that common but include hypertension, and involvement of blood vessels, brain, bone, and other tissues. In addition, various nervous system tumors may occur and, slightly more often, one type of chronic leukemia.

A definitive diagnosis is confirmed by DNA analysis of the *NFl* gene,[4] which will reveal a mutation in about 95% of all cases. In about 5% of individuals with the typical signs of NFl, a different gene (*SPRED1*) is the culprit. Hence, when a negative result is obtained after sequencing the *NFl* gene, the *SPRED1* gene should be analyzed. Once a mutation has been determined in either of these two genes, preimplantation genetic diagnosis or prenatal diagnosis can be offered. In addition, other family members at risk can simply be tested for this recognized single mutation.

The additional value of a precise diagnosis of NFl enables appropriate and careful surveillance to be established. Attention will be focused on all organs at risk and in particular require an annual eye exam by an ophthalmologist (beginning in early childhood), early developmental assessment in childhood on the lookout for learning disorders, annual blood pressure monitoring, and a careful annual physical examination.

There should be no confusion with neurofibromatosis type 2 (NF2). This disorder, caused by a different gene (*NF2*) is typically characterized by tiny tumors in the inner ear,[5] and usually in both ears, that herald their appearance by a ringing sound in the ears (tinnitus), hearing loss, or some loss of balance. Decreased visual acuity occurs in at least one-third of those affected, and up to 50% may develop usually benign tumors (meningiomas) in the brain. Analysis of the *NFl* gene enables a precise diagnosis.

---

3. Called plexiform neuromas or neurofibromas.
4. Both the *NF1* and *NF2* genes as well as the two genes involved in tuberous sclerosis (this chapter) have been found with similar DNA sequences (orthologs) in the fruit fly. Many other neurological disorders(including Tay-Sachs disease, limb-girdle muscular dystrophy, juvenile Parkinson's disease, Huntington's disease, spinocerebellar ataxia type 2, and others) have orthologs in the fruit fly.
5. Called vestibular schwannomas.

The diagnosis of NF1 and many other genetic conditions can be made by a physician using signs and symptoms as a guide, but where uncertainty exists or where a precise molecular diagnosis is necessary, consultation with a clinical geneticist[6] would be highly recommended. Once again, Peter's family history provided tell-tale information, besides his own manifestations of NF1. The frequent male tendency to avoid physicians does not diminish that individual's **chances** of illness but frequently removes **choices** that enable the prevention of untoward complications and even death.

Peter and Olga's lawsuit against their physicians concluded with a final settlement.

Mary was scared and happy. Her first child, May, then 5 years old, was autistic and suffered from a seizure disorder. Early indications were that there were also significant learning problems for which early intervention had already begun. She was happy because she had just learned that she was pregnant again. That happy feeling was quickly dissipated by a gnawing anxiety spawned by her sister Holly's recent experience, which was still fresh in Mary's mind. Holly had her first child, a son, who seemed perfectly well. During Holly's second pregnancy, the fetus was discovered to have a tumor inside the heart. Holly and her husband decided to terminate that pregnancy.

Armed with this information, Mary appeared for a genetics consultation, nervously and continuously rubbing rosary beads during the visit. Her concern as a single mother (her boyfriend had abandoned her immediately upon learning about the pregnancy) was whether she was at risk for having another child with autistic problems and seizures. She was also worried that she would have a child with a heart tumor (which she had never even heard of), as had occurred in Holly's second pregnancy.

Mary's mother had died in her late 30s from leukemia. The only medical information Mary could remember was that her mother had talked about having "cysts on her kidneys." She brought a photograph of her mother along to the consultation, and it showed an acne-like rash over the midportion of her face and nose. Mary said that her mother, who was "beautiful," was extremely upset and aggravated by this facial eruption, which was chronic and resisted all treatments.

---

6. Board-certified as a specialist by the American Board of Medical Genetics.

Mary admitted to having learning problems in school and attending some special education sessions. When asked about at least six whitish spots on her legs and thighs, she indicated that they had been present since at least her teenage years. She had not mentioned them to her previous obstetrician, and he had not asked either.

Mary was flabbergasted when I indicated the likely diagnosis for her daughter May, herself, her sister Holly, and her mother was tuberous sclerosis. Moreover, I indicated that the heart tumor[7] in the fetus was typical for this condition, which is best called tuberous sclerosis complex (TSC).

Her rosary beads fell to the floor when I told her of the 50% risks of transmitting this dominantly inherited condition to each of her offspring, including her current pregnancy. There was no relief from her anxiety when I indicated the availability of determining, by DNA analyses, whether a specific mutation could be found in one of the two known TSC genes. She readily agreed to this recommendation when it became clear that she would be able to determine whether the fetus was affected if a specific mutation could be determined in her DNA.

Molecular studies in our Center for Human Genetics at Boston University School of Medicine soon revealed by gene sequencing that she had a mutation in the TSC2 gene. This result became available in the nick of time, enabling her to have an amniocentesis and prenatal genetic studies that allowed us to show that the fetus was not affected. In due course, she delivered a healthy son.

Subsequently, we also showed that Holly harbored the same mutation and that Mary's other sister and brother did not. Mary's daughter May also had the mutation and TSC. MRI studies of the brains of Mary, May, and Holly revealed no abnormality.

Mary and her siblings grew up in a very modest home with a father only intermittently employed in construction. Her mother worked in a daycare nursery, and neither had medical insurance. Sadly, as a consequence, Mary's learning difficulties were never fully evaluated, and certainly no one paid attention to her white spots, which were small and appeared

---

7. Called rhabdomyoma.

unimportant. Mary, too, had done little to have her daughter May fully evaluated. Holly's doctor never mentioned the association of the heart tumor with TSC, and apparently Holly herself showed no signs of TSC. Fear was the father of action that drove Mary to seek a genetics consultation (advised by a nurse who was her neighbor). This fortunate referral made it possible for Mary to have prenatal genetic studies rather than terminating the pregnancy, and thereby (as is most often the case) securing the health of the fetus and facilitating the birth of a healthy child. More children by far are born healthy as a consequence of prenatal genetic studies compared to the very few pregnancies that end up with a termination.

TUBEROUS SCLEROSIS COMPLEX

Dominantly inherited disorders typically vary in their manifestations between families but also within families. The tell-tale signs of TSC were evident in Mary's family members, albeit not all present in the same person. Knowledge about medical matters among family members is almost invariably limited, whether by cultural norm, embarrassment, unwillingness to admit illness or weakness, interpersonal strife, or disaffection—to name but a few reasons. Recognition of the hypopigmented spots, the learning problems, the autistic behavior, seizures, kidney cysts, and eventually the tumor in the heart makes the diagnosis of this family disorder very obvious. The fact that the diagnosis was not recognized reflects a combination of medical inattention, lack of knowledge, and failure of the family to seek appropriate care.

A number of other major physical signs do occur, with some noticing small little growths (fibromas) around their nails, acne-like growths over nose and cheeks (angiofibromas), or a patch of shark-like skin more frequently on the back. Tiny nodules may occur at the back of the eye (in the retina), and benign tumors may be seen on imaging of the brain. Kidney cysts and even tumors may become evident over time, whereas the tumor in the heart may be seen in a fetus as early as 16 weeks of pregnancy by ultrasound imaging. These heart tumors may occur in as many as 60% of those affected, but the good news is that they are benign and slowly regress to disappear entirely over a period of months after birth. The only time that surgery is required is if the tumor gets in the way of a heart valve or of blood flow, at which time open heart surgery is required. However, it is possible that years later, this benign tumor may recur and, hence, at least an annual check-up would be recommended. This would also enable surveillance of the kidney and attention to neurologic function.

There may also be multiple minor signs that might include bone cysts, small growths along the gums, tiny pits in the teeth, and kidney cysts.

The precise diagnosis is established by sequencing both the *TSC1* and *TSC2* genes. Once a mutation is determined, other family members can be tested simply for that mutation (a much less expensive test). A family member at 50% risk and who apparently shows no signs, such as Mary's sister Holly, should still have a mutation analysis.

Bear in mind, however, that in about 20% of individuals with TSC, a mutation may not be recognized, suggesting that there may still be another gene to be discovered. In some of these individuals, samples of DNA from other tissues, besides blood, should be studied, including saliva, skin, or even hair follicles. If their blood studies were normal and the mutation was found in one or more other tissues, then they will be regarded as having TSC of the mosaic type. In about two-thirds of those affected, and not mosaics, the mutation is brand new and therefore not inherited. However, thereafter, they have a 50% risk of transmitting the mutation to each of their offspring.

Once the mutation in a family has been recognized, preimplantation genetic diagnosis or prenatal diagnosis becomes feasible. TSC is not rare, occurring in about 1 in 5,800 live births. The reason why the majority of families will consider prenatal studies in future pregnancies is the likely burden of this genetic disorder, especially as it relates to involvement of the brain and nervous system. At least 50% of those affected have developmental delay or mental retardation, and at least 80% have or have had seizures. Brain tumors have the potential for causing considerable grief, and some occur in up to 14% of those affected.[8]

In addition, behavioral impairments, including pervasive developmental disorder and autistic behavior, are common. About 25% of those with TSC have autistic behavior and 40% to 50% are considered to be within the autistic spectrum disorders. Aggression and ADHD are also common.

In an estimated 80% of children with TSC, kidney abnormalities may be seen that include cysts, benign tumors, and (rarely) kidney cancer. The *TSC2* gene and the dominantly inherited polycystic kidney disease gene (*PKDI*, as discussed in Chapter 18) are neighbors. As a consequence, and not rarely, a

8. Called giant cell astrocytomas.

deletion of both genes might occur, with both conditions manifesting in the same person.[9]

This brings to mind the urgent telephone call I received from a radiologist. While waiting for his next patient to have an ultrasound scan, he decided to lie down on the table and scan himself "just for fun!" To his horror, he discovered he had bilateral kidney cysts and a tumor in one kidney.[10] This sudden, unexpected discovery led to DNA tests and the recognition of a familial mutation in the *TSC2* gene. Involvement of the skin occurs in virtually 100% of those with TSC. That isn't too surprising since, after all, the skin is derived from the very same embryonic tissue origins as the brain. Indeed, the skin is a mirror to the brain and frequently yields a diagnosis of a neurologic disorder.[11]

Once a precise diagnosis has been made, long-term surveillance of critical signs and symptoms is established. A brain CT scan or MRI is recommended every 1 to 3 years for children and adolescents. Kidney ultrasound on the same schedule is wise and sometimes supplemented by a CT scan or MRI. Seizures are managed with anticonvulsant medications, and early intervention is instituted for those children with developmental delays or behavioral problems. Ultrasound of the heart (echocardiograms) would only be indicated if there had been earlier problems. Skin problems may require consultation with a dermatologist.

Brain and kidney lesions have the potential for causing significant health problems, which may prove fatal if unattended. Hence, knowledge of the family history, early anticipation of potential problems, and well-established surveillance schedules will enable affected individuals to secure their health and, not infrequently, save their lives.

---

9. Called a contiguous gene syndrome.
10. Fortunately, it turned out to be a benign angiomyolipoma.
11. Called a neurocutaneous disorder, of which there are many.

GENES WITH SIGNATURES

Brendan and his wife Maryanne had emigrated to the United States from Ireland and had set to work to establish a life for themselves and their future family. Brendan pursued a career in information technology and Maryanne followed her interests in social work. As do many immigrants to the United States, they worked hard, saved assiduously, and bought a small house in a nice suburb. "The clock was ticking," Mary would often intone, and eventually Brendan relented. Maryanne soon found herself pregnant and was sure to have been taking her folic acid supplementation prior to becoming pregnant. She had seen enough of the serious birth defect spina bifida in Ireland and knew that folic acid (which is a vitamin B), taken daily at least 3 months prior to becoming pregnant and for the first 3 months thereafter, helped prevent spina bifida some 70% of the time.[1]

Pregnancy was uneventful, and Maryanne looked spectacular throughout her pregnancy. Labor and delivery went off without a hitch, and Brendan and Maryanne were blessed with a little boy whom they named Derek. Although cranky at times, Derek seemed to be developing normally, and Maryanne was assured by her pediatrician that all was well. However, at age 7 months, Maryanne noticed that Derek could not maintain a sitting position, even when propped up with pillows. She became really worried when one of her girlfriends with a similarly aged child suggested that she should check again with her pediatrician. He did order a chromosome study, which yielded a normal result. Initially, the pediatrician tried to be

---

1. This is the figure we published in 1989 in a large study of more than 22,000 pregnant women and that made front-page headlines in the New York Times. Subsequently, the Medical Research Council in the United Kingdom published a multicenter study that confirmed our original findings.

reassuring and indicated that the range of normal development is wide and that some babies may sit supported only at 8 or 9 months and do fine thereafter. Unfortunately, this did not turn out to be the case. By age 1 year, Derek was still not able to maintain a sitting position, let alone stand, even holding onto the crib. Brendan noted that Derek was particularly floppy and both agreed that he had become "a happy bundle."

Over the ensuing year, no real improvements occurred, and Brendan and Maryanne continued seeing various neurologists and developmental specialists. None of the physicians they consulted were able to explain his increasingly obvious developmental delay, inability to walk, and absence of any words. Evaluations included high-resolution chromosome studies, which yielded normal results, and imaging of his brain by MRI, which revealed no abnormality.

Soon after his second birthday, Derek began having seizures, and a new neurologist observed that his head size was small. Checking back, the neurologist noted that his head circumference had been normal at birth. Maryanne pointed out that he was intermittently tremulous. Close to his third birthday, Derek began to walk but was noted to have a robot-like stiffness and seemed to maintain his balance by lifting his arms, flexed at the elbow, while he propelled himself forward with jerky movements, much like a puppet.[2] Derek would drool, stick out his tongue, and still say no words but would laugh even without provocation or in a room by himself. This clue led his neurologist to refer Maryanne to me for a consultation.

I confirmed all the features mentioned above and further noted that Derek required little sleep and would wake frequently through the night. In particular, he seemed to be hyperactive, happy, but speechless.

I suggested that the diagnosis may well be a condition called Angelman syndrome, pointing out that Derek had most of the typical features of this genetic condition. I initiated the necessary DNA tests, which, within a few weeks, confirmed the clinical diagnosis. Only then did Maryanne reveal that she was 6 months along in her second pregnancy and already too late to undergo any type of prenatal test. Either way, she said, she would not consider terminating any pregnancy. She asked whether her sister Megan, who had suffered three early miscarriages, could be at risk for having a child like Derek. She also mentioned that her brother Roy suffered from depression.

---

2. Originally, Derek's disorder was known as the Happy-Puppet syndrome.

In due course, Maryanne delivered their second son, John. Once again, he looked fine, but over the ensuing 8 months, they recognized that he had the same condition as Derek.

The diagnosis of Angelman syndrome rests primarily on the typical clinical features exhibited by Derek and subsequently by his brother John. Confirmation of the diagnosis rests on the DNA tests that focus on the chromosome 15 pair. (The reader will recall from Chapter 2 that each parent transmits a single chromosome 15.) Along the path of the long arm of chromosome 15 is the gene (*UBE3A*) and a closely adjacent critical imprinting center that, if abnormal, results in Angelman syndrome.[3] In Angelman syndrome, the focus falls on this very spot, but on the mother's chromosome 15.

Some remarkable things can happen at this location, all resulting in Angelman syndrome. First, and most common, a tiny piece of DNA may be missing (called a deletion). Second, a mutation may occur in the Angelman syndrome gene, and here is where a remarkable mechanism occurs and accounts for Derek's and John's Angelman syndrome.

Years ago, and with the help of experimentation in mice, it was noted that there is a functional difference between the father's and mother's chromosomes, in at least certain chromosome pairs. In those pairs, they behave differently and must be carrying some type of imprint that marks their parental origin. These imprints may functionally change on transmission. For example, in Maryanne's family, her father transmitted a mutation to her that was imprinted (inactive and silenced). However, when she passed that mutation along to her children, the imprinted silencer was lifted, exposing the mutated gene and resulting in a dysfunctional gene product leading to Angelman syndrome. Hence, this imprinting is reversible and can be erased and reimposed with each generation. Since Maryanne has a pair of #15 chromosomes and would be expected to pass along one of them to each of her children, there was and is a 50% risk of transmitting the faulty one in each pregnancy then and in the future.

---

3. Or Prader-Willi syndrome, discussed later.

Maryanne's sister was also at risk but tested negative. The reason for her miscarriages is not known. Her brother's depression is not known to be related to the *UBE3A* gene.

The third possible mechanism resulting in Angelman syndrome depended on major advances in genetics made about a quarter of a century ago, which enabled recognition of the parental origin of each member of a chromosome pair.

This critical development shook up our thinking since we always thought that each parent contributed one chromosome to every pair. The actual discovery in 1988 led to the recognition that inheritance of a *pair* of chromosomes could occasionally come from one parent (called uniparental disomy).[4]

When a *father* contributes both of his chromosome 15s to a child, the absence of the mother's chromosome 15 acts as though there is a gene deletion and results in Angelman syndrome. When a *mother's* chromosomes 15 pair is transmitted and the father's one chromosome 15 is absent, a different disorder emerges (called Prader-Willi syndrome, discussed below). The most likely mechanism leading to uniparental disomy comes into play soon after conception. In this situation it is thought that an early cell actually has three #15 chromosomes (Trisomy 15)—two from one parent and one from the other. Subsequent loss of the one parent's chromosome 15 leaves a pair from one parent, and uniparental disomy occurs as a result.

The causes of Angelman syndrome are gene deletions (65%–75%), a simple point mutation in 5% to 11%, and uniparental disomy in about 3%

---

4. The first disease example recognized was cystic fibrosis. As discussed in Chapter 14, cystic fibrosis only occurs when a mutation is passed by each parent to their offspring. If an individual carries a cystic fibrosis gene mutation (which is located on chromosome 7) and the partner does not, by sheer random chance a child may be born with both chromosome 7s from the carrier parent possessing the mutation, which is the equivalent of receiving the mutation from two parents. This mechanism remains an infrequent event in cystic fibrosis, accounting for less than 1% of all cases. A few other chromosome pairs are known thus far to be involved occasionally with uniparental disomy with a clinically determinable outcome. Included among these disorders are diabetes in the newborn (the chromosome 6 pair), an overgrowth syndrome called Beckwith-Wiedemann (the chromosome 11 pair), growth restriction (Silver-Russell syndrome), certain cancers (various chromosomes), and other rare conditions.

to 7%. A mutation in the imprinting center occurs in about 3% of cases. In about 11% of cases, no explanation has been forthcoming, even though the child has all the typical features of Angelman syndrome. Now we know that there is yet another gene (called *SLC9A6*), which we routinely analyze by sequencing in our laboratories and in which a mutation may occur, causing an Angelman-like syndrome.

The sheer complexity of our body's fine structure is again revealed by the intricate structure and function of the imprinting center adjacent to the Angelman syndrome gene. In the few cases in which an imprinting defect occurs and Angelman syndrome results, the maternal chromosome carries a <u>paternal</u> imprint. (The exact opposite occurs in the Prader-Willi syndrome discussed below.) These imprinting center errors provide insight into the mechanisms involved that result in imprint erasure, resetting, and maintenance. Remarkably, in the majority of patients with an imprinting center error, the incorrect imprint occurred without a change in the sequence of DNA. It is unclear how and why this happens.

ANGELMAN SYNDROME

Thankfully, Angelman syndrome is uncommon, occurring in between 1 in 12,000 and 1 in 20,000 of the population. Once the molecular diagnosis has been made confirming the symptoms and signs, treatment regimens can be followed to achieve and secure the best health possible. A long list of treatments varying with age includes attention to feeding problems, reflux, seizures, behavioral modification, educational training and enrichment, and care for orthopedic problems.

After a defined mutation has been discovered, future preimplantation genetic diagnosis or prenatal diagnosis will usually be possible. In less than 1% of cases, a chromosome translocation (*see* Chapter 4) involving chromosome 15 may be the cause of Angelman syndrome. Hence, chromosome analysis will usually be part of the evaluation when the diagnosis is being sought.

PRADER-WILLI SYNDROME

In precisely the same region, there is another gene (*SNRPN*) that acts and has similar characteristics as displayed by the *UBE3A* gene in Angelman syndrome.

There is one key difference. All the action is on the chromosome 15 contributed by the father. The genetic condition that emerges is dramatically different from Angelman syndrome. This disorder, called Prader-Willi syndrome,[5] is seen in about 1 in 10,000 to 1 in 30,000 of the population and is characterized typically by a child born floppy who exhibits considerable difficulty in feeding, only to be followed in early childhood by excessive eating, resulting in obesity.

In addition, delays occur in sitting, walking, running, and other motor milestones, as well as behavioral and cognitive impairments. Moreover, a striking pattern of behavior is frequently seen and includes temper tantrums, stubbornness, manipulative behavior, and obsessive-compulsive disorder. Affected males or females tend to be short; have light-colored hair, eyes, and skin; and have particular facial features that geneticists tend to recognize. Genital underdevelopment is usual, and infertility is common. Later, non-insulin-dependent diabetes develops, mostly in association with the obesity.

The diagnosis is confirmed by DNA analysis[6] that enables a precise diagnosis in at least 99% of affected individuals. This test once again allows recognition of the parent-specific imprinting that occurs, this time silencing or affecting the adjacent critical region of the *SNRPN* gene, which results in Prader-Willi syndrome.

Additional but inconstant features include a habit to pick at the skin; thick, sticky saliva; unclear speech; a high pain threshold; and, in teens and adulthood, a tendency to steal and lie. Psychosis occurs in 5% to 10% of affected individuals by young adulthood. In one case, I immediately suspected a diagnosis when observing a developmentally delayed child in the waiting room who had become fixated on a jigsaw puzzle.

Genetic evaluation by a clinical geneticist is advisable when the diagnosis of Prader-Willi syndrome is to be considered or when the diagnosis is made. In general, when a deletion is found in the father's chromosome 15 in the Prader-Willi syndrome region, the likelihood of recurrence in a subsequent pregnancy is less than 1%. This is similar for uniparental disomy. However, if there is a mutation in the imprinting center, the risk for having a second child with this disorder approximates 50%. The other possible causes are associated with less than a 1% risk of recurrence. However, given the complexities of inheritance

---

5. Prader-Willi syndrome was first described by pediatricians in Switzerland led by Dr. Andrea Prader and Dr. Heinrich Willi.
6. Called a DNA methylation test.

for both Angelman syndrome and Prader-Willi syndrome, genetic consultations are critically important. Note that it took some 3 years for Maryanne to be referred to a geneticist. Because about 50% of pregnancies are unplanned, couples should be fully aware of this need, more especially if they already have had a child with Prader-Willi or Angelman syndrome or a child with a genetic disorder in which a precise cause has not yet been established.

IMPRINTING DEFECTS AND ASSISTED REPRODUCTION

Imprinting is an acquired mechanism that results in the modification of one specific parental gene so that only one of the two genes is actually expressed. Imprinting centers for each of the genes subject to this mechanism control and impose the effects as these genes are transmitted in the sperm or the ovum. There are at least 100 genes subject to imprinting (*see* Appendix VII). Of particular concern, however, are reports indicating that the frequency of some disorders—such as Angelman syndrome, the eye cancer retinoblastoma (*see* Chapter 8), and Beckwith-Wiedemann Syndrome (BWS)[7]—may all occur with increased frequency following assisted reproductive technology (ART) using in vitro fertilization. The evidence implicating imprinting is compelling for both BWS and Angelman syndrome. Children conceived <u>without</u> ART who have BWS have imprinting defects in 40% to 50% of cases. In those born with the help of ART who are diagnosed with BWS, more than 90% have imprinting defects. The majority of children born after ART who have Angelman syndrome also have imprinting defects. The real additional risks, however, after ART are likely to be below 1%.

Multiple published studies do, however, document a small increase in the rate of birth defects, including mostly sex chromosome abnormalities, with ARTs. Notwithstanding these observations, it has proved difficult to distinguish whether the cause is due to the basic reasons for the infertility or from the ART itself. Meanwhile, those choosing ART are advised to have careful

---

7. This is mostly a sporadic disorder, but in 15% of cases it is transmitted as an autosomal dominant condition. The typical features include overgrowth, beginning with increased birth weight, a large tongue, enlarged intra-abdominal organs including liver, spleen, kidneys, adrenal glands, and pancreas. Overgrowth of one side of the body is common and more subject to development of various tumors on that side, including of the liver and kidney. A prominent hernia of the belly button or actual protrusion of the intestine through the belly button is also characteristic. Low blood sugar soon after birth is critically important because, if not recognized and treated, mental retardation could eventuate. Many other features also occur in this remarkable condition.

and sophisticated continuing care and surveillance, including consideration of prenatal diagnostic studies after pregnancy has been achieved.

Couples who have ART also need to be well-informed about the well recognized increased risks of their children being born prematurely or of low birth weight (with all the possible attendant serious complications) and increased perinatal mortality. Mothers, too, are at increased risk of complications, including diabetes in pregnancy, preeclampsia, placental problems, and more frequent cesarean sections. All of these issues of ART and infertility are not trivial. Between 1% and 4% of newborns in Europe are conceived after ART.

22

MATERNAL INHERITANCE AND INEVITABILITY

The parents of both Xiao and Xiuqu emigrated from a province (Guandong) in the south of China and settled in Boston. They were delighted when their children Xiao and Xiuqu decided to marry. As was customary, Xiao and Xiuqu worked hard and excelled in college. They continued to work hard at their chosen careers in business and accounting and only later began to plan a family. Xiuqu's first pregnancy ended prematurely at 34 weeks. Their first daughter almost died from the complications of prematurity and a life-threatening infection. Powerful intravenous antibiotics were used, and over a 2-month period, she recovered and was finally discharged from hospital. Upon discharge, however, there were questions about her hearing because the screening test was inconclusive. After almost 2 years and repeated hearing tests, it was clear that their daughter had a serious hearing impairment.

Early intervention was initiated, and other than hearing loss, her development was unimpaired. Meanwhile, they had learned that Xiuqu's sister, who had remained in China, had a son who was found to be deaf in early infancy.

A second pregnancy followed and once again ended prematurely, this time at 35 weeks. Fortunately, their second daughter was not as ill as their first but nevertheless was also treated with powerful antibiotics. A few months after discharge from hospital, she too was discovered to be hearing-impaired and by 4 years was determined to be deaf. A genetics consultation followed. The possibility of both Xiao and Xiuqu each being a carrier of a harmful deafness gene was considered the most likely reason for both of their daughters being born deaf. The guess was autosomal recessive inheritance, and they were counseled about a possible 25% risk of having an affected child in any future pregnancy. DNA tests were not then available.

About 4 years later, and without planning, Xiuqu found herself pregnant again. This time, they had a son who was born at term, weighing 8 pounds 2 ounces. The newborn period was uneventful, and his growth and development were entirely normal. The years passed without any health problems, and their son went off to college. In his second year, there was an outbreak of meningitis, and he became seriously ill. Powerful antibiotics given intravenously saved his life and he went home to recover. Shortly thereafter, it became clear that he had developed serious hearing impairment.

*I saw their college-aged son and the parents for a genetics consultation. I revisited the information in the family history and upon direct questioning quickly recognized that all three children had been exposed to a particular category of antibiotics.[1] DNA studies had become available, and within a few weeks it was clear that Xiuqu and her three children all harbored a specific mutation[2] in the mitochondrial genome (see Chapter 6). Mutations in the mitochondrial genome (and not from the cell nucleus) are transmitted by a mother to **all** her offspring. As Xiuqu aptly stated, "It was like checkmate*

Chapter 6 discusses how mothers, and not fathers, transmit their mitochondrial genes to every child. Notwithstanding this transmission of the same mitochondrial gene mutation (in this case, A1555G), variability in the age of onset of hearing loss, severity, and rate of progression is common. Since the first description of this specific mitochondrial mutation in an Arab-Israeli family, additional observations have shown that exposure to powerful antibiotics (*see* Footnote 1) could damage the exquisitely tiny hair cells in the inner ear (cochlea). This is what happened to Xiao and Xiuqu's three children, who were all exposed to one or more of these antibiotics. Their third child, albeit born with this gene mutation, only manifested the hearing loss after exposure to the antibiotic.

---

1. Called aminoglycosides. With typical antibiotics such as streptomycin, gentamycin, paromomycin, neomycin, kanamycin, and tobramycin.
2. A1555G

Of obvious interest is why Xiuqu herself showed no signs of hearing impairment despite harboring the same gene mutation that she transmitted to her children. This phenomenon, called heteroplasmy or homoplasmy, is discussed in chapter 6. In addition, modifying genes from one of the parents might also influence the appearance and severity of a mitochondrial disorder. More important, however, was the fact that she had never been exposed to this class of antibiotics.

A family history of deafness should alert couples planning a pregnancy, as there are now a considerable number of DNA tests available to determine at least some of the more common genetic conditions associated with deafness.

The tiny inner ear hair cells of individuals with the A1555G mutation appear exquisitely sensitive to exposure by known and unknown environmental factors. Now we know that the aminoglycoside antibiotics rank as an important cause of deafness after exposure, but not infrequently, those who harbor this mutation may develop progressive deafness precipitated by unknown factors. In some populations, such as the Black population of South Africa, the frequency of this mutation approximates 1 in 100. This is a potentially serious matter, because tuberculosis is common in that population and antibiotics that can prove harmful to the inner ear are frequently used. A study of Spanish families with this mutation found it as the most common cause of late-onset familial progressive deafness (56%). About 27% of all Spanish families with deafness had this mutation.

Hearing loss is one of the most common birth defects, affecting about 1 in 500 newborns. Bilateral permanent hearing loss increases in frequency, affecting close to 1 in 300 in their teens. More than 50% of congenital deafness is genetic and mostly transmitted as an autosomal recessive condition and usually without any other birth defects (called non-syndromic). By far, the most common gene involved in recessive deafness is Connexin 26, with about 1 in 33 individuals being carriers (about 1 in 26 Ashkenazi Jews are carriers).

Xiao and Xiuqu's experience was not easily avoidable then. Today, however, a history of deafness in the family serves notice on those who might want to check their carrier status. Unfortunately, there are at least several hundred genes involved in our hearing apparatus, the majority of which are not currently available for testing by DNA. However, the most common syndromic

and non-syndromic conditions are indeed testable. It is also important to recognize that the deaf community does not regard the inability to hear as an
"impairment" or a disability. Clearly, a deaf individual is not disabled and can
be highly accomplished.

As discussed in Chapter 6, Xiuqu was right in describing her futile efforts at
having an unaffected child as "checkmate." She transmitted her mitochondrial
gene mutation to all of her children. Her son, however, would not transmit his
mutation to any of his children.

MITOCHONDRIAL DISORDERS

Since the mitochondria are dispersed among almost all cells and tissues, a
wide range of disorders occur depending on the tissues involved. Curiously,
depending on the mutation, some tissues or organs will be severely affected,
while other tissues and organs remain uninvolved. Mutations in these floating
mitochondrial factories within the cells of the nervous system cause an entire
range of symptoms and signs that include balance problems, seizures, mental
retardation, migraine, partial paralysis, and blindness. Weakness and loss of
sensation in the limbs, exercise intolerance, paralysis of the eye muscles, and
droopy eyes represent further signs of different mitochondrial disorders. In
the heart, rhythm disturbances may occur as well as severe heart failure (resulting from so-called "cardiomyopathy"). A wide range of other signs may also
occur but may yield a diagnosis, as all 37 mitochondrial genes can be sequenced
and analyzed. An axiom that captures the essence of mitochondrial disorders
is "*any organ, any sign, any time*". Treatment, however, is currently focused on
alleviating symptoms in the absence of a cure.

The mitochondria floating in the fluid (cytoplasm) surrounding the nucleus
are transmitted by females through endless generations. This fact enables
extensive historical studies of female genetic history within human populations. Recovery of mitochondrial DNA has been of immense value in determining geographic origins of peoples and their migrations through history.
Because mutations occur in mitochondrial DNA, they provide the equivalent
of mile-markers and identification tags for individuals and populations.
Identifications of those who perished in the New York 9/11 catastrophe were
often made possible by using the mitochondrial "footprint."

Well over 1,300 mitochondrial genes **within** the nucleus (*see* Chapter 5) have
the propensity to cause a vast panoply of genetic disease. Transmission (discussed in Chapter 5) is autosomal dominant or recessive or X-linked. Nuclear

mitochondrial disorders might arise in virtually any organ, frequently with devastating outcome. About 1 in 250 children are born with a nuclear mitochondrial mutation, most having either few or no symptoms or signs. A more serious mitochondrial disorder occurs in about 1 in 6500. These diseases involve the brain, heart, muscle, eyes, liver, gut, bone marrow, inner ear, and kidneys. As a consequence and depending on the specific mutation and the mode of inheritance, there could, for example, be seizures, mental retardation, blindness, deafness, heart failure, muscle weakness, breathing difficulty, liver failure, anemia, and kidney failure. Once again, treatment is largely palliative and aimed at the relief of symptoms and signs. Where early diagnosis is possible, families may learn of their precise and high risks, which would then inform their plans for future childbearing.

Prenatal diagnosis for non-nuclear mitochondrial disorders is not a simple option, given the unpredictable occurrence and possibilities of mutations appearing in homoplasmic (meaning that all the mitochondria carry the mutation) or heteroplasmic (not all the mitochondria carry the mutation) form. These complex disorders require consultation with clinical or biochemical geneticists.

One hopeful glimpse into the future that could negate the "checkmate" has been provided by scientists in Oregon. The approach they used in monkeys aimed at avoiding the mother's mitochondrial mutation. They simply removed the normal nucleus from her egg and inserted it into a donor egg from which the nucleus had been removed. This secured the transfer of the mother's complete set of normal nuclear genes, leaving behind the abnormal mitochondria. Fertilization by the partner's sperm by in vitro fertilization enabled them to produce at least four healthy infant monkeys. Long-term follow-up will, of course, still be necessary. More recent are the successful efforts by researchers in Newcastle in the United Kingdom. They used two fertilized human embryos unsuitable for in vitro fertilization, removing the nuclei from both and interchanging them. While this experiment allowed these scientists to hone their technique, the hope is to place a mother's normal nucleus into a donated egg with its nucleus removed, thereby avoiding the abnormal mitochondrial mutation in the cytoplasm of her own egg. The future child would have all the nuclear genes of both parents, less than 2% of the abnormal cytoplasmic genes (not enough to cause disease), and 37 mitochondrial genes from the pre-tested donor.

23

HARMFUL MATERNAL EFFECTS ON THE FETUS

Krunal had her first epileptic seizure soon after her 13th birthday. She well recalled that day, not only because of the seizure, but because it heralded her first menstrual period. She had been in school when, out of the blue, she recalled a ringing in her ears and later finding herself on the floor in the classroom with her classmates staring at her. She was mortified when she realized that she had wet herself. During the ensuing 15 years, she had a number of major (grand mal) seizures, and her neurologists had worked diligently to find an anticonvulsant drug that would be most effective with the least side effects. Eventually, after trying multiple different drugs singly or in combination, her physicians settled on valproic acid (Depakene) tablets. As a consequence, her 6 to 10 seizures per year became much less frequent at 1 or 2 per year.

Extensive neurological evaluation, including repetitive imaging, genetic studies, and biochemical studies, revealed no recognizable cause.

Krunal related to me that she had "epilepsy of unknown origin," quoting her doctor. No one in her family had epilepsy or even a single seizure. She had also not suffered any head injury, nor any other illness that could have pointed to a cause.

The consultation with me was occasioned by her discovery of pregnancy after she had already missed two menstrual periods. She lived with her boyfriend and had no intention of becoming pregnant. However, once pregnant, she was thrilled and had been looking forward to having a baby. The obstetrician she consulted promptly sent her in my direction because of his concern about the potential effects of the valproic acid medication on fetal development. An ultrasound scan at 12 weeks of pregnancy had revealed normal fetal growth, and it was too early for assessment of any fetal anomalies. She had not been taking any vitamin or folic acid supplements.

She thought she had become pregnant on a night when she and her boy-friend had been binge drinking.

Krunal cried during my description of the increased risk of birth defects related to valproic acid being taken in those earliest weeks of pregnancy. In particular, risks of having a child with spina bifida[1] are up to 6% compared to background risks of close to 0.1%. Moreover, I explained that there was a condition called valproate embryopathy or the Fetal Valproate syndrome, characterized by some dysmorphic facial features, heart and blood vessel defects, and especially spina bifida. Growth and mental retardation as well as multiple other abnormalities in a whole range of organ systems may also occur.

Sure enough, obstetrical ultrasound scanning of the fetus around 18 weeks of pregnancy revealed a clear and distinct spina bifida, and the whole dis-cussion about the option for pregnancy termination was revisited. By this time, her boyfriend had left her, complaining that she had not taken appro-priate steps to prevent pregnancy. Because she was herself the product of a single mother with whom she had no contact, she remained alone in her decision-making. She elected to keep the pregnancy.

Soon after birth, Krunal's son had surgery to close the open, leaking spina bifida lesion. Sadly, a lack of movement in his legs was noted at birth and accurately predicted that he would be profoundly paraplegic and would never walk. Moreover, within weeks of the spinal surgery, the common complication of expanding fluid spaces in his brain (called hydrocephalus) was diagnosed. To diminish the pressure within his head and to hopefully prevent additional brain damage, a shunt was placed in the main space (ventricle) of his brain. Over the next few years, significant mental retarda-tion was noted and compounded the difficulties that he had with paraple-gia and lack of control of bowel and bladder. Because of blockage or injection, his shunt had to be neurosurgically replaced repeatedly, with fre-quent hospitalizations for brain infection (meningitis) and kidney infection from the catheter in his bladder.

I heard sometime later that Krunal had abandoned him in a hospital and disappeared.

---

1. A defect in the spine through which a portion of the spinal nerves and even spinal cord could extrude, forming a lump on the back and resulting in paralysis of the legs and possible lack of control of the bladder and even the bowel.

Although Krunal's son did not have some of the features of the valproic acid syndrome, he did suffer from the most feared complication. The future for those born with open spina bifida is filled with challenges and complications.

In a study of 117 children with open spina bifida followed for 25 years, only 7% had little or no disability. Within their first year of life, 21% had died; 41% had died by age 16 years. Of 59% who survived to age 16 years, 60 of 69 had been shunted for hydrocephalus and 2 had become blind as a consequence. Mental retardation was present in 19% and seizures in 17%. Close to half were incontinent and one-third were wheelchair bound. By age 25 years, 48% had died. On the positive side, 49% of those who had survived to age 25 years achieved university entrance, and 45% were employed. The prognosis for children surviving with spina bifida depends on multiple factors, including the severity of the lesion, its location along the spine (the higher, the worse the complications), the nature and expertise of the treatment provided, as well as the parental care given.

The brain equivalent of spina bifida is an awesome abnormality in which the top of the head is open and exposes the deformed brain in a disorder called anencephaly. Collectively, spina bifida and anencephaly are termed neural tube defects and, at least in the Western world, occur in between 1 in 500 and 1 in 1,000 births. In certain regions of the world, including China, India, and Egypt, the frequency of neural tube defects has approximated 1 in 125 births. This was similar to the incidence in the 1960s in Ireland. Recognition of the importance of folic acid (vitamin B9) supplementation in the prevention and avoidance of neural tube defects has made all the difference. We showed in a landmark study[2] published in 1989 that women who took folic acid supplements in the 3 months prior to becoming pregnant and for the first 3 months after becoming pregnant avoided a neural tube defect approximately 70% of the time. Subsequent studies confirmed our original observations.

Clearly, women in their reproductive years should be on folic acid, even if they do not plan to become pregnant. When anticonvulsant treatment is required, every effort should be made to switch to a safer drug, but only in consultation with a neurologist. Prenatal ultrasound and maternal serum screening for neural tube defects remain important, especially since about 95% of all cases occur without there having been the birth of a previously affected child. The highly experienced team at the University of Washington in Seattle have reported on the remarkable rate of abandonment by the parents of children with spina bifida, which is both poignant and telling and has further implications for the affected child and the unaffected siblings.

Krunal's epilepsy is not at all rare. In the United States, there are more than 2 million persons with epilepsy, and an estimated 3% of people in the general population will have a seizure at some point in their lives. Between 1 in 100 and 1 in 200 individuals have epilepsy. Failure to find a cause for seizures such as Krunal's is common, given that in 30% to 40% of individuals with epilepsy beginning before the age of 20 years the cause remains to be discovered. (See further discussion on genetic aspects of epilepsy in the section on Frequently Asked Questions at the end of the book.)

Women with epilepsy who are pregnant and on anticonvulsants have a 4% to 9% risk of having a child with a birth defect, mental retardation, or genetic disorder, which is two to three times greater than those who are unaffected by epilepsy. The most common anomalies are cleft lip or palate and heart defects.

Choice or change of anticonvulsant medication prior to conceiving is critically important for women with epilepsy. Once again, this is a step that should only be taken in consultation with a neurologist. It is especially important to avoid seizures during pregnancy, as their occurrence is associated with infants of lower birth weight and premature delivery, with all its attendant complications.

POTENTIALLY HARMFUL MEDICATIONS AND PREGNANCY

Women who are planning to become pregnant or who are already pregnant need to realize that they pose risks to the developing fetus by virtue of what they ingest, the status of their personal health, and the extent of their exposure to environmental hazards. This discussion focuses first on medication use during pregnancy and is followed by consideration of examples of maternal

---

2. Milunsky A, Jick H, Jick SS, Bruell C, MacLaughlin DS, Rothman KJ, & Willett W. (1989) Multivitamin/folic acid supplementation in early pregnancy reduces the prevalence of neural tube defects.*JAMA*.262: 2847–2852.

illnesses that endanger the developing fetus and then by examples of potentially hazardous environmental factors.

Despite the fact that thousands of medications are available, only a tiny fraction are known to indisputably cause birth defects. The most important of these drugs are listed in Table 23.1. You may have thought that no woman need be reminded of the dangers inherent in taking medications during pregnancy, especially in the first 3 months. However, it is remarkable that a majority of women take between 4 and 14 different prescription or over-the-counter drugs during pregnancy. Every woman planning a pregnancy who must take a specific medication should first consult a physician about the potential risks of birth defects, hazards of breast feeding, and possible complications in the newborn. Changes in a medication or a temporary period with no medication may be viable options, but only in consultation with a physician.

While the good news is reflected in the few medications that cause birth defects, the bad news is that there are remarkably few very rigorous scientific studies that have examined even common medications for their propensity to cause fetal anomalies or birth defects. Among the many factors and considerations in such studies is proof that exposure of the fetus occurred at a critical time in those earliest weeks of fetal development.

The drug thalidomide, taken for nausea in pregnancy, resulted in thousands of children in West Germany and England being born without arms and legs or with catastrophic deformities of the limbs as well as other serious birth defects. Mothers who took thalidomide on the 30th day after conception had children with the most deformed arms and legs, whereas those who took the drug on the 35th day had babies who only had lower limb defects. Many women who took this drug also had perfectly healthy babies. The timing turned out to be more important than the dosage in producing these defects. More recently, thalidomide has been reintroduced in some countries for the treatment of leprosy and AIDS. One can only hope that pregnant women are not again subject to the devastating experiences women have had with this drug in the past.

Genetic as well as other factors determine the way a drug is metabolized in the body. In some individuals, certain drugs are broken down more quickly than in others. The slower the breakdown, the higher the remaining concentration in the body and the greater likelihood that the drug will reach toxic levels. Although drugs are routinely tested in animals before use in humans, interactions in different species may vary. For example, no abnormalities appeared in the offspring of pregnant rats and mice that were give doses of thalidomide. However, the drug did cause serious defects in the offspring of

Table 23.1 Medications Conclusively Shown to Cause Birth Defects

Medication	Uses	Common Birth Defects and Consequences
Anticonvulsants (e.g., Dilantin, [phenytoin], Tegretol, carbamazepine, trimethadione, phenobarbital, valproic acid [Depakene])	Treatment of epilepsy	Multiple and variable serious birth defects; mental retardation; for valproic acid, spina bifida, heart defects, cleft palate and other defects
Anticoagulants (e.g., dicumarol, warfarin)	Prevention of blood clots	Underdevelopment of cartilage and bone (especially in nose); blindness; mental retardation; possible fetal or newborn bleeding
Anticancer drugs (e.g., busulfan, chlorambucil, cyclophosphamide, 6-mercaptopurine, aminopterin, (methotrexate)	Treatment of cancer	Fetal death; multiple and variable serious birth defects
Antithyroid preparations (e.g., propylthiouracil, methimazole, radioactive iodine)	Treatment of hyperthyroidism	Enlargement or destruction of fetal thyroid gland
Sex hormones (e.g., progesterone, estrogen, Progestoral, diethylstilbestrol [DES], methyltestosterone, Norlutin), Danazol	Oral contraceptives; formerly, prevention of miscarriage	Masculinization of a female fetus; for DES-vaginal cancers in adolescence, miscarriage, tubal pregnancy, and structural abnormalities of the genital tract
Antibiotics Tetracycline	Treatment of infections	Pigmentation of teeth and underdevelopment of enamel
Streptomycin	Treatment of infections (e.g., tuberculosis)	Deafness

(Continued)

Table 23.1 Medications Conclusively Shown to Cause Birth Defects *(Continued)*

Medication	Uses	Common Birth Defects and Consequences
Miscellaneous drugs		
Antimalarial medicines (e.g., quinine, chloroquin)	Treatment of malaria and certain heart rhythm disturbances	Miscarriage; marked reduction in the platelet count in the newborn; possible deafness or blindness
Misoprostol	Treatment of duodenal ulcers	If it fails to cause miscarriage, major risk of causing Möbius syndrome (congenital facial paralysis with/without limb defects
Accutane (Isotretinoin or other derivatives of Vitamin A), Etretinate	Treatment of serious acne or psoriasis	Hydrocephalus or microcephaly; deformed or absent ears; heart disease; abnormally small eyes; cleft palate; mental retardation; other defects and miscarriages
Vitamin A in excess	Harmful diet fads	Miscarriage; defects of head, face, brain, spine, and urinary tract
Penicillamine	Ridding body of excess copper	Hyperelastic skin
Angiotensin-converting-enzyme inhibitors	Treat hypertension	Kidney damage and failure in newborns; skull calcification defects
Thalidomide	Formerly used overseas for treatment of nausea and vomiting during pregnancy	Absent to profoundly deformed limbs; multiple and variable serious birth defects
Hypoglycemic drugs	Treatment of high blood sugar	Low blood sugar in newborns
Psychiatric drugs		
Antidepressants (Lithium, Sertraline, Paroxetine)	Treatment for depression	Heart and other birth defects

Note: Check with your physician about any medication with a different name that may be similar to those listed here.

monkeys and rabbits. Drugs may also interact with one another in damaging ways or might compete with the body for essential nutrients such as folic acid, depriving the developing embryo/fetus, with resultant birth defects such as spina bifida.

Even topical medications applied to the skin are potentially hazardous. Girls and women in their late teens battling acne frequently use the very effective accutane (isotretinoin) as treatment. Unplanned pregnancies while using accutane and providing the medication to a friend, who also unwittingly becomes pregnant, are two well-recognized scenarios. The outcome for the subsequently born affected infant is brain defects, absent or deformed ears, heart defects, cleft palate, mental retardation, and other anomalies.

The vast majority of women take multivitamin supplements during pregnancy, beginning after their second missed menstrual period, thereby missing the critical first 8 to 10 weeks of fetal development when all the organs are forming. The neural tube that forms the spine closes between 26 and 29 days after conception. Failure to close completely results in a neural tube defect. Unfortunately, too many fail to take folic acid supplements when planning pregnancy and continuing for at least the first 3 months after conceiving. There is little proven benefit to multivitamin intake after the first 3 months. Some pregnant women take too much of a particular vitamin and unintentionally jeopardize the health of the fetus. The idea that if some vitamins are good, then more are better is seriously flawed. In fact, excess doses of vitamin A taken in the earliest weeks of pregnancy are associated with a significantly increased risk of birth defects, as our research group discovered.[3]

The decision to take a medication during the first 12 weeks of pregnancy and especially between 2 and 8 weeks of pregnancy should be based on a careful assessment of benefits versus risk. Close attention should also be paid to the potential risks to the baby if breast feeding is planned in a mother taking a necessary medication.

Krunal's reported binge drinking may also have contributed to her son's defects. We don't really know whether there was in fact only one such episode or whether other illicit drugs were used. We do know that alcohol is the most common major agent (called teratogen) that can cause brain and physical defects in the exposed fetus. The effects of maternal alcohol ingestion causing functional and physical abnormalities in the child is common and reflected by

3. Rothman KI, Moore LL, Singer MR, Nguyen US, Mannino S, & Milunsky A. (1995) Teratogenicity of high vitamin A intake. *N Engl J Med* 23 (333):1369.

the 1 to 2 cases per 1,000 live births in the United States. The most important effect is on brain function, reflected subsequently by an average IQ of 65, together with various motor disabilities relating to weakness, tremor, hyperactivity, and incoordination. A smaller-than-normal head size and some subtle abnormalities of the facial features are common. Poor growth, joint and bone abnormalities, and heart defects are all common. For alcoholic women, the risk of their offspring having a serious problem approaches 50%. The precise minimum number of drinks per day that would be "safe" during pregnancy remains uncertain. The least significant effects have been noted after the use of two drinks per day in very early pregnancy. Obviously, women who care will not be drinking during pregnancy. The problem of course is being unaware that pregnancy has occurred. Hence, where that becomes a possibility, alcohol should be excluded.

Unplanned pregnancy poses risks to the fetus of a mother on a potentially teratogenic medication. Examples of mothers who have had a deep vein thrombosis in the veins of their legs who are taking an anticoagulant (blood-thinner) in the comarin group (such as warfarin) are well-recorded. This drug has an affinity for affecting developing fetal cartilage, such as the nose, pelvis, and thigh bones. The nose, for example, might be formed with only a single nostril. Other defects may also occur. For mothers on a comarin anticoagulant, when planning a pregnancy, it is important to consult with their physician and switch to the drug called heparin, which is not known to cause birth defects.

The extensive use of antidepressant medications remains a concern. All of these medications cross the placenta into the fetus and, for the most part, do not appear to significantly raise the risk of subsequent birth defects. However, accumulating data do point to an increased risk for a specific group of antidepressants[4] with special reference to heart abnormalities. In addition, later exposure in pregnancy from these antidepressants may cause some complications in the newborn, including jitteriness, respiratory distress, poor tone, and possibly the need to be admitted to an intensive care unit.

There is a veritable epidemic of obesity in the United States and elsewhere. By 2015, a worldwide estimate projects that there will be about 2.3 billion people overweight and more than 700 million adults actually obese. By 2004 in the United States, at least one-third of women age 15 years or older were obese. Seriously overweight women are at risk of developing diabetes, hypertension, clotting disorders, and being subject to higher rates of Cesarean

4. selective serotonin reuptake inhibitors

section and wound infection (*see* Chapter 27). Their infants are at greater risk of being damaged in the birth process, of being too large for gestational age, and for dying in the period just before, during, and after labor. Moreover, obese women have an increased risk of having babies with birth defects, which remain as the leading cause of stillbirth and infant death, accounting for at least 1 in 5 such deaths in the United States. Today, about 50% of women in the reproductive age group in the United States are either overweight or obese.

This new century has seen a rapidly accelerating epidemic of childhood diabetes, obviously followed by the increased prevalence of adult diabetes. Current estimates in the United States point to 9 in 100 people with diabetes. A country with the highest prevalence in the world is the Micronesian island of Nauru, where 31% of its 14,000 inhabitants have diabetes. For further discussion on the genetics of diabetes, *see* Chapter 26.

Prospective mothers with insulin-dependent diabetes need to have their diabetes under tight control **before** becoming pregnant. The medical literature is replete with data showing that mothers with poorly controlled diabetes have a 7% to 10% risk of having a child with a major birth defect, mental retardation, or genetic disorder. In contrast, mothers with tightly controlled diabetes have no greater risk than non-diabetic women for having a child with any of these problems. Typical birth defects in the offspring of mothers without well-controlled diabetes include spina bifida, abnormalities of the lower spine, heart defects, and kidney and intestinal defects.

Women with lupus erythematosis (a chronic disorder of the body's immune system, which affects virtually all tissues and organs) have an increased risk of having a child with heart block evident at birth (or even in the fetus). This condition, which is detectable on the electronic fetal heart monitor strip in late pregnancy, results from the blocked transmission of nerve impulses to the heart muscle. Affected children are otherwise normal but may suffer fainting spells or dizziness and may be subject to sudden death. Treatment after birth may involve implantation of a permanent pacemaker.

Throughout this volume, genetic disorders are discussed that may impact pregnancy, and where appropriate, parents are exhorted to see a clinical geneticist prior to pregnancy to secure their own health and that of a future child.

The types of environmental exposures prospective mothers may encounter include viruses, excess direct heat, X-rays, and toxins. The first 2 to 10 weeks of fetal development constitute the critical period of vulnerability to environmental exposures. Maternal illness due to German measles (rubella) could result in structural heart defects, deafness, and other abnormalities. Of course, immunization against rubella is a must **before** conception. My research group[5] found that use of the hot tub or sauna or the occurrence of high fever in those critical earliest weeks of pregnancy were all associated with an increased risk of having a child with a neural tube defect such as spina bifida. Hot tubs (or hot baths in some countries) should be avoided, as excessive heat increases the risk of conditions like spina bifida by two- to threefold. The problem is that in the first 4 weeks, women may not realize that they have become pregnant. Hence, if pregnancy is possible, the hot tub and sauna should not be used. High fever (called hyperthermia) in the first weeks of pregnancy is recognized as a cause of birth defects, not only in all animal species studied but also in humans. A range of birth defects from such exposed pregnancies have included not only spina bifida but facial anomalies, a small brain, eye defects, cleft lip with or without cleft palate, heart defects, ear abnormalities, and mental retardation. Most diagnostic X-ray exposure is not known to be harmful to the developing fetus. The dose delivered by the CAT scan is, however, much more significant and cannot be assumed to be safe. There is at present insufficient data on that subject.

Between 30% and 40% of birth defects still have unrecognized causes, with environmental factors suspected as having a significant role. About 90% of human cancers are thought to have environmental origins. Developmental pathways that lead to cancer as well as to birth defects may share a common route involving cell growth, proliferation, migration, and differentiation into specialized cells and organs. We should all worry that many toxic agents have been found in amniotic fluid surrounding the fetus, the newborn meconium (the first bowel movement), and the newborn's cord blood. There is a staggering list of environmental drugs and chemicals that pollute the fetal environment and that I have listed elsewhere.[6] This list incorporates the entry of these various chemicals and toxicants into meconium, amniotic fluid, and fetal blood, emphasizing not only pharmaceuticals and illicit drugs but also herbicides, pesticides, polychlorinated biphenyls (PCBs, which include dioxin), phytoestrogens, and phthalates. Many people now know that bisphenol A, which disrupts the female hormone estrogen and is used in the plastics industry, is found in amniotic fluid. This toxin apparently affects preimplantation

5. Milunsky A, Ulcickas M, Rothman K, Willett W, Jick S, & Jick H. (1992) Maternal heat exposure and neural tube defects. *JAMA* 268:7

6. Milunsky A & Milunsky JM (Editors). (2010) *Genetic Disorders and the Fetus: Diagnosis, Prevention, and Treatment*, 6Ed. United Kingdom: Wiley-Blackwell.

and alters postnatal development. Even organophosphates have been reported in meconium. One wonders which government will act to safeguard fetal futures, given the incredible exposures we have recognized for years.

Thyroid disorders occur in almost 3% of pregnant women. Multiple reports in the medical literature have indicated increased risks of birth defects in the offspring of mothers with a thyroid disorder and on thyroid hormone replacement therapy. The nature of these defects has been variable and inconsistent, involving various organ systems of the developing fetus, including brain and genital development.[7] There do, however, appear to be increased risks for various birth defects that are not yet able to be quantified. We know enough to advise women with thyroid disorders to have consultations with pregnancy specialists and have high-resolution targeted ultrasound studies between 16 and 18 weeks of pregnancy.

Smoking during pregnancy is linked to many adverse outcomes, including poor fetal growth, premature delivery, and an increased likelihood of death soon after birth. Smoking also decreases fertility and increases the risks of Sudden Infant Death Syndrome as well as child illnesses. Perhaps even more ominous was our 1999 discovery [8] of a tobacco-specific carcinogen (a cancer-producing agent) in the amniotic fluid surrounding the fetus of mothers who smoked in early pregnancy. Future implications of this early exposure to a cancer-causing substance remain unknown at present. Excess caffeine use in pregnancy is linked to an increased likelihood of miscarriage. Fewer than 4 cups per day might seem reasonable, but remember that caffeine is also present in tea, soft drinks, and chocolate.

Here are the most important steps prospective mothers can take to avoid having a child with a major birth defect or mental retardation:

1. Know yours and your partner's family history.
2. Determine your ethnic or racial origin and ask your doctor which carrier test(s) you and your partner should have.
3. Consult a clinical geneticist if you or your partner have a genetic disorder or concern about such a disorder in either of your families.
4. Seek obstetric consultation before conceiving.
5. Plan your pregnancy.

---

7. Hydrocephalus and hypospadias.
8. Milunsky A, Cannella SG, Ye M & Hecht SS. (2000) A tobacco-specific carcinogen in the fetus. *Prenat Diagn* 20: 307–310.

6. Change anticonvulsant drugs for epilepsy to the least harmful to the fetus in consultation with your doctor.

7. Control diabetes fully before becoming pregnant.

8. Lose excessive weight **before** becoming pregnant.

9. Check with your doctor about the safety of your medications before becoming pregnant.

10. Take folic acid (not less than 0.4 mg daily) for 3 months prior to and after conception.

11. Avoid excess doses of vitamins, especially vitamin A.

12. Avoid working with toxic chemicals such as organic solvents when planning and during pregnancy.

13. Limit caffeine intake.

14. Forgo alcohol use in the first 3 months of pregnancy and reduce intake during pregnancy.

15. Stop smoking.

16. Do not use illicit drugs.

17. Avoid the use of the hot tub and sauna and reduce fever promptly when planning pregnancy and in the first 3 months.

18. Schedule maternal blood screening tests at 11 to 12 weeks for Down syndrome and at 16 weeks for spina bifida.

19. Consider prenatal genetic diagnostic studies where indicated and after consultation with a clinical geneticist or genetic counselor.

20. Be sure to obtain the results of the newborn screening test.

There are few opportunities in life to prevent or avoid what might otherwise end in tragedy. Clear opportunities do exist to avoid such unnecessary outcomes. Remember, not knowing or caring to know may limit your choices but does not alter your chances!

PATTERNS OF ANOMALIES

I remember the day clearly, even though it was decades ago. It was a cold, blustery, and rainy day as I trudged up from the administrative buildings to the freestanding building containing one of the large wards of the Queen Mary's Hospital in Carshalton, in the south of London. I had been called to see a child who had been admitted earlier that week. The resident staff were puzzled about her presentation and without a diagnosis. The head nurse greeted me on entry to the ward and pointed to Jennifer's bed in the far right-hand corner. (In typical English style at the time, one could see all 25 or 30 beds at once from the entrance to the ward.) The head nurse said I would recognize the "large" child who was difficult to manage, then sitting on her bed.

As I walked through the ward with my eyes fixed on the child I planned to see and examine, I suddenly became aware of a child in the midst of a tantrum, bouncing up and down on her bed, as though on a trampoline. It must have only been a momentary glance because I never stopped walking toward the patient I was called to see.

I began my examination of Jennifer by simply looking and assessing her facial features, when I suddenly thought that the bouncing little girl that I had just seen looked exactly like Jennifer. I completed my full examination of Jennifer and asked if I could take a look at Michelle, the bouncer. I was immediately convinced that these two unrelated youngsters had the same features and disorder.

They both had mild-to-moderate mental retardation, and both were far taller than expected for their age. Their heads were large and their foreheads prominent. Their hair was a little sparse in spots and their eyes somewhat widely spaced. Their jaws were prominent and their cheeks flushed. Both had a history of early appearance of teeth. Both had a history of increased length at birth and rapid growth. They had large hands and feet but were poorly coordinated with considerable behavioral problems.

I was interested in their fingerprints and took them to one of England's most famous geneticists, Dr. Lionel Penrose. Among other things, he was an expert at dermatoglyphics and kindly agreed to see "this young, passionate pediatrician." My uneducated guess was that the ridges and whorls at the tips of Jennifer's and Michelle's fingertips were not normal, and to me, the number of ridges seemed to be present in greater than expected numbers. Dr. Penrose confirmed that consistent with their excessive heights, the ridge counts on their fingertips were also some two standard deviations above the norm.

By this time, I had concluded that these two unrelated girls had a newly described condition, then called cerebral gigantism, and together with colleagues, I subsequently published these two cases.[1] Both sets of parents were entirely normal, and neither had a family history of mental retardation or birth defects.

It took many years and hundreds more reported cases before discovery of mutations in a specific gene (*NSDI*) was discovered. Now we know that for this condition, better known as Sotos syndrome,[2] brain imaging invariably reveals enlargement of the ventricles (spaces) and X-rays show markedly advanced bone age. Other problems and features that occur include seizures, eye abnormalities, heart defects, spine curvature, and other orthopedic problems. Fortunately, the excessive growth spurt tails off before puberty, and those affected do not become giants.

I was keen to examine the fingerprints given the childrens' excessive growth, which was already evident by their increased length at birth. I thought it might be possible to show that whatever was stimulating their growth was already in action between 13 and 19 weeks of pregnancy

1. Milunsky A, Cowie VA, & Donohue EC. (1967) Cerebral gigantism in childhood. A report of two cases and a review of the literature. *Pediatrics.* 40:395.
2. In 1964, J.F. Sotos and his co-authors more accurately defined this syndrome of excessive growth and other features, which had been previously recognized.

when the fingerprints become apparent for the first time. This indeed turned out to be the case, given the abnormal increased ridge count.

Today we know that, for the most part, this disorder is sporadic and not inherited. However, for individuals with Sotos syndrome whose IQs are within the normal range, a dominant mode of inheritance will result in a 50% risk of having an affected child. Prenatal diagnosis or preimplantation genetic diagnosis would be available in such cases as long as a mutation has been recognized.

These cases illustrate the long, arduous, and ultimately successful search for the cause of this syndrome. It also illustrates the importance of remaining in contact with clinical geneticists over many years as we slowly unravel the cryptic causes of these intriguing, but worrisome, syndromes.

SOTOS SYNDROME

Sotos syndrome is rare, but other birth defects (better called congenital malformations) are not uncommon. Structural abnormalities such as heart defects occur in about 1 in 50 (2%) births, while all couples have an average risk of 3% to 4% for having a child with a birth defect, mental retardation, or genetic disorder. Malformations that occur with a recognizable pattern (e.g., a child born with a heart defect, a limb defect, and a genital abnormality) constitute a syndrome. Recognizable malformations occur in more than 2,000 disorders, and computer programs are necessary to assist clinical geneticists in distinguishing one syndrome from another. By the age of 7 or 8 years, the frequency of congenital malformations approximates 7% to 8%. The increased number relates to disorders that become apparent after birth or are diagnosed only later.

Canadian researchers, based on extensive population studies, estimated that about 8% of live-born individuals have some type of genetic disorder by about age 25 years. This is likely to be a rather marked underestimate given, for example, the frequency of undetected defects, such as bicuspid aortic valves, that occur in 1% to 2% of the population and are diagnosed mostly later in life (*see* Chapter 9). Heart defects at birth are, in fact, common; the prevalence being at least 0.8% among live births. Congenital defects represent a significant health burden and account for between 28% and 40% of hospital admissions in North America, Canada, and England. Premature infants are known to have about double the risk of being born with a birth defect compared to infants born at term. A study of 4,658 twins revealed an anomaly rate of 1 in 25 twins compared to 1 in 42 for singletons. Identical twins have nearly twice the frequency of birth defects than do non-identical twins. Birth defects remain a leading cause of infant death in the Western world.

Birth defects may have many causes. Chromosome abnormalities and mutations in single genes are important, and many examples are given throughout this book. Multiple susceptibility genes acting in concert with environmental factors (such as folic acid, alcohol, viruses, heat, X-rays, drugs, and toxins) are the root cause of some common defects (*see* Chapter 23). Birth defects may occur singly or in a particular pattern as a syndrome. Although more than 2,000 birth defect syndromes are known, the causes for many are still to be discovered.

Some birth abnormalities are caused by deforming pressure within the womb. For example, these so-called deformations might arise when there is a striking diminution of amniotic fluid surrounding the fetus. A potential consequence is that the head may be forced against the pelvis, resulting in obvious asymmetry of the skull at birth, or the legs may be cramped and constrained, with club foot or feet being the visible outcome at birth. These abnormalities do not usually recur in subsequent pregnancies as long as there isn't a continuing abnormality of the womb. This may occur when the womb is made up of two horns, which represent rather small compartments constraining a developing fetus.

On rarer occasions, a tear may occur in the inside lining of the sac in which the fetus is suspended. The sticky end of the torn tissue might adhere to the opposite end of the cavity within the sac, simulating a rubber band. This band tissue that traverses this inner space may ensnare a digit or even a limb, thereby strangling the distal tissue by cutting off its blood supply. There are records, for example, where birth was followed by the delivery of a digit. Rarely, such a so-called "amniotic band" might stretch across the face and cause horrific damage. These defects are categorized as disruptions.

Congenital defects may be minor and even subtle, whereas major structural defects involve vital and other organs. Most people have at least one imperfection, whether it be a slightly webbed second or third toe, a slight change in the configuration of the ear, an extra nipple, or some other example reflected in Table 24.1. The presence of at least three minor anomalies is associated with about a 20% likelihood that a major congenital defect is present, such as a heart defect or mental retardation. Syndromes are almost invariably combinations of

Table 24.1 Examples of Minor Congenital Anomalies

Cranium and Scalp
Triple hair whorl
Persistent fontanel
Malpositioned fontanel
Back of head flat/prominent
Prominent forehead
Ears
Very small
Lack of folds
Ear lobe crease/notch
Lop ear
Cup-shaped ear
Low-set ears
Skin
Shoulder dimple
Sacrum dimple
Prominent sole crease
Single palm crease
Skin tags (front of ears)
Birth marks
Pigmented spots
Hypopigmented spots
Trunk
Extra nipples
Two-vessel umbilical cord
Umbilical hernia
Face and Neck
Flat bridge of nose
Prominent bridge of nose
Eyes too close
Eyes too far apart
Eyes slant upward
Eyes slant downward
Cleft gum
Small mouth
Big mouth
Prominent tongue
Tongue-tie

(Continued)

Table 24.1 Examples of Minor Congenital
Anomalies (*Continued*)

Face and Neck (Continued)
Small chin
Webbed neck
Redundant neck skin
Droopy eyelids
Limbs
Tapered fingers
Overlapping fingers/toes
Broad thumb, great toe
Incurved fifth fingers/toes
Nails underdeveloped
Increased space between first and second toes
Webbed toes
Overlapping digits
Heel prominent

---

major and minor anomalies and mostly distinguished from one another by the presence of cardinal signs. Many of these syndromes are named for the individual who described the primary features. For example, a child with an IQ below the normal range who has a heart defect, a small head, and an elevated level of blood calcium in infancy as well as certain facial features and an amiable disposition has Williams syndrome until proved otherwise. Although there might be other minor facial features, teeth abnormalities, and short stature, it is the cardinal signs that point toward the diagnosis that can be confirmed by using FISH (*see* Chapter 2) to demonstrate a deletion in the long arm of chromosome 7 in this syndrome.

While I had diagnosed Jennifer and Michelle as having Sotos syndrome, it took 38 years for the precise gene to be discovered. Since the completion of the human genome project and spectacular advances in genetic biotechnology, however, there has been a significant escalation in the discovery rate of genes and their associated mutations that cause various syndromes and that had defied resolution for so long. I mentioned in Chapter 1 the consultation with a mother who adopted two siblings—a boy and a girl. She brought her son (age 45 years) to me to determine whether a cause for his severe but heretofore unexplained mental retardation might now be discoverable. She was prompted to seek this consultation by her adopted daughter, who was worried about her risk for having a child similarly affected as her brother. This severely retarded gentleman appeared syndromic[3] but without a definitive diagnosis. Sequencing genes on the X chromosome and known to be associated with mental retardation and performing a microarray study (*see* Chapter 5) facilitated a brand new diagnosis that revealed a deletion of a specific gene. We subsequently showed that his sister did not have a deletion on either of her X chromosomes and hence had no risk (beyond random) of having a child with the condition affecting her brother.

Parents whose child is mentally retarded, with or without other birth defects, frequently spend years in endless consultations searching for the cause and a possible remedy for their child's affliction. Exhausted physically, emotionally, and sometimes financially, their protracted search almost inevitably comes to an end in their child's teens. The fact is that for an increasing number of those with mental retardation, new technologies to analyze genes and chromosomes would now yield a precise diagnosis. For example, scores of genes on the X chromosome (in addition to others) linked to mental retardation can be analyzed in detail to yield a precise diagnosis. Although invariably treatment will not be forthcoming, a precise diagnosis may be critically important if future childbearing is planned or for siblings and other family members for their children or grandchildren.

Sometimes the quick recognition of a birth defect syndrome made soon after birth is critical. In the **Beckwith-Wiedemann syndrome,**[4] immediate clues that present themselves include a large, heavy baby with a big tongue, prominent eyes, and a strawberry birthmark on the central forehead above the nose. In this overgrowth syndrome, excess activity within the pancreas produces an abundance of insulin, which renders one-third to one-half of all of these babies hypoglycemic (low blood sugar). If the diagnosis is missed and hypoglycemia is present and severe, mental retardation could follow as a consequence of no timely diagnosis and treatment.

Faced with apparently unexplained developmental delay with or without other birth defects, careful consideration should be given to possible family relatedness (consanguinity). A markedly increased rate of birth defects and mental retardation is well-known for first cousins (7%–8% risk), uncle–niece unions, and following incest. Ancestral relatives held in common on both sides

---

3. A syndrome is a group of symptoms and signs.
4. Cardinal signs of **Beckwith-Wiedemann syndrome** include a large baby, prominent tongue, typical facial features, hernia or other abnormality through the navel, and low blood sugar.

of the family may be the likely explanation for a rare recessively inherited birth defects syndrome, such as seen in **Smith-Lemli-Opitz (SLO) syndrome.**[5] In this disorder, transmitted by a faulty gene from both parents, there is a severe defect in the synthesis of cholesterol, leading to a very low blood cholesterol level in the affected child/individual. This observation is a tip-off to obtain a precise diagnosis by sequencing the culprit gene (*DHCR7*). Between 1 in 50 and 1 in 100 people carry an SLO gene mutation. A couple has a 25% risk of having another affected child. Once a mutation is found in each parent, prenatal diagnosis in future pregnancies becomes possible. Other biochemical genetic disorders with associated birth defects are also well-recognized but fortunately are rare.

While physical defects mostly constitute the cardinal signs that facilitate a diagnosis of these syndromes, on occasion, certain behavioral characteristics alert the clinical observer. In the cases of Sotos syndrome that Jennifer and Michelle had, severe temper tantrums were typical. In **Williams syndrome,**[6] a loquacious, overfriendly, intellectually deficient person who likes or is good at music may be the behavioral tip-off to the diagnosis. In the presence of moderate-to-severe retardation in a young girl who is constantly wringing her hands, a diagnosis of **Rett syndrome** is suggested.[7] Episodic hyperventilation might be the clue to the diagnosis of a child with the rare **Pitt-Hopkins syndrome**[8] or in a girl with Rett syndrome. A child with significant mental retardation who bursts out laughing even when in a room alone against the background of a happy disposition, despite the severe intellectual limitation, raises the question of **Angelman syndrome.**[9]

---

5. Cardinal signs for **Smith-Lemli-Opitz syndrome** include moderate-to-severe mental retardation, low muscle tone, small head, heart defects, genital defects, droopy eyelids, and dysmorphic features.

6. Cardinal signs of **Williams syndrome** include mild-to-moderate mental retardation, heart defect, hoarse voice, prominent lips, and high serum calcium level.

7. Cardinal signs of **Rett syndrome** include moderate-to-severe mental retardation, loss of acquired purposeful hand skills, hand-wringing, and autistic behavior.

8. Cardinal signs of **Pitt-Hopkins syndrome** include developmental regression, seizures, episodic overbreathing, the vast majority affecting females. If males survive (most are not born), moderate-to-profound mental retardation is invariable. Typical dysmorphic facial features, seizures, and episodic overbreathing are also present.

9. Cardinal signs of **Angelman syndrome** include severe mental retardation with absent or little speech, paroxysms of inappropriate laughter, dysmophic facial features, and a jerky uncoordinated puppet-like walk.

The very obese teenager with intellectual disability, who literally is picking away at her skin (and drawing blood), immediately directs attention to the likely diagnosis of the **Prader-Willi syndrome.**[10] Some of these affected children have a surprising affinity, again despite their intellectual limitations, to do puzzles. Parents also report the enormous amount they eat (hyperphagia) and the need to put a lock on the refrigerator.

The **Smith-Magenis syndrome**[11] is a rare and complex multisystem disorder with moderate-to-severe mental retardation and multiple congenital anomalies, all resulting from a deletion in the short arm of chromosome 17. The behavioral features are nothing less than startling and include an inverted sleep pattern (awake all night and sleep during the day), self-injury including pulling out the nails and stuffing objects into all body orifices (called polyembolokoilamania), head banging, and aggressive behavior. The sleep inversion results at least in part from the hormone melatonin (which is produced by the pineal gland) being secreted mostly during the day, resulting in a desire to sleep. Besides the head banging, hyperactivity, and self-hugging, multiple other, mostly minor (but some major) congenital defects are encountered.

Earlier, I mentioned that common pathways exist for the development not only of congenital defects but also of cancer. There are, in fact, a host of birth defect syndromes where there is a specific propensity to develop various cancers. Examples include the Beckwith-Wiedemann syndrome, in which a liver or kidney cancer may occur. Much more frequent is the leukemia that occurs in Down syndrome (*see* Chapter 2). In **Poland syndrome,**[12] leukemia or breast cancer on the affected side may occur. In **Costello syndrome,**[13] various types of malignancy may develop. Kidney tumors may develop in a condition in which the iris of the eyes are absent (**Aniridia-Wilms syndrome**[14]). These are but a few of the examples that illustrate potential increased risks of malignancy

---

10. Cardinal signs of **Prader-Willi syndrome** include mild-to-moderate mental retardation, obesity, small hands and feet, low tone, and behavioral issues.

11. Cardinal signs of **Smith-Magenis syndrome** include mild-to-profound mental retardation, dysmorphic facial features, short broad hands and short fingers, speech delay, self-destructive behavior, and inverted sleep rhythm.

12. **Poland syndrome:** unilateral underdeveloped upper chest and muscles with possible absence of the nipple.

13. **Costello syndrome:** moderate to severe mental retardation, large head, typical features, heart defects,and abnormalities of skin, hair, nails, and teeth.

14. **Aniridia-Wilms syndrome:** moderate to severe mental retardation, short stature, small head, typicalfacial features, absent irises with other eye abnormalities, and kidney tumors in about 50% of patients.

and alert caregivers to the need for specific surveillance of children or adults with these specific syndromes. For each of these and all other syndromes, considerable variation is common and all have multiple other possible signs.

Finally, genes determine laterality, for example, that your heart is normally on the left side, your liver below the ribs on the right, and your spleen below the ribs on your left side. A mutation in a key laterality gene may lead to organ reversal with your heart on the right (dextrocardia), your liver on the left, and your spleen on the right (called total situs inversus). Not unexpectedly, this is likely to be a genetic condition inherited from both parents as an autosomal recessive disorder and hence found more frequently among those parents who are closely related.

Children or adults with unusual facial features or other observable physical abnormalities with or without mental retardation are best seen in consultation with a clinical geneticist. The need for and choice of specific genetic tests could then be determined. Families are advised to either remain in contact or revisit a clinical geneticist even years after their search for a cause has concluded. Families should be aware of possible consanguinity and make efforts to determine their ancestral origins. For a well-recognized number of different birth defect syndromes, surveillance for a lifetime would be important if there was a known increased risk of malignancy. All of this information would be important for the affected individual, their siblings, and their family.

25

TREATMENT OPTIONS

Jack and Katherine were exhausted and desperate. Their third child, Bryan, had become almost impossible to manage and care for at home. He was 18 years old, profoundly mentally retarded, and epileptic. He was fair-haired, with a fair skin showing signs of longstanding excoriation caused by persistent and seemingly resistant eczema. His small head was evident even to the casual observer.

Jack and Katherine first realized during his second year of life that Bryan was seriously delayed in his development. They consulted pediatricians and neurologists who, in turn, ordered various tests but did not succeed in making a definitive diagnosis. When, at 18 years, Bryan's behavior became intractably worse and almost impossible to manage, they sought the care of a neurologist who saw only adult patients. He reviewed the family history and noted that they each came from very large Irish families. Jack had five married siblings and Katherine had four married siblings, yielding a combined total of 37 nieces and nephews. None had any birth defect or mental retardation. In contrast, Jack had been born with a heart defect (a hole between the lower two chambers of the heart called ventricular septal defect), which required surgery toward the end of his first year of life. Bryan's parents felt certain that they were not related.

Their "new" physician started his inquiry and evaluation from "scratch." He obtained all the medical records from Bryan's previous doctors to determine what diagnostic tests had been done and whether he could find any important tests that still should be done.

His search for the laboratory result of the newborn screening tests were in vain. The pediatrician's medical record contained no such report. To his credit, he decided to seek a copy of that report from the state laboratories that had performed the newborn screening test, which covered a handful of biochemical genetic disorders. He was staggered to receive a call and then a copy of the report indicating that as a tiny infant on the fourth day of life, Bryan had tested positive for phenylketonuria (PKU), the first disorder to be tested routinely in newborn infants before hospital discharge.

Jack and Katherine were horrified to hear that Bryan had a biochemical genetic disorder that could have been treated by dietary restriction of protein, which would have enabled him to have developed normally and not be mentally retarded at all. My involvement began when I was consulted by the parents' lawyer, then engaged to sue their pediatrician, the hospital, and the state for medical negligence in failing to diagnose and treat Bryan's inborn chemical error.

It might seem incomprehensible in this day and age how such a grievous outcome could occur. It behooved the state laboratory to immediately and directly contact the child's doctor who ordered the test to inform about the abnormal result. This duty is especially compelling given the fact that PKU is very responsive to timely treatment, which, if started as soon as possible after birth, enables avoidance of mental handicap. It was the responsibility of the resident doctor in the hospital who wrote the order for the newborn screening test to be sure that the result was obtained. It was necessary for the child's pediatrician at the time of Bryan's first check-up a few weeks after birth to have immediately recognized the absence of the newborn screening laboratory report. The pediatrician claimed that he had never seen the report but admitted that his staff placed reports in the patient's file, which he would then read at the time of their visit. Apparently the lawyer was met with a blank stare from the pediatrician when he was asked about the possibility of improperly filed reports. This case, yet again, demonstrates compounding errors that are almost the rule in cases of medical negligence.

It was no surprise that there were no affected family members, given that PKU is inherited as an autosomal recessive disorder (*see* Chapter 6). Jack and Katherine had been lucky with their first two children as they had a 25% risk of having an affected child with PKU in every pregnancy. Subsequently, sequencing of the PKU gene (*PAH*) enabled recognition of each mutation in this gene in Jack and Katherine. Further testing revealed that both of their other children were carriers (they had a two of three likelihood). They informed their extended families and warned that there was a 50% likelihood that each of their siblings would be carriers. Sure enough, after testing, four of their siblings were indeed carriers of a PKU gene mutation. Their siblings who were carriers recognized the importance of later testing their growing children for their carrier status.

PHENYLKETONURIA

Phenylketonuria was first recognized as a biochemical genetic disorder in 1934. Once it became clear that there was an effective treatment that made it possible to avoid mental retardation and that a simple screening test could be used, widespread application was initiated. As a consequence, screening of all our newborns developed in the 1960s, and PKU was the first disorder to be tested. Newborn screening was subsequently adopted in most Western countries. Phenylketonuria is not uncommon among the Irish and their descendants, occurring in about 1 in 4,500 live births. About 1 in 33 individuals of Irish descent carry a mutation in the PKU gene (*PAH*). Curiously, the frequency of PKU among Turks approximates 1 in 2,600, with 1 in 26 of them being carriers, probably reflecting high degrees of consanguinity. Generally among White newborns, PKU occurs in about 1 in 10,000 live births, with 1 in 50 Whites being carriers. The disorder is much rarer among those of Japanese, Finnish, and African descent.

The actual diagnosis can be simply made by measurement in the plasma of the amino acid phenylalanine. Once a diagnosis is made, there is a need to analyze the *PAH* gene to determine the specific mutation in each parent and then to track and test that mutation in other linked family members. Prenatal diagnosis or preimplantation genetic diagnosis is also available for a couple facing a 25% risk of having a child with PKU, once the mutations have been determined.

The abnormal result of the newborn screen on Bryan should have alerted the caregivers to immediately initiate a low-protein diet and/or the use of a phenylalanine-free medical formula as soon as possible after his birth. This would have enabled avoidance of him developing irreversible and devastating mental retardation. For the child diagnosed in the newborn period, a low-protein diet, monitoring of blood levels of the culprit amino acid (phenylalanine), and continued surveillance (preferably by a health-care team) is best. Adherence to this necessarily strict diet in the early years is a challenge to all parents but unfortunately is a necessity.

While diet therapy for life is optimal, it is an absolute requirement for women with PKU who are planning a pregnancy. Well before conception, they should begin the phenylalanine-restricted diet in earnest and be monitored to determine that their plasma level of that amino acid is in a normal range for at least several months prior to conceiving. This care and attention should continue throughout their pregnancies because phenylalanine is toxic to the developing fetus and is potent in causing birth defects. Affected women who fail to pay attention to these details have a high risk of having a child with a damaged brain (including a small head, called microcephaly) with mental retardation, a heart defect, and growth restriction. Because at least half of all pregnancies are unplanned, women with PKU in their reproductive years who could become pregnant should maintain themselves on a phenylalanine-restricted diet with continued monitoring and surveillance.

Both men and women with PKU should avoid the artificial sweetener aspartane, which is in widespread use and contains the potentially damaging phenylalanine.

Nowadays, in some states in the United States (such as Massachusetts), 29 different disorders are screened for in our newborns, despite the fact that for some of them, optimal treatment is not available. However, making a prompt diagnosis at least enables couples to recognize their significant high risk (for most of these conditions) of having a second affected child. There are many biochemical genetic disorders, but none respond with the dramatic avoidance of mental retardation as seen in PKU.

The recognized negligence in the management of Bryan's newborn screening ended with a profoundly damaged life and all parties settling the claims made against them for negligence. Parents are reminded that they should be sure to be informed of the result of every test done on themselves or their children—especially the newborn screening.

Abe was a hypochondriac, according to his wife Zelda. Then at age 42 years, Zelda related that in all of their 18 years of marriage, Abe was always complaining of this pain or that. Rare visits to his primary care doctor had invariably concluded that the stress of his very successful business was the cause of his somatic complaints. True, he had been intermittently anemic, but the doctor said that it was due to iron deficiency, and sure enough, it did correct on iron supplementation.

When Zelda's cell phone rang unexpectedly during the consultation, Abe had a chance to get in a word edgewise.

He said that for as long as he could remember, the bones in his legs ached, as did some of his joints. A few weeks before our consultation, Abe related that he was in the process of fixing a gutter at their home when he slipped off the third step of the ladder. He immediately experienced severe pain in his right mid-thigh. Zelda drove him to the hospital emergency department, scolding him all the way.

The young, freshly minted emergency room physician examined Abe from top to toe, muttering along the way that Abe seemed somewhat anemic and that his spleen and liver were both enlarged. The X-ray he ordered revealed a pathologic fracture in Abe's mid-thigh, as well as marked degenerative changes in both hip joints.

The emergency department physician suggested that the pathologic fracture (a bone break at the site of disease or abnormality), the anemia, and the enlarged liver and spleen taken together with his Ashkenazi Jewish ancestry all pointed to a likely diagnosis of a condition called Gaucher disease,[1] and he referred Abe to me for a consultation.

The young physician was right on target. Biochemical genetic testing revealed that Abe had a specific enzyme deficiency,[2] confirming the diagnosis of Gaucher disease. He was indeed anemic, and moreover, his white blood cell count was below normal while his platelet[3] count was markedly depressed. The latter finding explained the ease with which he bruised. His enlarged spleen was literally gobbling up his circulating

---

1. Named for a French physician, Philippe Gaucher, who described the features of this disorder in 1882.
2. Glucocerebrosidase deficiency that results in excess accumulation of complex fats that are not broken down because of this enzyme deficiency
3. The tiny cells in the blood involved in forming clots to stop bleeding, among other actions. Very low platelet counts can result in serious bleeding.

blood cells (a process called hypersplenism). Moreover, his bones generally showed marked lack of density (osteopenia or osteoporosis) and his hip joints were in the process of crumbling (called osteonecrosis). There was indeed abundant evidence for his complaints of pain and discomfort over so many years.

I obtained a blood sample from him for DNA studies, which later revealed that he carried two different, but common, mutations in the Gaucher disease gene (GBA). Fortunately, Zelda proved negative following my testing of her DNA, but their three children, as expected, were all obligatory carriers of one or the other of Abe's mutations. For this autosomal recessive inherited disorder, carriers are healthy, and only if two mutations are inherited (one from each parent) is that individual affected. Only four mutations account for about 90% of cases among those of Ashkenazi Jewish ancestry; but this is true for only 50% to 60% among non-Jewish individuals. Sequencing the *GBA* gene, where necessary, can detect almost all other mutations.

Fortunately, enzyme replacement therapy to remedy his deficiency had become available, and Abe was referred to a comprehensive Gaucher disease treatment center. Much pain and discomfort could have been avoided if Abe had returned for a follow-up visit to his physician and for annual check-ups, which he missed solidly for all of his adult life.

GAUCHER DISEASE

Gaucher disease is generally rare, occurring about 1 in 57,000 in the population. However, among those of Ashkenazi Jewish ancestry, the frequency is considerably higher. For Ashkenazis, about 1 in 18 are carriers of a Gaucher disease gene mutation, with the disorder occurring in about 1 in 855 individuals. This form of Gaucher disease (called Type I) accounts for about 95% of cases. An estimated 1 in 1,296 is the frequency of births with Gaucher disease among Ashkenazis prior to the availability of carrier testing, which is now routinely available (*see* Chapter 15). Subsequent testing of Abe's three siblings revealed two who were carriers, as were each of their children. I heard subsequently that Abe eventually underwent surgical removal of his spleen, which continued to sequester his platelets in particular, placing him at risk of a life-threatening hemorrhage. Various other therapies were provided to remedy his bone loss, anemia, and other symptoms.

There are two other rarer major types of Gaucher disease (Types 2 and 3, accounting for about 5% of all cases) with onset of serious signs either soon after birth or in infancy. These more serious presentations invariably involve the brain and nervous system and, if untreated, cause early death.

Fortunately, by routine screening and detection of carriers, couples have the option of prenatal diagnosis in planned pregnancies, the choice of adoption, artificial insemination by donor, or preimplantation genetic diagnosis. Enzyme replacement therapy,[4] although extraordinarily expensive, has made a major difference in the lives of those affected.

Over the past decade, an association between Gaucher disease and Parkinson's disease (*see also* Frequently Asked Questions) has emerged. Detailed studies, including full sequencing of the Gaucher disease gene, have revealed that **carriers** have as high as a 28-fold increased likelihood of developing Parkinsonism. Not unexpectedly, those **with** Gaucher disease also have a higher than expected likelihood of developing Parkinson's disease. Moreover, the carrier state for Gaucher disease confers a higher risk of developing Parkinsonism at an earlier age. Carriers too seem to respond less well to the usual medications for Parkinson's disease and enzyme replacement therapy appears to be less effective, according to a French study. The precise mechanism causing brain cells to malfunction as a result of the enzyme deficiency is unknown but is the focus of intense research.

An increased risk of certain cancers, especially lymphomas/leukemias and multiple myeloma[5]—have been reported in those with Gaucher disease. Other named cancers include colon, lung, thyroid, and prostate. Although the risk may be increased, the actual odds are not large, approximating 1 in 50.

Other biochemical genetic disorders, in which excess and various substances accumulate because of enzyme deficiencies, are well-known. For a slowly increasing number of them, enzyme replacement therapy may become a reality,[6] with the promise of a much better quality of life, and can perhaps even be life-saving.

---

4. Using miglustat (taken by mouth), imiglucerase (given only intravenously at 2-week intervals), or velaglucerase alfa intravenously every 2 weeks.
5. Malignant involvement of plasma cells in bone marrow that bedevil the immune system.
6. Pompe disease, Fabry disease, Hurler syndrome.

OTHER THERAPIES FOR GENETIC DISORDERS

A remarkable array of therapeutic approaches are available and in development for the treatment and management of many genetic disorders. Some key examples have been discussed earlier in this book. Certainly advances in biotechnology and genomics have yielded new approaches, and together with those already established help save lives, extend life spans, dramatically improve the quality of life, and even result in cures.

Completion of the Human Genome Project has enabled identification of disease-causing genes that can be targeted for manipulation. Mice have been especially valuable for manipulation, as about 99% of genes in humans have counterparts in mice. Mice in whom a gene has been deleted (called knock-out mice)[7] have been especially bred.

Knock-in mice have been bred with a specific gene inserted. From these genetically engineered mice, an understanding of gene function has been facilitated, including an understanding of how genes are regulated or influenced by other genes. This gene targeting technology has created mice with specific mutations that cause certain genetic diseases in humans. There are, for example, knock-out mice bred for phenylketonuria, Huntington disease, cystic fibrosis, Fragile X syndrome, Tay-Sachs disease, obesity, hypertension, breast cancer, and many other diseases. These knock-out or knock-in mice have made treatment trials possible by providing representative models of human disease that are available in a continual supply. In addition to the innovations that have and will spring from these novel approaches, there are well-developed and new therapeutic avenues.

The range of therapeutic approaches include dietary modifications, use of specific medications, depletion of toxic elements, surgical repair and reconstruction, transplantation, and gene therapy. Recognition of genetic susceptibility coupled with identification of harmful factors has led to opportunities for the avoidance of health and life-threatening events. Various examples serve to illustrate these therapeutic approaches.

---

7. To help decipher the function of a gene, it can be targeted and knocked out of the genome (or inserted as a knock-in). These manipulations have been accomplished with at least 4,000 genes in mice.

Restriction and Substitution

Dietary modifications by restriction and substitution have achieved remarkable success and are best exemplified by the management of phenylketonuria discussed in this chapter. What must be restricted in such cases is the essential amino acid called phenylalanine, which is present in all high-grade proteins. Initiation of a low-protein diet that limits the production and accumulation of the brain-damaging toxic products and substitution of a synthetic supplement has enabled the avoidance of mental retardation. A similar but much rarer condition, called galactosemia, is also managed by dietary restriction. Untreated, this recessive disorder results in mental retardation, cirrhosis of the liver, cataracts, and early death. The cause is a deficient enzyme whose failure to break up a milk sugar leads to the accumulation of one of its components (galactose), which proves toxic especially to the brain, liver, and eyes of the fetus and infant. Dietary restriction is focused on the exclusion of milk and milk products. Once again, similarly to phenylketonuria, diagnosis in the newborn is critical and life-saving, and continued dietary treatment allows normal development. Women with galactosemia who plan to have children must avoid milk and milk products while planning and throughout pregnancy to have the best chance of the fetal brain not being damaged by the accumulation of galactose. Both biochemical and DNA methods are available to detect carriers as well as for prenatal diagnosis.

Avoidance of milk and milk products is also important in the management of the extremely common lactose intolerance— a disorder characterized by cramps and diarrhea after ingesting milk products.

Augmenting or excluding certain food or liquid intake in the face of various genetic disorders can help secure health and even save lives. Careful attention to water intake is essential for a number of disorders. In cystinuria, the genetic condition that produces kidney stones, water intake (even in the wee hours of the morning) is important if painful renal colic caused by stones is to be avoided. (Taking alkalis provides additional help in preventing stone formation in both kidneys and bladder.) Individuals with sickle cell disease (see Chapter 15) need to avoid dehydration that could otherwise result in sickle cell crises or strokes. Those with nephrogenic diabetes insipidus (a condition in which the kidney's fail to conserve water) could die from dehydration if undiagnosed and untreated. A number of genetic disorders involve low blood sugar (hypoglycemia), including the common diabetes mellitus. Simple sugar or candy may be vital in managing a sudden drop in blood sugar. Certain sugars, such as glucose, sucrose, and fructose (sugar in fruit), may individually cause serious problems for persons with rare hereditary disorders involving the body's carbohydrate chemistry. In the condition called fructose intolerance, the body is unable to digest the natural sugars in fruit. Dietary therapy is facilitated by the fact that the affected person often develops an aversion to sweet-tasting foods. A similar situation exists for some very rare disorders in which bizarre behavior and even coma may eventuate after a protein meal.[8] These individuals often have an aversion to meat. An obvious restriction is saturated fats and the use of low- or no-cholesterol foods as an aid in the treatment of heart and blood vessel disease.

Obvious restrictions apply to individuals with a serious allergy that could cause an acute reaction, shock, collapse, and death (called anaphylaxis)—for example, allergies to peanuts, penicillin, chestnuts, and red currants. Other drugs (e.g., sulfa drugs) or foods (e.g., shellfish) that result in allergic reactions obviously must also be excluded from the diet. All of these allergic responses are inherited either via a single dominant gene or multiple genes acting in concert with the extrinsic allergic factor.

In the disorder called acute intermittent porphyria, commonly seen in White South Africans of Dutch descent, barbiturates may precipitate severe attacks of abdominal pain and may prove fatal. This dominantly inherited disorder carries a 50% risk for the affected individual transmitting the disease to each of his or her offspring. Similar symptoms may be precipitated not only by barbiturates but also by many other medications, including sulfa drugs, anticonvulsants, hormones, and antifungal drugs.

Supplementation and Replacement

Dietary supplementation may be extremely important in preventing certain birth defects and treating some genetic disorders. The most prominent supplement discussed earlier (*see* Chapter 23) is the routine use of folic acid (0.4 mg daily) as a supplement for women planning pregnancy and also taken through the first 3 months of pregnancy. The aim is the avoidance of spina bifida and other neural tube defects, which is successful in at least 70% of such pregnancies. Dietary supplementation using fat-soluble vitamins A, D, E, and K are critically important in the management of disorders in which there is fat malabsorption (e.g., cystic fibrosis).

---

8. Such as Ornithine Transcarbamylase Deficiency.

Supplementation and replacement are necessary for the common form of diabetes mellitus, with the provision of insulin that is necessary when the pancreatic cells fail to produce a sufficient quantity or when the body builds a resistance to the available insulin.

In the treatment of the water-losing nephrogenic diabetes insipidus, hormone replacement in the form of a fine powder inhaled through the nose is health-preserving and life-saving. The hormone vasopressin is absorbed through the nasal membranes into the bloodstream and circulates to the kidney, where it helps concentrate the urine, thereby preventing excessive water loss. The infant born with a non-functioning thyroid gland (called congenital hypothyroidism) is usually diagnosed by routine newborn screening. Early diagnosis is critical if mental retardation is to be avoided. Treatment with thyroid hormone should be initiated promptly and continued for life. All parents should be certain to obtain the results of the newborn screen and NOT assume everything is normal if they have received no specific results. I have seen desperately sad consequences (avoidable lifelong mental retardation) when results were not obtained and treatment not begun in the first few weeks after birth.

A steadily increasing number of disorders characterized by absence or deficiency of specific enzymes are being treated by enzyme replacement. These disorders are otherwise progressive and characterized by systematic accumulation of complex fats, proteins, or carbohydrates, almost invariably leading to chronic illness, mental retardation, and/or death. Earlier in this chapter, I discussed Gaucher disease, typical of this category, but other conditions that are now treatable by enzyme replacement therapy include Fabry disease, Hurler syndrome, and Pompe disease.

Hemophilia A is a typical example of the value of replacement therapy (see chapter 17). In this disorder, the affected individual is deficient in the critical clotting Factor VIII.

Administration of Factor VIII concentrates have secured the health and saved the lives of many with Hemophilia A (*see* Chapter 17).

Retinitis pigmentosum is a disorder that ends in blindness and that is caused by various gene defects that may be recessive, dominant, or sex-linked. The initial symptom is visual difficulty at night or at twilight, followed by progressive loss of peripheral vision. Most are legally blind by age 40 years. The use of high-dose vitamin A supplements (15,000 IU daily) has been shown to slow the annual decline of visual loss by about 20%. An important caution for those with retinitis pigmentosum is to avoid taking high-dose vitamin E supplements—a practice that seems to hasten visual loss.

Table 25.1 Examples of Medication Types Used to Treat or Avoid Selected Genetic Disorders

Genetic Disorder	Type of Medication	Purpose
Biotinidase deficiency	Vitamin (Biotin)	Newborn diagnosis avoids mental retardation, seizures, vision loss, hair loss, balance problems, skin eruptions
Congenital adrenal hyperplasia	Steroids (e.g., cortisone)	Save life; remedy growth and other problems
Coronary heart disease	Anti-inflammatory (e.g., aspirin)	Reduces frequency of heart attacks
Cystic fibrosis	Pancreatic supplements	Remedy malabsorption of fats
Diabetes mellitus	Hormone (insulin)	Controls blood sugar
Diabetes insipidus	Hormone (antidiuretic)	Concentrates urine to stop water loss
Factor V Leiden gene mutation	Anticoagulant	Prevents thrombosis
Familial hypercholesterolemia	Statin drugs	Reduces blood cholesterol and frequency of heart attacks
Familial polyps of the colon	Anti-inflammatory (e.g., cyclooxygenase inhibitor)	Reduces polyp formation in the colon
Growth hormone deficiency	Hormone	Remedies lack of growth hormone, restores growth
Hemochromatosis	Chelating agent	Rids body of excess iron
Hypothyroidism	Hormone (e.g., thyroxine)	Remedies underacting thyroid gland
Long QT syndrome	Beta-blockers	Reduce the frequency of heart rhythm abnormalities
Malignant hyperthermia	Muscle relaxant (e.g., Dantrolene)	Prevents death from very high fever during anesthesia
Marfan syndrome	Beta-blockers	Reduce risk of rupture of the aorta
Osteogenesis imperfecta	Biphosphonate pamidronate	Improves bone density
Prothrombin gene mutation	Anticoagulants	Prevent thrombosis
Retinitis pigmentosum	Vitamin A	Mega doses delay visual loss
Sickle cell disease	Increases fetal hemoglobin production (e.g., hydroxyurea, vaccine)	Reduces painful crises and frequency of blocked arteries. Reduces frequency of bacterial infection (by pneumococcus)
Smith-Lemli-Opitz syndrome	Cholesterol	Improves growth and behavior
Spina bifida/anencephaly	Folic acid (Vitamin B complex)	Prevents about 70% of cases if taken before or within days of conception
Tyrosinemia	Enzyme inhibitor	Improves liver and kidney function and prevents eye and skin complications
Wilson's disease	Chelating agent	Rids body of excess copper

Many other examples exist in which replacement of proteins are critical to health and survival, including the use of gamma-globulin for those whose bodies fail to manufacture these proteins that protect against infection.

Medications

An arsenal of medications exists for the treatment, albeit non-curative, of a huge number of genetic disorders (*see* Table 25.1). Hormone treatment for genetic deficiencies in the endocrine glands (thyroid, pituitary, pancreas, adrenal, parathyroid) are all remedied by administration of the necessary deficiency hormone. Certain forms of gout are inherited, and specific drugs available will block the formation of the accumulating uric acid that leads to excruciating attacks of pain.

Although most drugs available are dedicated to remedying troublesome or worrisome symptoms and signs, those that interdict or prevent the most serious consequences or complications are really valuable.

Excessive accumulation of toxic elements may cause irreversible damage to certain organs in the body and eventually prove fatal. Discussed earlier is the accumulation of iron in hemochromatosis (*see* Chapter 14) and copper in Wilson disease (Chapter 26). The **depletion** approach for hemochromatosis is a schedule of blood-letting by routine phlebotomy until toxic body iron stores are returned to a normal range of values. Chelation therapy is used to rid the body of copper in Wilson disease and also to rid the body of iron in hemochromatosis using different chelating agents.

Repair and Reconstruction

Repair and reconstruction are surgical modalities of therapy that play an important role in the treatment and correction of a wide range of birth defects and genetic disorders. Surgical approaches to repair, reconstruct, or limit damage to virtually all body organs play a key role in securing the health of those with a wide range of genetic disorders. Examples include surgical operations on the head (for hydrocephalus—enlarged head, excess fluid accumulation); the heart (ventricular septal defect or "hole-in-the- heart"); cleft lip or palate; exposed bowel (called omphalocele); genital abnormalities; and limb defects. Surgery to remove cancers of genetic origin may well be life-saving.

Transplantation

Transplantation plays a vital life-saving role in specific genetic disorders. For example, the adult form of polycystic kidney disease (*see* Chapter 18), if not complicated by cysts or aneurysms elsewhere in the body, can be treated effectively by removal of the diseased kidneys and transplantation of a healthy one. Similarly, transplantation has been valuable for certain hereditary heart disorders, such as cardiomyopathies (*see* Chapter 9), of the liver (for cirrhosis or cancer), bone marrow (leukemias and lymphomas), and corneas (various eye diseases). More recent techniques involving the growth of connective tissue cells (fibroblasts) in sheets in the laboratory have been used as grafts to cover burns and skin defects or even to "manufacture" bladders.

Bone marrow transplantation has been used for decades in treating severe subacute combined immunodeficiency disease and has been successful in treating this otherwise fatal disorder. Bone marrow transplantation for various genetic storage diseases has had variable, but mostly unimpressive, results. More promising have been the enzyme replacement therapies now in use and in development. In contrast, stem cell transplantation holds promise not yet realized. These so-called pluripotent cells are found in the embryo and eventually in the blood from the umbilical cord and in the bone marrow and tissue of the fetus. These cells retain organ-specific destinies and the hope is that they will be able to repair or replace organs or tissues impaired by illness such as diabetes, heart disease, stroke, burns, or arthritis and help repair injury, for example, of the spinal cord or brain. Equally hopeful is their use in degenerative diseases of the brain, including Huntington's disease, Parkinson's disease, or Alzheimer's disease. Because embryonic stem cells can be grown in the laboratory, there is much hope for their effective use in the many disorders and injuries not currently amenable to other cures. Hope has been spawned among paraplegics by reports of successful experiments in which paraplegic rats were able to walk again after embryonic brain stem cells were implanted in their spinal cords below the level of the injury.

Surgical implantation of devices—for example, cardioverter-defibrillators—for life-saving treatment for individuals with the Long QT syndrome (*see* Chapter 9) have been successful. The use of in-dwelling pumps have revolutionized the care in some chronic disorders.

Harmful Factors

Given the fact that we all harbor various genetic susceptibilities, attention to the avoidance of harmful factors can be important not only for securing health but also saving life. For example, individuals with albinism should avoid sun exposure because of the increased risk of skin cancer. Persons with alpha-1-antitrypsin deficiency, a recessive disorder, must absolutely not smoke or work in polluted environments because of the danger of lung disease. Those with pseudocholinesterase deficiency need to avoid certain muscle relaxants given during general anesthesia, as they fail to resume breathing on their own for 2 to 3 hours after the cessation of anesthesia. This is a recessive disorder that is particularly common in certain populations, such as Eskimos, many of whom have a family history of such problems following surgery and general anesthesia. In the Alaskan Eskimos, about 1 in 10 carry the gene for this disorder. Generally, about 1 in 30 Whites are carriers. Infants born with a specific mitochondrial gene mutation are especially susceptible to becoming deaf if they are treated with a particular class of antibiotics called aminoglycosides (*see* Chapter 22).

Gene Therapy

Repair and reconstruction, transplantation, medications, devices, and dietary modifications play important roles in mostly maintaining health and sometimes effecting a cure of a genetic disorder. Gene therapy, by repairing or replacing a defective gene, is a whole other matter. Not only is the mutant gene in every cell of the body (for almost all single-gene disorders), but access to brain cells is effectively blocked at the blood–brain barrier. Various strategies have been employed in laboratories, including the use of enzymes to unfurl the DNA helix and repair the defective strand using normal repair mechanisms within cells. Another approach has been to use small molecular drugs to override the gene defect.

If a defective gene cannot be repaired, perhaps it could be replaced by a normal copy. But how and by which method could a normal copy of a gene be introduced to every cell (or at least a sufficient number of cells) to be of therapeutic benefit? Moreover, not only would it be necessary for the normal gene to function (express itself), but safety would need to be ensured. One important solution has been the use of an engineered virus used as a transporter (called a vector) of the needed gene into cells. The engineered virus is unable to replicate and is not able to cause any known illness. The viral vector and its normal gene passenger gains entry into the cells and tissues of a host. This has been achieved by injection of the viral vector[9] carrying the normal gene under

---

9. Called Adeno-Associated Virus.

the retina[10] in Briard dogs, in which a spontaneously occurring gene mutation results in blindness. These dogs have had the equivalent of a human genetic disease causing blindness called Leber Congenital Amaurosis. Clear evidence of vision improvement in these dogs led to human trials of individuals with this form of blinding retinal disease, the onset of which occurs in the very first few years of life or even from birth. Clear evidence of vision improvement has been recorded in the small number of people with Leber Congenital Amaurosis[11] treated thus far. Since dogs treated early in life and for more than 9 years maintained visual function, there is great hope that this form of gene therapy will be the forerunner of heretofore unsuccessful efforts at remedying blindness.

Advances in gene transfer technology have led to the use of lentiviral vectors. These viruses, once rendered non-infectious, can deliver a significant gene load into cells. In a truly remarkable and ironic twist of fate, this virus that ordinarily devastates the immune system in HIV-AIDS, can be rendered safe (but not absolutely) as a gene transporter, even in treating immunodeficiencies as well as AIDS. Cells that have been taken from an affected individual and genetically corrected by having a lentivirus carrying the normal gene have been infused back into the circulation and used successfully in boys with adrenoleukodystrophy. This is a severe X-linked demyelinating brain disease[12] resulting in loss of intellectual ability and early death. In the first boys treated and followed for at least 2 years, the progressive brain destruction ceased. A similar approach is being tried for the treatment of thalassemia (*see* Chapter 15), with early tentative success.

An abiding concern remains about the difficulty of homing a gene into a location within the genome while maintaining safety. Grim experience attended the use of DNA that integrated into an untoward site in the genome during the treatment of subacute combined immune deficiency disease, subsequently resulting in leukemia in some. The protein product of an introduced gene may have the potential of fusing with another protein product of another gene to become a cancer-causing protein. Moreover, another challenge to overcome is our body's immune defense response, which may recognize the vector or the new (normal gene) protein product as a foreign invader.

---

10. The light-sensitive tissue that lines the inner rear surface of eyes receiving all the images we see.

11. Named after Theodore Leber, a nineteenth century German ophthalmologist who described this autosomal recessive disorder in blind children born to normally sighted parents.

12. A disorder of the nervous system in which the insulating sheath around nerves is damaged, severely impairing function.

The result could be inactivation or an actual immune disease reaction. Another concern has been that the donated gene that integrates into the genome will be passed to subsequent daughter cells and of course, if either ovaries or testes are involved, to a subsequent generation.

Notwithstanding these concerns, much optimism attends the increasing use of stem cells and safe viral vectors for the successful treatment of serious-to-fatal genetic disorders. Moreover, the ability to employ site-specific and even mutation-specific targeted gene therapy, will almost certainly create dramatic new treatments for the damaged heart muscle (after a heart attack) and ultimately in curing cancers.

THE FUTURE: PERSONALIZED MEDICINE

New advances in technology have revealed that cancerous tumors harbor many mutations in multiple different genes, providing new insight into the ominous labyrinth that leads to uncontrolled cell growth. This new knowledge has opened up possible drug design strategies based on the newly recognized genetic flaws. Meanwhile, genome-wide association studies, explained in Chapter 5, are revealing for virtually every disorder and characteristic evaluated and caused by gene–environmental interactions (the vast majority of common diseases), molecular signatures (biomarkers) that indicate our predisposition or susceptibility to one or other (or more) disorder. Much greater refinement in genotyping is anticipated that will enable recognition of an individual's likely response to a specific medication (such as an anticoagulant, a statin drug, or a cancer drug). Ultimately one hope is to analyze a tumor, recognize the mutations contained therein (and there are usually many), and devise a tailored chemotherapy for the affected person. All these advances will truly usher in a gene-based era of personalized medicine. We can safely anticipate that in the not-too-distant future, these genetic susceptibilities (e.g., to diabetes), will be established from umbilical cord blood collected at birth. A veritable cascade of therapeutic advisories, measures, and interventions are sure to follow and are aimed at avoiding ill-health.

Unfortunately, however, direct-to-consumer genetic laboratory services have prematurely gained traction, leading directly to confusion instead. Commercially offered gene-association studies are frequently based on flimsy or unreliable evidence. Results may indicate the statistical likelihood of a particular disorder, whose actual risk may well be less than 1% despite a many-fold reported increased risk. Unnecessary anxiety will then likely spawn a population neurotic about their health. Avid commercial interests driven by venture capitalists will need to be regulated to safeguard individuals and families at risk. Serious risk communication, without genetic evaluation and counseling by board-certified genetic counselors or clinical geneticists, is patently unwise.

The dramatic pace of advances in genetic biotechnology has enabled sequencing of all the genes of an individual (called next-generation sequencing). The current estimate is that we each harbor about 100 mutations in our genome. If it took only 5 minutes to discuss each mutation, more than 8 hours would be needed. The ability (let alone the wisdom) to interpret the mass of ensuing data is still developing. Nevertheless, in a few short years we will be able to glean a wealth of information about our genetic health, susceptibilities, and future risks. Published guidelines will be necessary, and counselors will need great sensitivity, clinical wisdom, and experience in helping individuals seeking guidance about their genomes.

SUGAR AND METALS

Sophie was a single mother. At age 25 years, she already had two children from different unions, receiving no support from either man, both of whom had disappeared after brief liaisons. Sophie worked as a computer programmer and on weekends she worked as a hostess at a posh restaurant. She had little time to care for herself, and her children were largely cared for by her mother—also a single mom.

Late one Saturday evening, Sophie's mother received a frantic phone call from a coworker at the restaurant. Sophie had suddenly collapsed and was extremely drowsy, but rousable. They had called an ambulance, and she was on her way to the local hospital. Later, additional facts emerged. By the time Sophie reached the hospital in the ambulance, she had lapsed into a deep coma with very heavy breathing. It was the first week of July, and new junior doctors had just begun. They had difficulty finding a vein to start intravenous fluids, and because the emergency department was so crowded, considerable delay occurred in making a precise diagnosis and achieving intravenous entry. Early the next morning, Sophie died.

During the night, the physicians had made a diagnosis of diabetes and treated her appropriately but in vain. Apparently a serious imbalance in her potassium levels coupled with the extensive chemical changes led to cardiac arrest.

In retrospect, her mother told of her daughter's frenetic efforts to earn a living and look after her children, systematically ignoring her own health. In the past year, she had gained an enormous amount of weight and become seriously obese. She had mentioned to her mother about her frequent waking at night to urinate and that she was constantly thirsty. Occasional episodes of dizziness, her mother said, she had ascribed to fatigue and overwork.

Sophie's mother said that Sophie's birth weight was 9 pounds 4 ounces and that she had otherwise been healthy throughout her years. Sophie's maternal grandmother developed diabetes in her 40s and was also obese. One other maternal uncle also had adult-onset diabetes. Both Sophie's children were heavy at birth, each weighing more than 9 pounds, with her requiring a Cesarean section each time.

Sophie's social and socioeconomic situation was and still is a common problem. Worse still was her systematic way of ignoring very important signs of deterioration as reflected by her enormous weight gain, her constant thirst, episodes of dizziness, and frequent waking at night to urinate. The latter three symptoms are the ones that commonly alert the physician to the diagnosis of diabetes. Sophie also chose to ignore her family history of diabetes, which was also unwise. A further sign of likely future diabetes, which she was probably told about, was the birth of both her babies weighing over 9 pounds each. Sophie herself weighed more than 9 pounds, a fact we now know predisposes to future development of diabetes.

In the United States, at least Sophie's rapid deterioration and death is decidedly uncommon, except for undiagnosed and untreated diabetes. Worldwide, diabetes is the fifth leading cause of death, resulting in almost 3 million deaths annually. Unfortunately, as many as 50% of those with Sophie's type of diabetes remain undiagnosed. This is particularly sad since treatment may make a huge difference to the quality of life and long-term survival. For very obese diabetics, surgically reducing the size of the stomach (called bariatric surgery) or by-passing the stomach, may literally banish the diabetes and save lives.

DIABETES

Our bodies maintain a steady level of blood sugar whether we are at rest or on the run. After a meal, blood sugar levels rise and are slowly returned to normal levels within a 1- to 2-hour period. Many genes orchestrate this fine adjustment, preventing blood sugar from rising too high or falling too low. Therein lies the potential problem in that any defect among these many genes may interfere with the regulatory control of blood sugar. Not only is there the potential for one or more gene defects, but also various environmental factors further challenge the system. Exercise, stress, infection, illness, medications, fever, alcohol, diet, pregnancy—to name but a few factors—may all interfere with blood sugar control. Failure of the body's regulatory mechanisms to return blood sugar levels to their normal range result in persistent high blood sugar concentrations, causing diabetes mellitus.

Diagnosis

You may have thought that the diagnosis of diabetes could simply be achieved by determination of a specific level of the blood sugar taken when fasting. In fact, the American Diabetes Association advocates the use of a blood test measuring glycated hemoglobin for diagnosis. This test has the advantage of not requiring fasting and is also preferred for monitoring blood sugar levels. Moreover, higher levels of glycated hemoglobin are associated with coronary artery disease and serve as a warning that should not go unheeded.

Many physicians still use the oral glucose tolerance test, which involves fasting overnight (for 10–14 hours) until a blood sample is taken in the morning and then drinking a very sweet liquid. Blood samples are then drawn for blood sugar measurements at 30- to 60-minute intervals for 3–5 hours. This is called the oral glucose tolerance test (OGTT). The body's response to a sugar load is to primarily secrete insulin, which drives the sugar level back to normal. Failure or a lag of the blood sugar to return to normal at 2 to 5 hours reflects inadequate insulin production (or resistance to insulin), persisting high blood sugar, and hence a diagnosis of diabetes. An abnormal OGTT consists of a fasting glucose level equal to or above 126 mg/dL, and a 2-hour level greater than 200 mg/dL. Before a final diagnosis of diabetes is made, a repeat OGTT is recommended to be sure. The reason for this caution is the realization that multiple factors may affect the blood sugar. For example, a low carbohydrate intake for several days before the OGTT may blunt the body's insulin response. Individuals on certain diets may fall into this category. Coffee or smoking before or even during the test is to be avoided.

Interpretation of the OGTT is complicated and probably unreliable in the face of acute or chronic illness, immobilization, prolonged bed rest, infection, or while taking any one of a number of different medications (including diuretics, certain vitamins, anticonvulsants, steroids, aspirin, and other drugs) . The test should be performed first thing in the morning since the blood glucose levels vary cyclically during the day. Age may need consideration because tolerance to glucose decreases with advancing years. Interpretive levels for the OGTT are different during pregnancy. Hence, a mistaken conclusion could be reached if pregnancy is not mentioned (or recognized) when an OGTT test is done.

An OGTT is recommended for the following reasons:

1. a urine tests positive for sugar;
2. a fasting blood sugar level obtained during a screening test is elevated (*see* discussion below);
3. to identify the diabetes of pregnancy (gestational diabetes);
4. identification of diabetes in individuals without symptoms, but who are either obese or have a strong family history of diabetes;
5. for diagnosis in those with coronary artery disease, other problems with their circulation, eye problems (retinopathy), and those with unexplained symptoms and signs in their lower extremities (neuropathy), including prickling sensations, pain, and weakness; and
6. for diagnosis in those with abnormal blood sugar levels found in the course of surgery, trauma, stress, heart attacks, or while on steroid medications.

The diagnosis of diabetes is usually simply made by the OGTT. However, screening tests for diabetes are usually administered as part of routine annual care. This involves analysis of a fasting blood sugar level, which both the American Diabetes Association and the World Health Organization suggest a level less than 126 mg/dL.

Types of Diabetes

Diabetes is a genetic disorder involving multiple genes (for the most part) interacting with multiple environmental factors. It involves the body's handling (metabolism) of carbohydrates, protein, and fat and is associated with relative or absolute insufficiency of insulin secretion, or the body's tissue resistance to insulin.

Two types of diabetes are recognized, both being characterized by the body's failure to maintain normal levels of blood sugar (glucose). Type 1 diabetes is caused by a virtually complete or near total deficiency of insulin. Type 2 diabetes occurs in a whole range of different disorders, which either cause resistance to insulin, interfere with insulin secretion, or increase glucose production.

While type 1 diabetes begins more often among the young and type 2 occurs among adults, both types may occur at any age. Equally, insulin may be required in either type, earlier or later. Typically, type 1 diabetes begins in childhood and often has an abrupt onset. Immediate insulin treatment is necessary to prevent the rapid development of coma that may lead to death. This type results primarily from destruction of the cells in the pancreas that manufacture insulin. These so-called "beta cells" are progressively destroyed by antibodies (proteins called auto-antibodies) that mistake beta cells as a foreign invader to be destroyed. This auto-immune destruction appears to be due to susceptibility genes on the short arm of chromosome 6 that are linked to the human leukocyte antigen (HLA) blood groups.[1] These beta cell auto-antibodies are present in more than 75% of individuals diagnosed with type 1 diabetes. Hence, it is not the diabetes that is inherited but, rather, the genetic susceptibility to specific environmental factors (most probably viral infections) that lead to antibody formation and destruction of the pancreatic cells.

Much less common is the occurrence of auto-antibodies to other glands that secrete hormones, including the thyroid, adrenal, ovaries, and testes. Affected persons may not only have diabetes but also thyroid disease or other disorders affecting the hormone-secreting glands.

A majority (60%–80%) of those with type 2 diabetes are overweight or obese. In these genetically predisposed individuals, increasing insulin resistance develops, resulting eventually in overt diabetes. Sophie would have been advised that her positive family history for diabetes put her on notice not to become obese. Those who are overweight and who have developed diabetes can often improve or even correct the situation by losing sufficient weight as to return to an overtly nondiabetic state. Exercise increases insulin sensitivity, while a sedentary existence does the opposite and makes insulin resistance worse.

Diabetes may also occur in association with a host of other disorders in which insulin secretion is decreased or where insulin resistance develops. Various medications may precipitate diabetes and include drugs for hypertension, diuretics, estrogen hormones, antidepressants, and others. A long list of genetic syndromes may be complicated by diabetes.

---

1. HLA system refers to cell-surface proteins from genes located on chromosome 6. Among many roles, these proteins are critical in auto-immune diseases, susceptibility to infection, and in organ transplant rejection.

A Common Disorder

Over the past two decades, there has been a veritable explosion in the number of people with diabetes. According to the International Diabetes Federation, by the year 2007, 250 million people had diabetes; the federation estimated that 380 million would be affected by 2025, primarily of type 2, largely due to increasing obesity and less exercise.[2] In the United States, 9% of the population have diabetes. Among those older than age 60 years, the frequency of diabetes exceeds 20%.

Interestingly, Scandinavia has the highest frequency of type 1, while countries along the Pacific Rim (including Japan and China) have a very much lower rate. However, the prevalence of type 2 diabetes has reached epidemic proportions in China. An estimated 92.4 million adults older than age 20 years have diabetes, more than 60% undiagnosed! High rates of diabetes are found among American Indians and Alaskan natives, as well as among African-Americans and Hispanics. However, the highest prevalence of diabetes is found in the Micronesian island of Nauru, where almost 1 in 3 of its 14,000 inhabitants are affected. Highlighting the effect of environment (diet) on those with a genetic susceptibility is the observation that immigrants from low-frequency countries develop much higher rates of diabetes after they settle in developed countries.

The telephone call from Boston left Luisa sinking to the floor in a faint while her husband Pierro, standing close by, caught her in time before she hit the stone floor. They had just heard from the hospital in Boston to which their third child, Alicia, had been admitted the night before. Pierro could only grasp the essential bits of information from the doctor who called. He remembered hearing that Alicia was semi-comatose and that every effort was being made to determine the cause while supportive measures were being taken.

It took Pierro and Luisa a full day to organize their household and to seek permission from their employers to absent themselves from work for an uncertain period while they rushed by air to the United States from their home on the Italian island of Sardinia. They had last seen Alicia 8 months earlier when she had visited during a college break at Christmas. Their shock at the cost of the airfare for an immediate ticket was compounded by

2. In 2010, 285 million people had diabetes worldwide.

the long security lines at the Rome airport. When eventually in-flight, they anxiously recalled Alicia's last visit. Pierro had noticed that she had become "clumsy," which was surprising to him, as she was quite athletic. He also thought that her personality had changed and that she had become "difficult." Luisa thought that Alicia had become anxious and depressed, and both were dismayed to hear that Alicia's academic performance had deteriorated in the last year. She also seemed to have no energy.

On arrival at the hospital, they were stunned to find their daughter Alicia drowsy, confused, and tremulous. They learned that the doctors had obtained a battery of tests and discovered that Alicia had an extremely low serum copper level and a low level of a protein[3] that ferries copper around the body. They also noted abnormal values that reflected disturbed liver function. They concluded that Alicia had a condition called Wilson disease.[4] When it was explained that this was a genetic disorder (autosomal recessive), Pierro was incredulous, insisting that there was no one in the family with any such disorder and that longevity was characteristic for both his and Luisa's families. Moreover, he exclaimed, "My other three children are perfect and that there must be a mistake in the laboratory!" Pierro's angry denial of the diagnosis for Alicia did not help Luisa's desperate anguish.

The next 10 days saw Alicia steadily improve and emerge from her impaired state of consciousness. Pierro returned to Cagliari, his home town in Sardinia. Luisa remained in Boston in the home of a friend while seeing Alicia slowly recover on treatment aimed at removing copper from the body.

Notwithstanding Pierro's refusal to accept the fact that Alicia had a genetic disorder for which he was also a carrier of a culprit gene, Luisa was able by telephone to convince her other three children to each send a blood sample for testing the Wilson disease gene. They were all dismayed when it was discovered that one of the other three children was also a carrier. But more important, their pregnant younger daughter had two copies of the Wilson disease gene mutation and was therefore affected. They were initially bewildered by the fact that she showed no symptoms or signs of this disorder. Subsequent testing of her husband, who had a random 2% risk of

---

3. Ceruloplasmin.
4. Also called hepatolenticular degeneration, and first described in 1912 by Dr. S.A. Kinnier Wilson, a neurologist in England.

being a carrier, in fact showed him to harbor a mutation in the Wilson disease gene. This young couple were counseled immediately and informed they had a 50% risk of having a child with Wilson disease. Also, that pre-natal diagnosis was still available to them even though the pregnancy was already 18 weeks in duration. After careful consideration, they elected not to have prenatal diagnostic studies for this treatable condition.

The appearance of an inherited disorder for the first time in a family is typical for autosomal recessive disorders (see Chapters 6 and 15). While Pierro and Luisa were unaware of any consanguinity, their great-grand-parents came from the same village. There was a strong likelihood that unbeknown to them both, they probably had an ancestor in common. Proof came later when DNA analysis of blood samples drawn from Pierro, Luisa, and Alicia revealed that they both had the same tell-tale mutation[5] in the Wilson disease gene. Pierro and Luisa each carried one copy of this mutation, while Alicia had inherited the mutation from both parents. For each of Luisa's pregnancies they had not known their 25% risks of having a child with Wilson disease. It was expected that there was a two out of three likelihood that each of Alicia's three siblings would be carriers once they were tested. At least one of each of the parents of Pierro and Luisa would also be carriers. Strong recommendations were made for tests to be performed, especially for Alicia's siblings, given that one sister had recently announced her first pregnancy.

The onset of Alicia's symptoms and signs of Wilson disease in her early 20s was not unusual. Her history of having no energy, having personality changes, experiencing problems with coordination (clumsiness), and depression were typical for this disorder.

WILSON DISEASE

For most Western countries, the frequency of Wilson disease is about 1 in 30,000. About 1 in 90 people are carriers of a mutation in this disease gene. However, in Sardinia, China, and Japan, the frequency of Wilson disease approximates 1 in 10,000, and about 1 in 50 people are carriers of a Wilson

---

5. Called ATP7B

disease gene mutation. Carriers are healthy and remain so for life. Routine carrier testing would be recommended for families with consanguinity and for those living in countries where the carrier frequency approximates 1 in 50.

The symptoms and signs of Wilson disease typically involve the nervous system and the liver. Mental health issues are common, and early indicators of this disease include depression, personality changes, neurotic behavior, and, as seen with Alicia, some intellectual deterioration. Frequently tremors, clumsiness, and involuntary movements or muscle rigidity make their appearance and may be noticed by changes in the way a person walks. Liver involvement may be signaled by lack of energy, malaise, jaundice, or severe overwhelming liver failure leading to death. The basic problem in this disorder is the excess deposition of copper in tissues, especially in the liver and specific areas of the brain.[6] Copper that deposits in the cornea of the eye will, in about 50% of cases, be seen as a ring.[7]

Precise diagnosis is achieved by DNA analysis of the Wilson disease gene, this test being the one of choice for carrier detection as well as for determination of the diagnosis in an individual with no symptoms or signs.

Treatment

The primary purpose of treatment is to rid the body of excess copper and should be instituted as early as possible, preferably before any symptoms appear. The two valuable drugs used in this chelation therapy aimed at ridding the body of copper are penicillamine and, where necessary, Trientine. Usually after one or other of these primary drugs have been used, zinc tablets taken daily are added. Zinc interferes with the absorption of copper from the bowel. Affected individuals are advised to restrict their intake of foods containing high concentrations of copper, including liver, brain, chocolate, mushrooms, shellfish, and nuts. Those who fail to respond to treatment develop more serious liver disease or severe nervous system involvement and may have to consider removal of their liver and liver transplantation.

---

6. In the basal ganglia.

7. Called a Kayser-Fleischer ring and mostly seen only by slit lamp examination. Symptoms and signs of this disorder can become apparent as early as age 3 years and even after age 50 years.

Pregnancy

Treatment with penicillamine through pregnancy is recommended because of the risk of sudden and overwhelming liver failure. There is, however, less than a 5% risk of birth defects related to the use of penicillamine. Insufficient data exist about the use of Trientine in pregnancy. Prenatal diagnosis or preimplantation genetic diagnosis is available once mutations are known in both parents. However, this appears thus far to be an uncommon choice, as was the case for Alicia's sister and her husband. They recognized that their child would be born with Wilson disease and would require lifelong treatment. Moreover, it would not be possible to stop treatment because discontinuation may lead to liver failure, which may then not respond to medical treatment.

The decision to continue the pregnancy, while recognizing the requirement for future lifelong treatment, is extraordinarily difficult. Although the psychological and economic burden of taking a medication for life is obvious, the inability to predict complications from penicillamine, which occur in about 25% of cases, is a serious concern. These include intolerance/hypersensitivity, kidney disease, drug-induced lupus erythematosis, oral ulcers, and bone marrow depression. The side effects of penicillamine may be severe enough to force suspension of its use, leading to the need for liver transplantation. In one Italian study, 6 of 23 subjects with Wilson disease had to abandon penicillamine treatment because of side effects. Once again, painful uncertainty will give prospective parents at risk considerable pause in deciding to have a child who would require lifelong treatment. Thankfully, there are not many genetic disorders that have parents face the anguish of uncertainty. Happily, Alicia recovered and remains in reasonably good health on treatment. Her sister is still asymptomatic, on treatment, and has a child who has begun medical therapy.

OBESITY

A WEIGHTY BURDEN

It was a dreary, misty, and rainy day, which began with a distressing consultation. I knew, as Antonio and Connie entered my office, that this was not going to be an uncomplicated visit. Connie entered first, occupying most of the portal with her massive frame that held all of her 350 pounds. Antonio, initially obscured by his morbidly obese wife, entered next and appeared as thin as a rake. Once seated, they held each others' hand tightly and continually. Connie wept throughout the 1-hour consultation.She had much to cry about. She began first recounting her early childhood when she was described as "chubby." In retrospect, she remembered that her mother and all of her four sisters and grandmother were "very heavy women." She knew that some of them had diabetes but did not take insulin. She maintained that for all of her 40 years she had tried not to gain weight. Her efforts had always been in vain.

Some 10 years previously and at a similar weight, she had given birth to their only child, a son named Dominic, who was born with severe spina bifida (see Chapter 23). He had been paralyzed from the waist down, had no control of his bowel or bladder, developed hydrocephalus that required a shunt in his head for decompression, and was mentally retarded. Dominic died before he was 5 years old. Antonio and Connie were devastated to lose the only child they had and whom they had conceived after many years of trying.

This office visit was recommended by their primary care physician, following Connie's surgery for cancer of the inside lining of her uterus (endometrial cancer). The doctor had become concerned about the risk of recurrence of cancer in another organ given the history of colorectal cancer in her mother and breast cancer in one maternal aunt. Connie said that she was weeping because of the loss of her uterus, her cancer, the loss of Dominic, and her uncontrollable weight.

I explained that the cause of her endometrial cancer was uncertain but could be related to her family history. I offered, and she accepted, testing of the four genes involved in causing hereditary nonpolyposis colon cancer, which includes cancers in some other organs (*see* Chapter 8). I stressed the importance of continuing at least annual surveillance with her primary care physician, as well as annual mammography. A colonoscopy had been performed at the time immediately prior to her surgery and no abnormality was found.

Although there was no future possibility of having children, Antonio persisted in asking about the cause of Dominic's spina bifida. Once again, I indicated that the precise cause was unknown but that multiple genes are thought to interact with environmental factors (such as folic acid and diet). I did acknowledge, to a direct question, that obese women had a clearly increased risk of having children with structural birth defects, including spina bifida.

Some weeks later, I was able to at least transmit the happier news that Connie did not have a mutation in any of the four genes that we had sequenced.

Given the serious complications that obesity engendered, I recommended that Connie see a bariatric surgeon with the aim of dramatically reducing her body weight.

A COMMON PROBLEM

Obesity is not a new problem, women having been immortalized as such in stone-aged sculptures.[1] Hippocrates also noted the adverse effects of obesity.[1] However, obesity has become a worldwide scourge, with an estimated 1.6 billion adults (older than age 15 years) being overweight and 400 million being obese

---

1. Haslam D. & Rigby N. (2010) The art of Medicine – A long look at obesity. *Lancet* 376: 85.

(a body mass index [BMI] greater than 30).[2] Connie was morbidly obese with a BMI greater than 40. Current predictions are that there will be 2.3 billion people overweight and more than 700 million obese adults worldwide by 2015. More than one-third of women in the United States are obese. The health implications for such women are startling. There are highly significant increased risks for obese women developing diabetes and/or gestational diabetes, hypertension, clotting disorders potentially resulting in sudden death or strokes, increased Cesarean section rates, and wound infection. Moreover, the infants of obese mothers have a clearly increased risk of difficulties in delivery because of their size associated with an increased risk of death in the period just before, during, and immediately after delivery. Very well-known is the increased risk obese mothers have for bearing children with a whole range of structural birth defects that include spina bifida, heart defects, cleft lip and/or palate, anal abnormalities, hydrocephalus, and limb defects.

COMPLICATIONS

Being overweight or obese (BMI greater than 30) is associated with a diminished life expectancy. Cancer is the cause for many of the obesity-related deaths. One estimate indicates that overweight and obesity are responsible for 14% of all cancer deaths in men and 20% of those in women in the United States. The medical literature now clearly indicates that an increased BMI is associated with an increased rate of multiple and different cancers that include endometrial (uterine), colorectal, and postmenopausal breast cancer. New evidence points to poorer outcomes in obese women with breast cancer. More recent literature also points to an increased risk of other cancers, including those of the esophagus, thyroid, kidneys, gallbladder, pancreas, ovaries, leukemia, and non-Hodgkin's lymphoma. As much as double the risk of multiple myeloma (an immune system cancer) is recognized. The point has been made that excess body weight in adolescence carries an increased risk of colon cancer deaths later in life.

Obese women are at an increased risk of gestational diabetes (discussed in Chapter 23). They also have an increased risk of fetal demise or stillbirth, toxemia of pregnancy, blood clots, pregnancy induced hypertension, labor

---

2. The degree of obesity is measured by the body mass index (BMI), which is calculated as weight (lbs or kg)/height (inches or meters squared) x 703. Overweight is regarded as having a BMI of 25–29.9 and obesity is regarded as having a BMI greater than 30.

induction, cesarian delivery, wound infection, and late-life dementia. The heavier a woman's weight is prior to pregnancy, the more likely she is of having a pregnancy last too long (post-term pregnancy), which in turn is associated with an increased set of complications for the child, including an increased death rate.

HOW DOES IT HAPPEN?

The millions of diet books sold attest to the desire of many overweight people, while reflecting the intractable problem of obesity. Central to the reality of obesity is the fact of excess calorie intake over the number of calories expended. Keep on stuffing a closet and it will become over-full. This analogy has biological underpinnings in the understanding of obesity. It is thought that the number and size of fat cells are established toward the end of pregnancy and in early infancy. This early "programming" of fat cells is tantamount to providing the number and size of closets available to fill later. In experiments with rats whose calorie intake was markedly reduced during suckling, a permanently reduced number of fat cells were found later. The matter, however, is very much more complex than this.

Invariably, it is what we do to our genetic constitution that causes the problem. Obesity results from an excess of body fat, which in turn is directly caused by an excess intake of calories exceeding those used for energy expenditure. While there are a host of different syndromes—genetic and otherwise—that result in obesity, the overwhelming majority of those who become obese have a chronic energy imbalance—they simply and continuously take in more calories than they use. An excess of only 2% of calories per day over energy expenditure results in a weight gain of about 5 lbs. (2.3 kg) in a year. The average American man or woman gains about 20 lbs (9.1 kg) between ages 25 and 55 years. This represents a tiny imbalance between energy intake and expenditure amounting to only 0.3% extra calories ingested.

The complex orchestral arrangements that lead to obesity include the brain, all the hormone-producing glands (such as the pituitary, thyroid, adrenal, insulin-producing cells of the pancreas), the intestines, fat cells, muscles, and the nervous system. Multiple genes and a few dozen hormones and proteins (all the products of individual genes) have been identified thus far, which function as chemical signals to target organs or cells. Such signals are responded to by reciprocal signals in the form of secreted hormones or proteins, which in turn provide feedback responses to the original source as well as to other organs or cells. Hence, there is normally a continuous balanced to-and-fro interplay via signals between all organs involved in responding to food intake and calorie expenditure.

One particular central site with a key role is in the brain (called the hypothalamus). A critical role in the regulation of energy intake and expenditure is exercised by the hypothalamus by control of hunger and satiety, as well as for the regulation of hormone secretion involved in depositing energy stores. There is likely to be "satiety" and "hunger" centers within the hypothalamus. The hypothalamus may signal "hungry" and be aided and abetted by visual cues (walking past a deli) or favorite smells (walking past a bakery), thereby activating the whole system. Fat cells themselves are not inert closets, but secrete products such as the protein leptin (from the *ob* gene), which we know from original experiments in mice influences body weight and energy stores through actions on the brain that regulate food intake and energy expenditure.

Moreover, it appears likely that fat cells in different regions of the body (e.g., the abdomen and the thighs) may not have identical operations. Loss of fat decreases leptin levels, thereby stimulating food intake. An increase in body fat raises leptin levels, reducing food intake. Rare cases with mutations in the leptin gene (making it ineffective) have resulted in morbid obesity. Also, only rarely does a person produce too little leptin, with obesity as a consequence. Obese individuals may also be leptin-resistant. Leptin interacts with brain cells and a whole network of chemical connections with feedback circuit control, ultimately balancing and modulating weight gain. Genetic, environmental, hormonal, psychological, and other factors have the potential to disturb the delicate balance.

Complicating this vast interplay of cell–cell signaling is the recognized effect of programming that begins in the womb and in early infancy. It is thought that the appetite center in the hypothalamus is set in relation to body size early in pregnancy. Pertinent to this view is that males born in the Netherlands, toward the end of World War II (in the winter of 1944–1945) and exposed to famine in the first half of pregnancy, became obese as adults. In contrast, those whose mothers starved during late pregnancy and the first month after birth subsequently remained thin. It is also likely that the number of fat cells is established in late pregnancy and early infancy and that these males may have been born with a permanently smaller number and size of fat cells.

In a study of the children of Pima Indian women with diabetes, a higher prevalence of obesity was found compared with the offspring of non-diabetic mothers, despite similar maternal weights in the two groups. Although obesity can begin at any age, when it becomes apparent in early childhood or adolescence, it tends to be lifelong. Clearly the gene machine that powers the signaling cycle for hunger, satiety, and fat storage is subject to dysregulation at any one of enumerable sites. With few exceptions, the overwhelming number of those who become obese do so primarily because of an excess calorie intake over expenditure. Regardless of where in the chain of signals there is dysfunction, it is the calorie intake that has to be controlled first, while energy expenditure through exercise is increased. Drug control of the appetite center is the dream of every pharmaceutical company. Ultimately it is personal long-range lifelong discipline that will make the difference rather than adherence to one or other misleading dietary fad.

"FAT" GENES

Several genes, when mutated, may cause obesity in humans and animals. However, these single genes account for only 5% to 10% of those with morbid obesity (BMI greater than 40). In these rarer cases where a mutation in a single gene causes morbid obesity, a 50% risk applies to the offspring of the person with that gene alteration.

For the most part, however, many genes are involved in the signaling pathways described above. Thus far, more than 250 locations of such genes in our genomes have been identified. For the overwhelming majority of those with obesity, the interaction of genes and environment is considered to be the basis. Not only are there genetic factors at work, but common experience confirms common cultural, environmental, and dietary factors operating within families. In combined studies covering 2,002 obese children, one or both parents were obese 72% of the time. Mothers were obese more often than fathers. The risk of extreme obesity is about six to eight times higher in families of extremely obese individuals. Moreover, first-degree relatives of individuals who had childhood-onset obesity were twice as likely to be obese compared with relatives who developed obesity as adults. In some 30% of families, both parents of obese children are obese. Up to age 5 years, having two obese parents gives a child a 10-fold increased risk of becoming an obese adult. If the child is obese between ages 10 and 17 years, regardless of parental obesity, there is a 20-fold increased risk of becoming an obese adult. The familial risk of obesity increases with the degree of obesity. Studies of adopted children in Denmark and of twins who were reared apart in Sweden showed that adopted children were more closely related to their own parents than to their adopted parents so far as measures of their body weight chemistry was concerned. Identical twins have similar weights when reared apart, with a concordance rate of about 70% for men and 66% for women. From all these studies, the degree of heritability of the BMI has ranged between 40% and 70%.

There are well-known, but thankfully relatively rare, syndromes associated with obesity,[3] some already obvious through overgrowth at birth and ultimately associated with mental retardation and other features. Technical descriptions of the approximately 30 single-gene syndromes would not be appropriate here. However, if within your family there is an individual with obesity and mental retardation with or without other features, consultation with a clinical geneticist is recommended.

A frequently recognized disorder—the polycystic ovary syndrome—is characterized by obesity, hairiness, infertility, and failure to ovulate. The reason for multiple cysts developing in the ovaries is uncertain. Dominant inheritance with very variable signs even in the same family is common. Other modes of inheritance and similar conditions are known, which therefore require specialist consultation to reach a precise diagnosis. Obese women having in vitro fertilization experience a higher failure rate in achieving a pregnancy than non-obese women.

The consequences of obesity include serious medical problems, frequent psychological difficulties, and invariable changes in behavior. To make matters worse, the observations in a Kent State University study provided strong evidence that chronic obesity was associated with poorer cognitive performance, including memory, word fluency, attention, and visuospatial ability.

MEDICAL CONSEQUENCES

Obesity is second only to smoking as the leading cause of preventable death in the United States. In extremely obese men, the risk of dying is 12 times higher between ages 25 and 34 years compared to men in the general population. Increased death rates among the obese continue throughout life. Cardiovascular disease, hypertension, diabetes, lung problems, and gallstones all occur more frequently among the obese. There is also an increased mortality from cancer, as noted earlier. Even with moderate obesity, there is an increased risk of

---

3. Examples of syndromes include Prader-Willi, Alstrom, Bardet-Biedel, Cohen-Albright hereditary osteodystrophy, and Borjeson-Forssman Lehmann.

hypertension, diabetes, gallstones, kidney stones, and stroke as well as heart disease. Common problems of osteoarthritis, varicose veins, and gout are also more frequent in the obese.

Psychological consequences of obesity are common and reflect the individual's personal feelings to self and to the reaction by others. Negative self-images are commonly reported, some to the point of self-hate. Because of the way they feel about themselves, the very obese often experience anxiety, depression, hostility or guilt. Behavioral consequences of obesity usually result from the effects of excessive weight.

Hence, limited ability to have exercise, shortness of breath, pain in the joints, swelling of the legs, and easy fatigue often lead the obese person to withdraw from social contact. There is also evidence that excessively obese individuals may lose out on employment or be rejected in situations that require interviews.

There are extensive consequences of obesity on women's reproductive systems. Obesity is present about four times more often in women with menstrual disturbances than in those with normal cycles. Failure to ovulate is strongly associated with obesity. Teenage obesity is frequently followed by abnormal menstrual cycles and excessive facial and body hair growth years later. Ample published data show higher rates of infertility among obese women as well as an increased risk of miscarriage. Those obese women who become pregnant have increased risks of hypertension, toxemia of pregnancy, gestational diabetes, and urinary tract infection and more often need Cesarean section.

TREATMENT AND PREVENTION

The treatment of obesity has, to a large extent, been a dismal failure. Some diets actually work—mostly for a short time. The overwhelming majority who begin their efforts at weight loss are almost certainly going to be back at their previous weight in 5 years or even heavier. Regardless of the special diets, behavior modification therapy and various anti-appetite drugs, successful treatment of obesity has proved elusive.

What can work over the long haul is a strict limitation of calorie intake together with a change in the dietary habits of the whole family. Basic to that effort is a drastic reduction in fat intake, which is also good for the entire family. In addition, a persistent alternate-day aerobic exercise of at least 30 minutes with additional exercise on the intervening days is recommended. This approach is not a program but a lifestyle change without end.

Appetite suppressant drugs have had very limited success. The hope is for a drug that effectively interrupts the body's biochemical "obesity pathway." Meanwhile, for the morbidly obese, there is bariatric surgery, which encompasses various techniques such as surgical bypass—which connects the upper intestine to the lower small intestine—or a procedure that reduces stomach volume by a stapling technique. Complications of these procedures are not uncommon and may even lead to death. They are procedures that are mostly offered only to those whose BMI exceeds 30 and are at serious risk of dying from other complications.

Given the intractable nature of obesity and the dismal record of failure in its treatment, avoidance and prevention are critical. The development of a national policy aimed at the strategic prevention of obesity is long overdue. A public health initiative, such as the one that resulted in the decline of tobacco use, is required. Fundamental to any such program would be the plan to increase awareness of the many health consequences of obesity. The educational elements of such a policy should already aim at effective lifetime eating habits from early childhood. We already know that about 60% of overweight 5- to 10-year-old children have at least one associated biochemical or clinical cardiac risk factor such as high blood fat levels, high blood pressure, or raised levels of insulin. Indeed, 25% have two or more of these risk factors. It is these risk factors that become chronic diseases in adults. Close to 80% of the obese suffer from diabetes, high cholesterol levels, high blood pressure, gallbladder disease, osteoarthritis, and, of course, coronary heart disease. In fact, 40% of obese adults have two or more of these problems.

Major policy initiatives aimed at educating the public are necessary since it is clear that physical activity may prevent obesity, lessen the effect of the complications mentioned, reduce the death rate, and have other good effects on health generally.

Because we know that 8 out of 10 overweight children become overweight adults, we should all be ashamed that we allow our school systems to serve such high-fat offerings in their cafeterias. Equally disturbing is the move by an increasing number of school systems not to support physical education programs. We are in the midst of a worldwide scourge that needs urgent attention. Thankfully the direct culprits are not our genes, which simply (and mostly) aid and abet our inability to strike a balance between caloric intake and expenditure.

Antonio and Connie's pain and suffering were largely avoidable. Her colon cancer analysis of the four genes for hereditary nonpolyposis colon cancer proved negative, raising the greater likelihood that her obesity had a causal role in the development of her cancer. Failure to take folic acid supplements for at least the 3 months prior to becoming pregnant and for at least 3 months thereafter removed the 70% opportunity for avoiding spina bifida. Obstetrical ultrasound studies performed prior to 16 weeks of pregnancy may not always detect spina bifida in the presence of maternal morbid obesity. Suboptimal visualization of the fetus because of the mother's enormous fat pad would suggest a detailed ultrasound after 18 weeks of gestation, recognizing, of course, how late in the pregnancy this is.

Obesity is best avoided beginning in infancy. Clearly, no one becomes overweight if they are starved, regardless of any genetic predisposition. Excessive calories and limited exercise make it likely that our common genetic predisposition to become obese is facilitated. We now know from genetic research that the drive to eat and overeat is signaled by powerful biological mechanisms and is not entirely a voluntarily controllable phenomenon. For certain, obesity is not a moral failure but needs to be addressed with the necessary understanding that we are all possessed by various genetic predispositions to environmental factors that could be controlled.

HYPERTENSION

I was moved by the caring and careful manner in which Nadia assisted her mother into my office. Nadia's mother, Mina, had suffered a stroke one year previously and was left with severe weakness on the left side of her body. Fortunately, being right-handed, she had retained her intellectual abilities but did have some problems with speech and swallowing. Nadia's doctor had recommended this consultation in view of the fact that her mother and other relatives had hypertension. Nadia was concerned about transmission of this trait, even though at age 30 years, she had a normal blood pressure.

Nadia's mother, who had lived in India for most of her life, had sought very little medical attention at any time and was, in fact, unaware of her own high blood pressure. Two of her brothers and her late mother apparently had hypertension. One other brother and two other sisters were known not to have hypertension. Nadia's mother was felled by a stroke when she was running for a bus.

Based on what we currently know about developing a disorder because of the interactions of multiple genes and environmental factors, Nadia's probable risk of developing hypertension was likely between 3% and 5%.

Nadia, being a biologist and fully familiar with modes of inheritance, was worried that her family history was consistent with a dominantly inherited type of hypertension. Before responding, I inquired about when her relatives became aware of their hypertension. For two of her uncles, treatment for hypertension had begun around age 50 years.

No other information was available on this point. I also determined that Nadia's mother, then in the United States, had been fully evaluated and no cause had been found for her hypertension.

Because there was no direct test to determine an individual's predisposition to develop hypertension, a reliable statement about Nadia's risk was not possible. I did mention that those who have a strong family history of two or more first-degree relatives with hypertension prior to age 55 years have between two and five times higher likelihood of developing hypertension themselves than someone without such a history. This would represent the common form of hypertension—called essential hypertension—and would result from the action of multiple genes with certain environmental factors, such as salt intake.

FACTORS THAT RAISE BLOOD PRESSURE

The heart and blood vessels (arteries and veins) are essentially a pump with outgoing and returning vessels, which unlike rigid pipes, are affected by the pump pressure, the flow of blood, and the environmental and other factors that influence the tone of the smooth muscles that line these channels. It is indeed this tone in the arteries (called peripheral resistance) that is particularly important in raising the blood pressure. There is an orchestral-like arrangement among all of these factors that functionally harmonize to produce our blood pressure. Factors that change any part of this balanced arrangement have the potential of raising the blood pressure. For example, substances that raise the arterial tone may elevate the blood pressure. These include some anti-inflammatory drugs, some medications for asthma, oral contraceptives, caffeine, nicotine, and cocaine, as well as other illicit drugs.

The blood pressure is recorded by two figures, one (systolic) over the other (diastolic). Blood pressure is recorded by a pressure cuff being placed around the upper arm, inflating the cuff, and then listening with a stethoscope at the site of the brachial artery at the elbow joint just below the cuff. As the cuff is deflated, tapping sounds are first heard, at which level the mercury measurement can be made to assess the systolic reading. When the sounds disappear, the reading made then is the diastolic pressure. The normal systolic blood pressure is 120 or less (expressed as millimeters of mercury) over diastolic pressure of 80 or less.

While descriptions of mild, moderate, and severe hypertension have been used for decades, new advances have made it clear that hypertension is best staged by assessment of the levels of systolic and diastolic pressures. This change has come about because of the realization that the word "mild" has conveyed an idea of unimportance. In fact, about 70% of those with diastolic hypertension, and more than half of the deaths and disability that are attributable to hypertension, have occurred with levels of diastolic blood pressure between 90 and 104. The level of systolic blood pressure is also important, especially since it is a major contributor to complications that occur because of hypertension, which include mortality, coronary heart disease, strokes, heart failure, and kidney failure.

However, there is no absolute threshold where definitive risks become clear. Instead, in adults, there is a continuous, steadily increasing risk for heart disease, stroke, and kidney disease with rising levels of both systolic and diastolic blood pressure. Studies involving about 1 million adults show that risks, small initially, rise slowly and steadily from a beginning blood pressure of 115/75mmHg. It is clear that cardiovascular disease risk doubles for about every 20mmHg increase in systolic and 10mmHg increase in diastolic pressure. Among the elderly, systolic blood pressure and the difference between systolic and diastolic levels (called pulse pressure) are more powerful predictors of heart disease than diastolic blood pressure. The implication is that the larger arteries are more rigid because of atherosclerosis. Certainly, hypertension can accelerate complications of diabetes such as cardiovascular and kidney disease. In turn, the risks of hypertension can be aggravated by the presence of diabetes, high blood fat levels, obesity, and smoking. About 60% of those with hypertension are more than 20% overweight. Some 12% to 16% of hypertensive individuals have familial blood fat abnormalities. Not infrequently, an earlier stage of hypertension can be successfully managed by weight loss, exercise, alcohol reduction, and salt restriction.

A WORLDWIDE PROBLEM

It is a staggering realization that an estimated 972 million adults (about 26.4% of the world's adult population) had hypertension in 2000. This number is expected to increase by as much as 60% and reach 1.56 billion by the year 2025. In the United States, the National Health and Nutrition Examination Survey of Adults reported that 28.7% (about 58.4 million) individuals have hypertension. That is almost 1 in 5 adults with high blood pressure. The prevalence varies among different ethnic groups, led by 33.5% in non-Hispanic Blacks and followed by 28.9% in non-Hispanic Whites and 20.7% in Mexican Americans. Among individuals ages 60 years and older, the prevalence is at least 65.4% and almost certainly rising as a consequence of the epidemic of obesity. Hypertension appears earlier in African-Americans, is often more severe, and consequently results in higher rates of morbidity and death from stroke, heart failure, and terminal kidney disease than seen in Whites. Current estimates point to hypertension as the cause of 6% of adult deaths worldwide.

GENES AND BLOOD PRESSURE

These awesome epidemiological data make simple and direct inheritance highly unlikely. Indeed, close to 95% of all cases of hypertension have been explained as a consequence of the interaction of multiple genes and environmental triggers.

The many genes that control, regulate, or modify blood pressure do so by a very large number of interactive mechanisms. There are a veritable cascade of factors that include control of kidney function, with special reference to the handling of salt, and the kidney's secretion of and response to specific hormones; blood pressure and oxygen supply; the nervous system and secretion of stress hormones, such as adrenaline and other hormones secreted by brain cells (so-called "neurotransmitters"); geometric design of the blood vessels including layout, elasticity, and contractility of the smooth muscles within the wall of these vessels, as well as the size and thickness of the vessel wall and its diameter; the permeability of blood vessels and cells allowing the movement of salt and other molecules (ions) to and fro across cell walls; the structure, power, and function of smooth muscles within the wall of arteries and veins and the multiple growth factors required for the growth and maintenance of these smooth muscles within arterial walls; molecules (such as nitric oxide) released by the internal lining cells of blood vessels that interfere with circulating platelets to cause clotting as well as effectively relax the smooth muscle within the arteries; and associated high levels of circulating insulin, which dilates blood vessels as well as the involvement of multiple other hormones that, in addition to their other actions, may cause dilatation or constriction of blood vessels. Not surprisingly, then, it has been extremely difficult to recognize culprit genes that collectively aid and abet the development of hypertension. Even genome-wide research has had limited success in consistently identifying such genes.

Perhaps the most frequently invoked environmental factor is salt intake. In fact, superb studies have been unable to confirm a <u>consistent</u> relation between dietary salt intake and blood pressure. Researchers in Utah located a gene (called angiotensinogen) that may explain difficulties in the interpretation of the relationship between salt and hypertension. This gene contains at least three common variations, possessing one of which makes a person more prone to hypertension as well as responsive to a low-salt diet.

Very rarely, severe hypertension occurs as a consequence of a defect in a single gene. These rare cases stem from defective genes that cause dysfunction or tumors in the kidneys, adrenal glands, or tissues of the autonomic (involuntary) nervous system.

We do know that a person develops a characteristic blood pressure pattern in infancy that tends to remain for life. So, if your blood pressure is on the high side at one month of age, then it is likely to remain on the high side throughout your life (and, similarly, to stay low if it was low initially). Those who begin with higher levels appear to be more likely to develop essential hypertension in adulthood. Since Blacks tend to start with higher blood pressures, their pressures, not surprisingly, rise faster as they age than do those of Whites. Certainly, the frequency of strokes caused by hypertension is highest among people who, as children, had the highest blood pressures.

Hypertension within families like Nadia's is common. We know that the blood pressures of related individuals have clearly been shown to resemble one another more closely than those of unrelated individuals living in the same house. For example, the blood pressure of parents has been shown to be much more closely related to their natural than to their adopted children. In twin studies, the genetic contribution to the cause of hypertension has been estimated to be between 30% and 60%. Attesting further to likely genetic factors in hypertension is the significant concordance found between identical twins (both affected) compared to non-identical pairs. A study of 1,003 identical and 858 non-identical male veteran twins with hypertension showed concordance of 62% and 48%, respectively.

ASSOCIATED DISORDERS

Unfortunately and not infrequently, a number of unwanted disorders are found in association. Hypertension and high cholesterol and other circulating fats in the bloodstream are often associated with resistance to the body's insulin. As a consequence, insulin levels rise and have the effect of stuffing the body's cells, resulting in obesity—especially abdominal obesity. The elevated insulin levels cause further mischief and interfere not only by enhancing blood clotting but also by affecting the tone of blood vessels. As a consequence, when these players operate in association, a brisk increase in the risks for heart attacks, stroke, diabetes, and death occur. This constellation of disorders is designated as the metabolic syndrome. Once again, multiple genes and environmental factors interacting together are regarded as causal.

GENETICS AND ENVIRONMENTAL CAUSES OF HYPERTENSION

Only about 5% of cases with hypertension have an identifiable cause. The list of genetic disorders that constitute this 5% is extensive, but the conditions are individually unusual or rare.[1] However, it is very important to consider and exclude the so-called secondary causes of hypertension because their discovery may lead to a cure. For example, discovery of a severe narrowing (stenosis) of one kidney artery can be remedied by surgery and the hypertension cured. Another disorder associated with hypertension called obstructive sleep apnea is being increasingly recognized. More than 50% of individuals with this disorder, in which obstruction to the airway occurs during sleep, develop hypertension. The more severe the sleep apnea, the more serious the hypertension. At least 70% of patients with obstructive sleep apnea are obese. Individuals who do not sleep alone frequently have a partner recognize this disorder from their sudden cessation of snoring—they literally stop breathing for a few breaths. Affected individuals rarely recognize the disorder but will frequently complain of daytime sleepiness and fatigue. Weight loss and continuous positive airway pressure given during sleep constitute the cornerstone of treatment. Many people with hypertension are unaware that licorice—for example, in candy or tea—raises the blood pressure. Some herbal medicine may also contain licorice. In fact, licorice ingestion may produce hypertension in a person without a previously elevated blood pressure. The mechanism is likely to be a mutation in a particular gene.[2] Licorice is best avoided or used sparingly for those with

---

1. Includes disorders such as polycystic kidney disease, disorders of the adrenal gland, the tumor called pheochromocytoma, multiple endocrine neoplasia types 2A and 2B, Von Hippel-Lindau disease, and neurofibromatosis type 1.
2. HSD11B2.

high blood pressure.[3] Surprisingly, licorice may also be in chewing tobacco, which therefore should also be avoided, because it causes an elevation of blood pressure. It is especially important to discover any identifiable cause, since conventional antihypertensive treatment is frequently ineffective until the cause is remedied.

The original suggestion that adult blood pressure might be related to fetal growth was based on an English study of individuals born in 1946 and followed for 36 years. Those who had lower birth weights had higher systolic blood pressures. Subsequent studies have confirmed that observation and sharpened the focus to reveal that small-for-gestational-age babies (rather than simply low-birth-weight and premature babies) have increased risks of future hypertension, insulin resistance, type 2 diabetes, and chronic kidney disease. Various factors were, of course, considered in these analyses. Studies concluded that blood pressure was associated with disproportionate growth of the placenta related to fetal size, indicating undernutrition of the fetus. Maternal protein malnutrition during pregnancy can result in major changes in the fetal kidney hormones (renin; angiotensin) that influence blood pressure. Animal experiments support the hypothesis that undernutrition in the mother leads to persistent elevation of blood pressure in the offspring. A 1999 U.S. National Institutes of Health prospective analysis of subjects in the Danish Perinatal Study concluded that 11.3% of pregnant women who were small for gestational age at birth developed hypertension, compared to 7.2% who weren't small for gestational age.

Some other curious observations have been made in the context of fetal development. Fingerprint patterns (whorls and loops) have also been related to subsequent blood pressure levels. Fingerprints are established between the 13th and 19th week of pregnancy. Apparently low-birth-weight babies tend to have whorls more often as a result of swollen finger pads in early fetal development. A number of studies have concluded that more people with a whorl on one or more fingers have raised blood pressure in adult life compared with those without whorls. Further, babies who are short at birth in relation to their

---

3. Heraclitus of Ephesus, the pre-Socratic philosopher of the fifth century B.C. died at age 60 years, following his decision to withdraw to the desert and eat only herbs and roots. C. Fiore and colleagues at the University of Padua in Italy have hypothesized that Heraclitus became ill from consuming an excess of the licorice root. They pointed out that the prolonged intake of licorice may have led to salt and water retention, causing severe hypertension and edema, resulting in his death.

Table 28.1 Steps You Can Take (Besides Prescribed Medications) to Reduce Your Blood Pressure

Alcohol	Two or less drinks/day (2 glasses of wine, 2 ounces of liquor, or 24 ounces of beer); total abstinence if hypertension still uncontrolled
Obesity	Lose weight by cutting calories and exercising
Saturated fat	Total fat should be less than 30% of all calories; saturated fat should be less than 10% of total calories; no more than 100 milligrams of cholesterol per day.
Smoking	Stop smoking
Exercise	Regular progressive aerobic exercise; avoid weight-lifting
Salt	Avoid very salty foods and reduce salt intake
Potassium	Eat a potassium-rich diet (high in vegetables, fruits), low-fat dietary products
Licorice	Avoid licorice candy, tea, chewing tobacco, etc.
Blood pressure	Check annually or as recommended by your physician
Medication compliance	Do not stop your hypertension medication

head size generally have narrow palms, whereas adults whose hands are long in relation to their breadth have raised blood pressure.

Hypertension is not a disease but rather a dysfunction in normal body processes that increase the likelihood of cardiovascular complications or stroke. The Joint National Committee on Detection, Evaluation, and Treatment of High Blood Pressure recommend that blood pressure be measured every 2 years if the diastolic pressure has been below 85 and the systolic blood pressure has been below 130. Annual measurements are necessary if the diastolic pressure has been between 85 and 90 or the systolic blood pressure has been between 130 and 139. Obviously those with higher blood pressures require much more frequent measurements, as well as care. Although hypertension is rarely cured, it is almost invariably successfully treated. In combination with antihypertensive drug therapy, certain lifestyle modifications are extremely important (*see* Table 28.1).

For the most part, low blood pressure in an otherwise healthy person probably reflects, just as in high blood pressure, the interacting effects of multiple genes and certain environmental factors. However, while seeking genes that cause high blood pressure, Dr. Clinton Baldwin and colleagues at our Center for Human Genetics at Boston University School of Medicine discovered the location of a single gene on chromosome 18 that causes low blood pressure (hypotension[4]), which segregated within a large family. Those who had low blood pressure all had the same genetic makeup (haplotype) for what apparently is a dominantly inherited condition in that family. Subsequent identification of this mitochondrial gene for hypotension will shed further light on the biochemical pathways regulating blood pressure. Variations in a number of different genes involved in the body's handling of salt may predispose to hypertension or low blood pressure. One such gene,[5] for example, may also increase sensitivity to the commonly used thiazide diuretics for the treatment of hypertension.

TREATMENT

Treatment of hypertension is usually successful and often dramatically so. The importance of early and effective treatment cannot be overemphasized. By having your blood pressure checked on the schedule discussed, you will best secure your health and even save your life. This is especially so since hypertension is a key cause of strokes and a major contributor to heart attacks, as well as heart failure. The prime purpose of treatment and control is to prevent or limit damage to key organs (heart, kidneys, and brain) rather than trying to remedy or reverse the largely irreversible changes. There are still a remarkable number of individuals (up to 50%) who are unaware that they have hypertension. Even more startling is that only about 50% of people who know they are hypertensive pay sufficient attention to remain consistently controlled. Be sure you are in neither of these two groups.

Blood pressure is invariably higher when taken in the doctor's office than at home. This well-known "white-coat hypertension" is due to arousal of the sympathetic nervous system, which also increases the heart rate when anxious or frightened or makes us sweat in those situations. Similarly, very large studies have shown that framing the information about hypertension in a negative

---

4. DeStefano A, Baldwin C, Burzstyn M, Gavras I, Handy D, Joost O, Martel T, Nicolaou M, Schwartz F, Streeten D, Farrer L, & Gavras H (1998) Maternal component in the familial aggregation of hypertension. *Am. J. Hum. Genet* 63:1425–1430.
5. NEDD4L.

way induces adverse psychological consequences such as absenteeism and marital strife. The important message beyond "labeling" is that hypertension is readily controllable, and all adults with normal blood pressure should have it checked at least every 2 years. Early detection and treatment provides reassurance for a long life.

FREQUENTLY ASKED QUESTIONS

1. **I am 40 years old and with my wife have two children. I am concerned about my risk of developing Alzheimer's disease[1] since my father was diagnosed with this disorder at the age of 65 years.**

Alzheimer's disease (AD) is characterized by memory loss, uncharacteristic forgetfulness, misplacement of items, and inability to remember conversations or newly learned information. Memory may not, however, be impaired for complex material from the past, which may be recalled with great clarity. Fortunately, only about 10% of all cases of AD are directly inherited and transmitted via a single gene mutation. Dominant inheritance accounts for these early onset cases that have appeared in individuals as young as 25 years of age, but more commonly in the mid-40s. This clearly genetic form of AD involves a mutation in any one of four different genes,[2] and the alpha-2 macroglobulin gene. Within the APOE gene, there are three common structural variations (called polymorphisms) termed E2, E3, and E4. The E4 polymorphism occurs in about 14% of Whites but in about 40% of those who develop AD. For individuals who receive the E4 variation from both parents, the onset of AD was earlier than in those who received only a single copy, and the risk of developing AD was about 15 times greater. This increased risk translates into about a 95% likelihood of AD by the age of 80 years.

Individuals with the E4 variation have other risks as well. When the E4 polymorphism has been found among individuals with head injury, brain hemorrhage, and those having cardiac bypass surgery, all had a relatively worse outcome. Moreover, there is evidence that the combination of a history of head injury and the possession of the E4 variation increases the risk of future AD 10-fold. Certainly, it would be judicious not to take up boxing if you possess the E4 polymorphism.

Individuals who have a single E4 polymorphism have an increased risk of developing AD in their lifetimes, that risk approximating 20%. Those who have inherited two E4

---

1. Named after the German psychiatrist Alois Alzheimer, who first described the case of a 51-year-old woman with dementia in 1906.

2. These genes are *APP, APOE, Presenilin-1*, and *Presenilin-2*. The *presenilin-1* gene has been highly conserved through evolution, and a gene corresponding in structure has also been found in the simple worm (*C. Elegans; see* footnote in Chapter 9) and the fruit fly.

polymorphisms have about a 30% risk. Even in the absence of the APOE-4 variation, African-Americans up to age 90 years are four times more likely than Whites to develop AD. Hispanics even without the APOE-4 variation have double the risk. Four other susceptibility genes that increase the likelihood of developing Alzheimer's disease have been identified, and more are likely to be recognized as research continues. Identical twins more frequently develop AD but not 100% of the time, indicating other gene and environmental factors that must play a role.

Although the E4 polymorphism is a recognizable risk factor in more than half of all AD cases, 70% to 80% of individuals with this variation will develop AD. Genetic testing, therefore, for a condition for which there is no definitive treatment is not recommended. There is also little wisdom in getting to "know the future", but considerable sorrow that can be anticipated. Studies have shown that memory decline tends to begin earlier in those with the E4 variation than in those without this feature. Moreover, physical inactivity appears to be a risk factor for cognitive decline in those with the E4 polymorphism. Each of us has an overall lifetime risk of developing dementia that approximates 10%-12%. In your case, with one parent affected, the usual risk communicated is somewhere between 15%-25%.

Enormous research efforts are underway and there is good reason to hope that advances in genetic research will result in meaningful treatment and opportunities for prevention. Meanwhile, it would be judicious to bank the DNA of your father in the event the anticipated new advances will enable a more precise diagnosis that could guide preventative steps for you, if necessary.

Mutations in any one of the three genes (*APP, Presenilin-1, and Presenilin-2*) are likely to result in early onset Alzheimer's disease. However, current estimates indicate that some 400 genes at least are involved that may play a role in disease causation. Very significant associations were more recently noted for three additional genes.[3]

Incidentally, there have been studies that measured individuals' purpose in life. Perhaps, not unexpectedly, those with a greater purpose in life, had a reduced risk of Alzheimer's disease or of developing mild cognitive impairment. Setting goals and deriving meaning from life's experiences may be truly beneficial.

2. Is Parkinson's disease inherited?

Fortunately, Parkinson's disease[4] appears to occur sporadically, with about 1 in 800 individuals affected without relation to race. The exception is early onset Parkinson's disease, which is inherited as a recessive disorder and characterized by onset before age 40 years. About 10% of people with this disease are younger than age 45 years. Parkinson's disease is the second most common degenerative disease of the brain after

---

3. The three genes are known as *CLU, PICALM,* and *Crl*.
4. Named after an English pharmacist James Parkinson, who described this condition in "an essay on the Shaking Palsy" in 1817.

Alzheimer's disease. About 1 in 50 people develop this disorder after age 75 years. Typical features include tremor and the ability to only move slowly with rigidity.

Curiously, people who have never smoked are twice as likely to develop Parkinson's disease, while those who don't take much or any caffeine have a significantly greater risk. A history of having had the dreaded skin cancer melanoma is known to be associated with an increased risk of later developing Parkinson's disease. Moreover, individuals with red hair and others with blond hair have increased risks of developing Parkinson's disease compared to those with black or brown hair. Various other environmental risk factors have been reported, but the associations have been weak. The increased risk for individuals who carry a gene mutation for Gaucher disease was discussed in Chapter 25.

Needless to say, genome-wide association studies have already revealed eleven susceptibility genes that predispose to the development of Parkinson's disease.

The most frequently mutated gene (*LRRK2*) causes a dominantly inherited form of Parkinson's disease and is the most common genetic cause of this disorder recognized thus far. Mutations in this gene, especially in familial cases, are especially common among Portuguese, Ashkenazi Jewish, and North African Arab ancestries.

3. My sister has Restless Legs Syndrome. Is it genetic?

This is a common neurological disorder characterized by intense restlessness with an unpleasant prickling sensation in the legs. Constant moving of the legs begins at rest and tends to be worse at night.

More than 50% of cases have a family history of Restless Leg Syndrome, which is thought to be transmitted as an autosomal dominant disorder. Although a dominant form of inheritance may exist in some cases, at least six genes have been identified that suggest this disorder is due to an inherited susceptibility conveyed by multiple genes.

4. My younger sister, now 25 years old, was recently diagnosed with multiple sclerosis. Is this a genetic condition, and am I at risk?

Multiple sclerosis (MS) is a demyelinating disorder in which the ensheathing insulating fatty material around nerves and nerve fibers undergo destruction, resulting in a whole range of neurological problems. The best evidence indicates that MS occurs as a consequence of the interaction of susceptibility genes and one or more environmental triggers. At present, no one knows for certain whether viruses, other infectious agents, or some other factor are the root cause of this disabling disorder. Evidence that there is at least a significant genetic basis to MS is reflected in this disorder being linked to genes in the human leukocyte antigen (HLA) locus (*see* Chapter 26) and elsewhere in the genome. Linkage to HLA genes indicates a key role for auto-immune mechanisms in MS.

Important Canadian studies have pointed to a complex gene, environment, and gender interaction. First, women appear to be twice as likely as men to develop MS, and further, the MS risk is twice as high if half-siblings had a mother in common rather than a father in common. The Canadian studies also revealed that the rate of MS in twins is higher than that for non-twin siblings, implying some effect related to either birth or pregnancy. Also, the concordance is 30% for MS in identical twins (both affected) and occurs almost entirely in female pairs only! In contrast, the concordance in non-identical twins is only 2%, which is the same for siblings. For a disorder with a frequency of about 1 in 500 to 1 in 1,000 individuals in a lifetime, precise understanding of the cause(s) remains illusive. Notwithstanding this quandary, the risks you and others have is based on current data and reflected in the table.

Incidentally, in a study of 7,600 pregnancies in women with MS, the risk of Cesarean delivery was increased 30% and the risk of fetal growth restriction was increased by 70% compared with women without MS. Generally, however, pregnancy and breast feeding has a beneficial effect on MS.

The Risks of Developing Multiple Sclerosis

If this Relative has Multiple Sclerosis	Then the Risk (_in Percent_) of Developing Multiple Sclerosis is:
No family history of MS	0.2 for a child
One adopted sibling	0.2 for an adopted sibling
One step-sibling	0.2 for a step-sibling
One parent	2.7 for each offspring
Both parents	30.5 for each offspring
One sibling	3.1 for another sibling
One sibling (and parents are related— e.g. uncle–niece union)	9.0 for another sibling
One maternal half-sibling	2.4 for another maternal half-sibling
One paternal half-sibling	1.3 for another paternal half-sibling
One of identical twins (female)	34.0 for the other twin
One of identical twins (male)	6.5 for the other twin
One of non-identical twins	5.4 for the other twin

Personal communication from Dr. Dessa Sadovnick, University of British Columbia Hospital, Vancouver, B.C., Canada.

5. **I had great difficulty learning to read in school and they told me I had dyslexia. My son has attention deficit hyperactivity disorder (ADHD), but I did not. Is there any relation between these two conditions, and could I have transmitted his ADHD to him without having that condition myself?**

A specific reading disability in someone of normal intelligence is called dyslexia and reflects an unexpected difficulty in learning to read and/or spell in an otherwise healthy child. A typical estimate is that dyslexia occurs in 5% to 10% of children in the third grade or beyond. Males are more frequently involved but not to the extent originally believed. Both ADHD and dyslexia each have an incidence of 5% to 10% in school-age populations. Considerable overlap in these conditions is reflected by the fact that between 15% and 35% of children with dyslexia are also diagnosed with ADHD, while 25% to 40% of children with ADHD also have dyslexia. Indeed, speech, language, and learning disabilities including ADHD are all intertwined. Multiple genes are indisputably involved with great variation in inheritance patterns. Therefore, there is no great reliability in predicting risks of transmission for any one form of these impairments. In some families, there appear to be risks that approximate 50% for having a second affected son and about 28% for having a second daughter. In some families, the original risk may approximate 50% for having either an affected son or daughter. There is no definitive genetic test for any of these related learning disorders.

6. **I used to stutter as a child, but with some therapy my speech disorder slowly melted away before puberty. Is this a genetic disorder, and will my children inherit stuttering from me?**

Family histories of stuttering are well-known, but the precise pattern of inheritance is yet to be elucidated. The best evidence, thus far, is that multiple genes are likely to be involved that endow a susceptibility to develop this speech impediment. Different causes are also likely, as exemplified by one remarkable study of a Pakistani family in which a single gene with large effect was recognized. However, less than 5% of cases are likely to be related to that particular gene.

At present there is no reliable genetic counseling that can provide a satisfactory and scientifically based risk assessment with reference to future children. It is not particularly useful to know that your risks are increased but not currently quantifiable.

Boys are about twice as likely to stutter compared with girls at the preschool stage. At about age 9 years, boys are about four times more likely than girls to have a stutter. Among biologically related families, the frequency of stuttering is increased. Identical twins are more often concordant compared to non-identical twins. The frequency of stuttering upon entry to high school is about 1 in 100, which is the figure for adults.

7. **In my teens, I constantly had episodes of diarrhea that my doctor initially thought might be caused by stress—more especially since my mother had a diagnosis of ulcerative colitis. Later, they changed her diagnosis to Crohn's disease. In my early 20s, I had a biopsy of my small intestine, which they said was withered (atrophied) and which led to a diagnosis of celiac disease. Are these disorders related, and can they be inherited?**

Celiac disease is caused by the body's immune response to dietary gluten in individuals who are genetically susceptible. Most signs develop in early childhood or closer to middle age. Eating foods that contain gluten (derived from wheat, barley, and rye cereals) results in abnormalities of absorption in the small intestine. Typically there is diarrhea, weight loss, weakness, and even anemia. However, early diagnosis will interdict the development of some of these symptoms and signs. Blood tests that demonstrate auto-antibodies to a component of gluten, called gliaden, also assist in the diagnosis, which is really made by intestinal biopsy. Fortunately, treatment with a gluten-free diet usually leads to complete remission of symptoms and signs. About 1 in 100 people have celiac disease. Unfortunately, the majority of affected individuals remain undiagnosed.

Women with celiac disease have an eight to ninefold higher risk of recurrent miscarriage, than women without this disorder. Celiac disease is also about 4 times more frequent in infertile women than in the population-at-large.

Concordance of celiac disease between identical twins is strikingly high (at 75% compared with non-identical twins at 11%). Celiac disease occurs in 8% to 12% of siblings of diagnosed individuals.

Among those with celiac disease of European ancestry, close to 90% have involvement of a very specific region of involvement in the cluster of HLA genes (*see* Chapter 26). There are, however, at least 27 other genes not involved in the HLA cluster that together predispose to the development of celiac disease. Celiac disease occurs in up to 15% of children with type 1 insulin-dependent diabetes mellitus and in about 6% of adults with this form of diabetes. The reason is the shared and common mechanism involving genes in the HLA cluster and probably other genes elsewhere.

Crohn's disease[5] and ulcerative colitis represent the most common chronic inflammatory disorders and result from the intestine being the battleground between antibodies mounted by the immune system and some mostly unrecognized environmental factors. Susceptibility genes, shared in part by both these disorders, predispose an individual to one or other of these inflammatory disorders. A few dozen genes and gene locations have been identified in addition to the very well-established association in the large cluster of 200 genes in the HLA region (*see* Chapter 26). Both Crohn's disease and ulcerative colitis have HLA associations in common, but clearly multiple other genes are also involved in the predisposition to develop these chronic intestinal disorders. A positive family history of inflammatory bowel disease is found in 5% to 10% of affected individuals. Siblings or children of affected family members have a 10- to 15-fold increased risk of developing either of these disorders, but more especially Crohn's disease. Identical twins are concordant for Crohn's disease in 35% of cases compared with 7% for non-identical twins. For ulcerative colitis, 11% are concordant compared with 3% who are not. That clearly shows a significant genetic basis for these disorders.

From the extensive genome studies done thus far, there is recognizable overlap between these three disorders.

8. **My mother's brother and his wife have twin boys (my first cousins) who both exhibit facial tics mostly associated with a movement of the neck and head while they simultaneously emit a squeaky high-pitched sound. Because they are**

---

5. Named for Dr. B. B. Crohn who in 1932 with colleagues described this disorder.

identical twins, I have begun to be concerned that there is a genetic disorder in the family. Is that the case?

The condition you describe is almost certainly the Gilles-de-la-Tourette syndrome.[6] The main components of this syndrome variably include socially inappropriate behavior (such as sudden involuntary exclamations of obscene words or derogatory remarks (called coprolalia), sudden motor tics (such as sudden uncontrolled movement of a limb or twisting motion of the neck and head), or simple tics (such as shrugging of the shoulders, twitching of the eyes or facial grimaces, or compulsive behaviors or touching themselves). Estimates are that between 1 and 10 children per thousand have this condition.

There are clearly established increased familial histories that make this one of the most heritable childhood-onset neuropsychiatric disorders. Identical twins are concordant in 77% to 100% of cases, whereas non-identical twins are concordant only in about 23% of cases. Notwithstanding the clear familial nature of this disorder, the mode of inheritance remains to be established. It is already clear that the basis of this disorder rests in a number of susceptibility genes. Moreover, there is also an association with obsessive-compulsive disorder, and it is thought that there may be a common underlying susceptibility to these chronic conditions. In a few families, there also appears to be a familial connection between Tourette syndrome, obsessive-compulsive disorder and ADHD. Tourette family studies show a 10- to 100-fold increase in the rates of this syndrome in first-degree relatives, compared to rates in the population at large.

Although the mode of inheritance of the Tourette syndrome is clearly complex and remains to be clarified, recent data show that close to 10% of individuals affected have copy number variants (explained in Chapter 5), including deletions and duplications the same as or similar to those observed in schizophrenia and autism (*see* Chapter 19).

9. **My mother tells me that when I was a toddler I had two episodes of high fever associated with ear infection and at both times had a seizure. Now that I am 24 years old, am I at risk of developing epilepsy and of having children subject to convulsions?**

Seizures in association with high fever (called febrile convulsions) occur mostly in infants and children prior to age 7 years and almost invariably do not indicate an acute illness of the nervous system. In the absence of any family history of seizures (with or without fever), there is probably no increased likelihood—or at most a slightly higher possibility—of developing epilepsy later. Febrile convulsions are the most common form of seizures in childhood, occurring in about 1 in 20 children. A family history of febrile seizures is noted in about 7% of individuals who have such convulsions.

---

6. Named for Georges Gilles de la Tourette, a French neurologist, who described this disorder in 1885.

The likelihood of seizures is increased if a parent was similarly affected, with figures that range between 12% and 25%. For non-identical twins, the concordance rate ranges between 14% and 18%, whereas for identical twins the rates reported range between 31% and 70%.

Despite remarkable advances in genetic biotechnology, more than half of all cases with epilepsy remain, with cause(s) unknown. On average, about 1 in 155 people have some form of epilepsy. There are many forms of seizures besides the jerking and twitching of the limbs and body with loss of consciousness (called grand mal epilepsy). For example, there are absence seizures (a sudden staring into space or glazing over of the eyes that may only be momentary).[7] Some may experience auditory or visual symptoms. Of course, the vast majority of these disorders do not occur following brain injury, alcohol, drugs, or other acquired illnesses.

In recent years, discovery of more than 15 different genes and their associated mutations have facilitated the recognition of specific epilepsy syndromes in some families. For the most part, however, epilepsies resulting from a single gene mutation remain clearly in the minority.

10. **I am 51 years old and extremely worried about my mother, now 71, who is gradually losing her eyesight. A diagnosis of age-related macular degeneration (AMD) has been made, and her primary care physician told her to prepare for becoming blind. Is there no meaningful treatment?**

Age-related macular degeneration is in fact the third-leading cause of blindness worldwide. Given that this disorder largely affects older individuals, the number affected is likely to double over the next one or two decades. Age-related macular degeneration leads to progressive and irreversible loss of central vision, affecting the critically sensitive area of the eye called the macula, which is part of the back of the eye called the retina. As a consequence, a profound disruption of daily living occurs, with affected individuals being unable to read their mail, pay their bills, drive, or shop for their groceries.

The cause for this older onset disorder is regarded as multifactorial, involving a genetic predisposition and environmental factors. Two triggering factors include smoking and obesity. A complex process within the retina causes structural and biochemical changes that result in the growth of new blood vessels, which in turn damages the macula, leading to vision loss and blindness.

Most recently, new therapeutic interventions have been developed that not only stop the disease progression but also may reverse vision loss and restore considerable visual acuity, thereby allowing those affected to lead a more normal life. Highly significant

---

7. Curiously, even in mice, there are seizure types whose names describe the manifestations and include stargazer, tottering, and lethargic. All result from specific gene mutations.

benefits have been achieved by the use of newly developed agents[8] that have to be injected into the rear cavity of the eye. Thus far, it appears that the risks of serious side effects are extremely low. More experience and a longer follow-up time are still necessary, but there is now great promise afforded by this new approach. The earlier the diagnosis of AMD is made, the sooner treatment can begin. Your mother should make haste and seek an urgent appointment with an ophthalmologist.

---

8. Two of these agents that may reverse the new blood vessel formation are RANIBIZUMAB and BEVACIZUMAB.

APPENDIX 1

Cancer Susceptibility Syndromes[1] for which Preimplantation Genetic Diagnosis have been Performed[2]

Ataxia telangiectasia	*Strong predisposition to leukemia and lymphoma*
Breast/ovarian cancer	
Basal cell nevus syndrome (Gorlin)	Skin and brain cancer (medulloblastoma)
Fanconi anemia	Leukemia risk
Familial adenomatous polyposis	Colon and liver cancer
Familial posterior fossa brain tumor	Also highly malignant Rhabdoid and teratoid tumors
Hereditary non-polyposis colon cancer	Cancers of uterus, ovary, kidney, ureter, pancreas, stomach, intestine, bile duct
Li-Fraumeni syndrome	Cancers of bone, breast, brain, adrenal, and leukemia
Multiple endocrine neoplasia— Type 2A	Medullary thyroid cancer, pheochromocytoma
Neurofibromatosis type I	Tumors of nerve sheaths, brain, optic nerve; leukemia
Neurofibromatosis type 2	Tumors of inner ear (schwannomas), spinal cord, brain, and skin
Retinoblastoma	Cancers of eye, bone, skin (melanoma)
Tuberous sclerosis complex	Tumors of kidney, brain
Von Hippel-Lindau disease	Cancers of brain, kidneys, eye; pheochromocytoma

[1] Other birth defects may be present in some syndromes.

[2] Prenatal diagnosis by CVS or amniocentesis is also available.

APPENDIX 2

Selected Single-Gene Disorders with Germline Mosaicism

Disorder	Inheritance
Achondrogenesis type II	AR
Achondroplasia	AD
Adrenoleukodystrophy	X-L rec
Albright hereditary osteodystrophy	AD
a-Thalassemia mental retardation syndrome	X-L
Amyloid polyneuropathy	AD
Aniridia	AD
Apert syndrome	AD
Becker muscular dystrophy	X-L rec
Cantu syndrome	AD
Central hypoventilation syndrome	AD
Cerebellar ataxia with progressive macular dystrophy (SCA7)	AD
Charcot–Marie–Tooth disease type 1B	AD
Coffin–Lowry syndrome	X-L dom
Congenital contractural arachnodactyly	AD
Conradi–Hunnermann–Happle syndrome	X-L dom
Cowden disease	AD
Danon disease (lysosome-associated membrane protein-2 deficiency)	X-L rec
Dejerine–Sottas syndrome (HNSN III) with stomatocytosis	AD
Duchenne muscular dystrophy	X-L rec
Dyskeratosis congenita	X-L
EEC syndrome (ectrodactyly, ectodermal dysplasia, orofacial clefts)	AD
Epidermolysis bullosa simplex	AR
Fabry disease	AR
Facioscapulohumeral muscular dystrophy	AD
Factor X deficiency	AR
Familial focal segmental glomerulosclerosis	AD
Familial hypertrophic cardiomyopathy	AD

Disorder	Inheritance
Fibrodysplasia ossificans progressiva	AD
Fragile X syndrome (deletion-type)	X-L
Hemophilia B	X-L rec
Herlitz junctional epidermolysis bullosa	A rec
Holt–Oram syndrome	AD
Hunter syndrome	X-L rec
Incontinentia pigmenti	X-L dom
Karsch–Neugebauer syndrome	AD
Lesch-Nyhan syndrome	X-L rec
Lissencephaly (males); "subcortical band heterotopia" (almost all females)	X-L rec
Multiple endocrine neoplasia I	AD
Myotubular myopathy	X-L rec
Neurofibromatosis type 1	AD
Neurofibromatosis type 2	AD
Oculocerebrorenal syndrome of Lowe	X-L
Ornithine transcarbamylase deficiency	X-L rec
Osteocraniostenosis	AD
Osteogenesis imperfecta	AD
Otopalatodigital syndrome	X-L dom
Pseudoachondroplasia	AD
Severe combined immunodeficiency disease	X-L rec
Spondyloepimetaphyseal dysplasia	AD
Renal-coloboma syndrome	AD
Retinoblastoma	AD
Rett syndrome	X-L dom
Tuberous sclerosis	AD
Von Hippel–Lindau disease	AD
Von Willebrand disease (type 2b)	X-L rec
Waardenburg syndrome	AD
Wiskott–Aldrich syndrome	X-L rec

AD=autosomal dominant; AR=autosomal recessive; X-L rec=X-linked recessive; X-L dom=X-linked dominant.

APPENDIX 3

Genetic Diseases in which Dynamic Mutations with Triplet Repeat Expansions do Occur

---

Dentatorubral pallidoluysian atrophy
Fragile X syndrome
Fragile XE syndrome
Friedreich ataxia
Huntington disease
Kennedy disease (spinal bulbar
muscular atrophy)
Myotonic dystrophy type 1
Myotonic dystrophy type 2
Spinocerebellar ataxia type 1
Spinocerebellar ataxia type 2
Spinocerebellar ataxia type 3 (Machado–Joseph disease)
Spinocerebellar ataxia type 6
Spinocerebellar ataxia type 7
Spinocerebellar ataxia type 8
Spinocerebellar ataxia type 10
Spinocerebellar ataxia type 12
Spinocerebellar ataxia type 17[1]

---

[1] There are at least 10 other types of spinocerebellar ataxia caused mainly by gene mutations without triplet repeat expansions. The common features are unsteadiness and lack of balance. Onset ages vary as do the associated symptoms and nervous system signs (e.g., spasmodic cough, tremor, cognitive impairment).

APPENDIX 4

Selected Genetic Disorders with Anticipation or Suspected Anticipation

---

Disorders with anticipation

All disorders with triplet repeats (exception: Friedreich ataxia) listed in Appendix 3.

Disorders with suspected anticipation

Adult-onset idiopathic dystonia
Autosomal dominant acute myelogenous leukemia
Autosomal dominant familial spastic paraplegia
Autosomal dominant polycystic kidney disease (PKD1)
Autosomal dominant rolandic epilepsy
Behçet syndrome
Bipolar affective disorder
Charcot-Marie-Tooth disease
Crohn disease
Dyskeratosis congenita
Facioscapulohumeral muscular dystrophy
Familial adenomatous polyposis
Familial amyloid polyneuropathy
Familial breast cancer
Familial chronic myeloproliferative disorders
Familial intracranial aneurysms
Familial pancreatic cancer
Familial paraganglioma
Familial Parkinson's disease
Familial primary pulmonary hypertension
Familial rheumatoid arthritis
Graves' disease

Disorders with suspected anticipation (Continued)

Hereditary nonpolyposis colorectal cancer
Hodgkin's and non-Hodgkin's lymphoma
Holt–Oram syndrome
Lattice corneal dystrophy type I (LCDI)
Li-Fraumeni syndrome
Meniere disease
Obsessive-compulsive spectrum disorders
Oculodentodigital syndrome
Paroxysmal kinesigenic dyskinesia (PKD)
Restless Legs Syndrome
Schizophrenia
Total anomalous pulmonary venous return
Unipolar affective disorder

APPENDIX 5

International Huntington Association and the World Federation of Neurology research Group on Huntington's Chorea

Guidelines for the Molecular Genetics Predictive Test in Huntington Disease

Excerpted and modified from the *Journal of Medical Genetics* 1994; 31:555. The complete guidelines, recommendations, and commentary are available online and should be read by not only those providing genetic counseling but also individuals planning or considering predictive testing. The key recommendations are as follows:

- All persons who may wish to take the test should be given up to date, relevant information to make an informed voluntary decision.

- The decision to take the test is the sole choice of the person concerned. No requests from third parties, be they family or otherwise, shall be considered.

- The test is only available to persons who have reached the age of majority (according to the laws of the respective countries).

- Each participant should be able to take the test independently of his/her financial situation.

- Persons should not be discriminated against in any way as a result of genetic testing for Huntington disease.

- Extreme care should be exercised when testing which would provide information about another person who has not requested the test.

- For applicants with evidence of a serious psychiatric condition, it may be advisable that testing should be delayed and support services put into place.

- Testing for HD should not form part of a routine blood investigation without the specific permission of the subject.

- Ownership of the test results remains with the person who requested the test.

Legal ownership of the stored DNA remains with the person from whom the blood was taken.

- All laboratories are expected to meet rigorous standards of accuracy. They must work with genetic counselors and other professionals providing the test service.

- The counselors should be specifically trained in counseling methods and form part of a multidisciplinary team.

- The participant should be encouraged to select a companion to accompany him/her throughout all the different stages: the pre-test, the taking of the test, the delivery of the results, and the post-test stage.

- The counseling unit should plan with the participant a follow-up protocol that provides for support during the pre- and post-test stages, whether or not a person chooses a companion.

- Testing and counseling should be given within specialized genetic counseling units knowledgeable about molecular genetic issues in Huntington disease, preferably within a university department. These centers should work in close collaboration with the lay organization(s) of the country.

- The laboratory performing the test should not communicate the final results to the counseling team until very close to the time the results are given to the participant.

- Under no circumstances shall any member of the counseling team or the technical staff communicate any information concerning the test and its results to third parties without the written permission of the applicant.

- Neither the counseling center nor the test laboratory should establish direct contact with a relative whose DNA may be needed for the purpose of the test without permission of the applicant and of the relative. All precautions should be taken when approaching such a relative.

- It is essential that prenatal testing for the HD mutation should only be performed if the parent has already been tested.

- The couple requesting prenatal testing must be clearly informed that if they intend to complete the pregnancy if the fetus is a carrier of the gene defect, there is no valid reason for performing the test.

- Test centers may still perform an exclusion test for a future pregnancy if a 50% at-risk person specifically requests it. For this test, the person at risk, partner, parents, and fetus are tested only with adjoining DNA probes.

- Excluding exceptional circumstances, there should be a minimum interval of 1 month between the giving of the pre-test information and the decision whether to take the test. The counselor should ascertain that the pre-test information has been properly understood and should take the initiative to be assured of this. However, contact will only be maintained at the applicant's request.

- The result of the predictive test should be delivered as soon as reasonably possible after completion of the test, on a date agreed upon in advance between the center, the counselor, and the person.

- The manner in which results will be delivered should be discussed between the counseling team and the person.

- The participant has the right to decide, before the date fixed for the delivery of the results, that these results shall not be given to him/her.

- The results of the test should be given personally by the counselor to the person and his/her companion. No result should ever be given by telephone or by mail.

- The frequency and the form of the post-test counseling should be discussed between the team and the participant before the performance of the test, but the participant has the right to modify the planned program. Although the intensity and frequency will vary from person to person, post-test counseling must at all times be available.

- The counselor should have contact with the person within the first week after delivery of the results, regardless of the test result.

- If there has been no further contact within 1 month of the delivery of the test result, the counselor should initiate the follow-up.

- It is essential that post-test counseling is made available regardless of the person's financial situation.

- The lay organization has an important role to play in the post-test period. The information and support that it can provide should always be offered to the participant, whether or not he/she belongs to that organization.

APPENDIX 6

Genetic Disorders in which Dilatation of the Aorta May Occur

- Marfan syndrome
- Loeys-Dietz syndrome
- Familial aortic aneurysms
- Contractural arachnodactyly
- Stickler syndrome
- Turner syndrome
- Fragile X syndrome
- Cockayne syndrome
- Pseudoxanthoma elasticum
- Cutis laxa
- Chromosome 17q21.31 deletion syndrome
- Bicuspid aortic valve (in about 50%)
- Chromosome 22q11.2 deletion (Velocardiofacial syndrome)
- Adult polycystic kidney disease

q = long arm of a chromosome

APPENDIX 7

Examples Of Imprinting in Genetic Disorders

Syndrome	Chromosomal location	Parental origin
Angelman syndrome	15q11–q13	Maternal
Autism	15q11-q13	Maternal
Beckwith–Wiedemann syndrome	11p15.5	Paternal
Birk Barel mental retardation syndrome	8q24	Maternal
Congenital hyperinsulinism	11p15	Maternal
Congenital myotonic muscular dystrophy	19q13.3	Maternal
Early embryonic failure	21	Maternal
Familial paraganglioma	11q23	Paternal
Hereditary myoclonus–dystonia	7q21	Maternal
Intrauterine and postnatal growth restriction	7	Maternal
Intrauterine growth restriction or miscarriage	16	Maternal
Mental retardation and dysmorphism	14	Paternal
Prader–Willi syndrome	15q11–q13	Paternal
Progressive osseous heteroplasia	20q13.3	Paternal
Pseudohypoparathyroidism	20q13.3	Paternal
Rett syndrome	Xq28	Paternal
Russell-Silver syndrome	7p11.2	Maternal
	11p15	Maternal
Short stature	14	Maternal
Transient neonatal diabetes	6	Paternal

p = short arm; q = long arm

APPENDIX 8

Genetic Resources And Support Organizations

The GENETIC ALLIANCE, the world's leading nonprofit advocacy organization, has an enormous network that includes more than 1,000 disease-specific advocacy organizations.

Their website (http://www.geneticalliance.org/about) contains almost 550 e-mail addresses of disease-specific support organizations.

INDEX

Page numbers followed by "f", "t", or "n" indicate figures, tables, and notes, respectively.

supplementation, of diet, 320–23
surgery, 323
survival motor neuron (SMN), 152–55
systemic lupus erythematosus
    birth defects and, 297
    coronary artery disease and, 133
    copy number variations and, 52
    Fragile X syndrome and, 145
    Wilson's disease and, 338

T. *See* thymine
TAAD. *See* Thoracic Aortic Aneurysm
    and Dissection
Tamoxifen, 111–12
Tarceva, 123
TATA Box, 56
Tay, Warren, 196n3
Tay-Sachs disease, 70, 193–201, 199t,
    207t, 208t
    deletions with, 196
    knock-out mice for, 318
    mutation and, 193–94
    preconception planning and, 201
    prenatal diagnosis of, 88
Tegretol, 293t
teratogen, 295–96
teratoid tumors, 368
testicular cancer, 19
tetracycline, 293t
thalassemia, 95, 197t, 199t, 200t, 201–5,
    207t, 208t
    chelation for, 203–4
    with sickle cell disease, 210
thalidomide, 292, 294t, 295
thiazide diuretics, 357
Thimerosal, 252, 252n2, 257
Thoracic Aortic Aneurysm and Dissection
    (TAAD), 245
thrombosis, 13
thymine (T), 51
thyroid cancer, 368
thyroid disease. *See also* hypothyroidism
    Down syndrome and, 21
    with multiple endocrine neoplasia,
        148–50
    of mothers, birth defects and, 299

Turner syndrome and, 33
thyroxine, 322t
tobacco
    birth defects and, 299
    coronary artery diease and, 134
    cystic fibrosis and, 188
    mutations and, 56
    pancreatic cancer and, 123
tobramycin, 284n1
transcription, 54, 56, 57
translocation, 17
    balanced, 41–42
    bone marrow and, 47
    cancer and, 47–49
    Down syndrome and, 21, 42
    leukemia and, 47
    lymphoma and, 47
    mental retardation and, 40–41
    sex chromosomes and, 42–43
    unbalanced, 42
    X chromosome and, 42–43
transplantation
    of heart, for HCM, 138
    of kidneys, 242
    of liver, 337
    as treatment, 324
transvaginal ultrasound, 110–11
transvestism, 30n4
TRAPS. *See* tumor necrosis factor-receptor-
    associated periodic syndrome
treatment, 311–28
    with diet, 319–23
    for Gaucher disease, 314–17
    gene therapy, 325–27
    for hypertension, 357–58
    medications as, 322t, 323
    personalized medicine and, 327–28
    for phenylketonuria, 311–14
    with reconstruction, 323
    with repair, 323
    transplantation as, 324
triglycerides, 132
trimethadione, 293t
triplet repeats, 144, 371, 372
    age of onset for, 81
    Huntington disease and, 167–68

DATE DUE